A.AMANTONIO

TO
VACCINATE

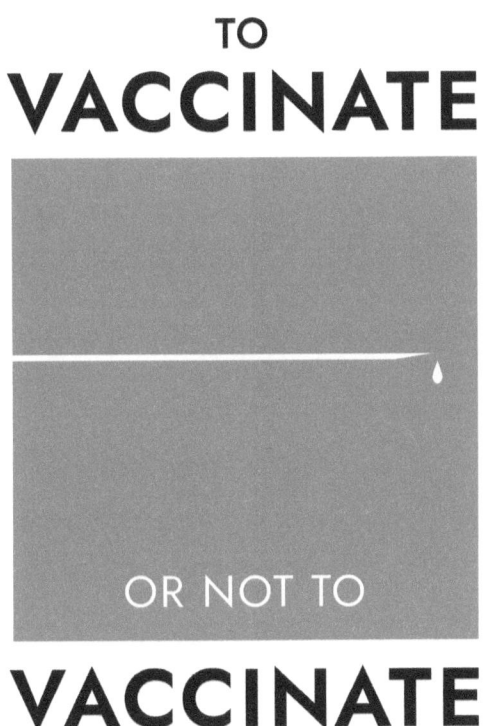

OR NOT TO

VACCINATE

A Review Of Scientific Literature On Vaccines

Note: This book is for educational and informational purposes only and is not intended to be a substitute for medical care and advice.

Library of Congress Control Number: 2020911145
ISBN: 979-8-6536-6322-2

Cover design by Ilia Sokolov, www.sisart.ru

First printing edition July 2020.
SciBook Publishing
en.scibook.org

To Emily

I would rather have questions that can't be answered than answers that can't be questioned.

— **Richard Feynman**

CONTENTS

CONTENTS

CONTENTS

FOREWORD

In recent years, we've heard more and more about the safety and effectiveness of vaccination in the media. This causes a widespread cognitive bias called "availability cascade": the more often a statement is repeated in society, the stronger the collective faith in it becomes. Other voices that cast doubt on this statement, and provide information that contradicts it, are not covered and get drowned out. Social networks are also increasingly blocking accounts and hashtags that provide information that doubts whether vaccination actually is the absolute good. The same happens in the scientific community: the scientists doing research that proves vaccines to be unsafe lose their funding and get ostracized.

In this book, you will find information about scientific studies, which the media and health authorities keep quiet about. Only scientific facts about vaccination are given here, with virtually no comments from the author.

The book is intended primarily for parents who want to personally understand whether or not they should vaccinate their children and get vaccinated themselves. Medical professionals who want to broaden their understanding of this topic will also find this book useful.

INTRODUCTION

Vaccination is the leading cause of coincidences.
— **Brett Wilcox**

A long time ago, when I was young and still enjoyed reading newspapers, I came across a long article published in one of the Friday issues, which talked about two lesbians. As it was a long time ago, I cannot remember exactly what it was about, but it had something to do with them not being able to legalize their relationship.

Among other things, the article said that the son of one of them had developed autism after getting vaccinated. It was mentioned in one sentence, after which they went on to discuss other affairs. I was struck by both this line and the fact that they were discussing such nonsense, instead of discussing what was the most important—that the child developed autism, and even more so, after getting vaccinated. I kept this article for a long time as a reminder that this topic needs to be thoroughly researched.

Over the past three years, after I became a parent, I spent thousands of hours researching vaccines. I have fully read over two thousand scientific studies, and I can now confidently tell you that unless you deliberately studied this topic, virtually everything you know about vaccination is a lie—from beginning to end.

> Almost everything written on this topic in the media is propaganda, fake news, and none of it has anything to do with neither science nor reality.

I really do not want to engage in reverse propaganda since it is a completely thankless task. However, first of all, I simply cannot keep quiet about it, since it is a question of life and death. Secondly, my excessive time investment into researching the topic of vaccination could perhaps help other parents make the right decision. If you are completely sure that vaccines are important, safe, and effective, and you want to keep that opinion, then this book is not for you. If you get even a little understanding of the topic, you will not be able to hold on to this belief.

I recently spoke to a relative, who told me that when his first child was born, he spent quite some time choosing a stroller, a crib, a car seat, etc., but he had not spent a single minute figuring out which vaccines his child should or should not get. Most parents delegate the right to this decision to others. They believe that other people—scientists, doctors, or nurses—have already examined this topic and made the best decision.

Parents make hundreds of decisions related to all aspects of a child's life in order to raise a healthy and happy baby: what to eat during pregnancy, where to give birth, how and what to feed the baby, whether to use a pacifier, etc. However, I am convinced that the most important parental decision is whether to vaccinate their child or not, and this most important decision is delegated to someone else by most parents. After all, the child's health is what is crucial for any parent, and there is virtually nothing else that would affect it more than the decision whether to vaccinate the child or not.

Some of the parents I have talked to are so convinced of the importance of vaccination that even knowing that there are people who consider vaccines to be unsafe, they simply do not want to investigate the subject. Instead, they aggressively defend their point of view, while not having read a single scientific article on the subject. They do not want to hear anything about the possibility of some vaccines not being very effective or even safe and that it has been proven by many scientific studies. It is possible to calmly discuss any other topic with them, but as soon as the topic of vaccination comes up, it is as if they become completely different people. They do not want to hear any reasoning and almost yell about the importance of vaccinating children and how blessed humanity is that medicine has given us vaccinations.

At first, I could not understand how it could be that these well educated and intelligent people become so fanatical and unreasonable as soon as this purely scientific subject is brought up. Then I seem to have understood it. All of them have already vaccinated their children, and, like most parents, they relieved themselves of the responsibility for this decision and delegated it to others. Subconsciously, they feel that if vaccines turn out to be not completely harmless, then it will mean that they have put their children's health and maybe even life in danger. Something like this is difficult to accept.

> It is much easier to live thinking that the child was born this way: with allergies, developmental delays, persistent ear infections, some autoimmune disease, or even a bunch of diseases.

It is very hard to live with the knowledge that they are the ones responsible for their child's disease. By delegating their right and responsibility for this decision and zealously defending vaccination, while not knowing anything about it, these parents protect themselves from strong cognitive dissonance. Therefore, if you have already fully vaccinated your children, are not planning on giving them more vaccines, and grandchildren are far in the future, you probably should not get into this topic. On the other hand, some consequences of the vaccination can be treated if you realize that they are acquired and not congenital.

The topic of vaccination is very extensive. It is impossible to completely understand it in a couple of hours or even days. In the time that I devoted to studying the subject, I could have learned a couple of foreign languages or mastered the guitar. However, as I look back, I can honestly say that the subject of vaccination is the most important one out of all I have ever been interested in. Conclusions drawn from the undertaken research go far beyond the topic of vaccination itself and even beyond medicine. Studying vaccines has changed my worldview more than anything else has.

Many parents believe that they are incapable of getting to the bottom of the vaccination topic, giving two reasons. The first reason is that "to delve into this topic, one needs to be educated in biology or medicine." That is not true. Vaccines are not rocket science, and any sensible person can understand them. I do not hold a biomedical degree, though my wife is a doctor, which did help me a lot when I was studying this subject. There are many biological concepts and terms that one would need to understand, and if someone is there to explain them, it will save a lot of time. However, understanding all of these biological processes is completely optional in learning whether vaccines are safe or not.

My wife also helped me to develop a very important skill: the ability to critically read medical studies. It turns out that reading medical research is very different from reading research on exact sciences, which I already knew how to read.

> There are many ways to design a study, choose a control group and placebo, and play around with data so that anything could be proven.

Second reason: "No one can understand this topic better than the scientists from the FDA (US Food and Drug Administration) or the CDC (US Centers for Disease Control and Prevention). So, if these scientists claim that vaccines are completely safe and effective, then any other opinion is, by definition, an opinion of a less qualified person."

First of all, this is an appeal to authority, which is a logical mistake in itself. Second, the question that the CDC scientists are facing is very different from the question that is facing parents. The CDC, perhaps, tries to answer the question of "How can the number of infectious diseases in the population be reduced with minimal risk, minimal cost, and maximum efficiency?" The question that parents are facing is, "How do I raise a healthy child?" Those are two completely different questions, and the answers to them might turn out to be completely different as well. Third, the CDC and FDA representatives do not have skin in the game.

You, as a parent, is the only one interested in the health of your children. It is of no interest to doctors, nurses, and especially the pharmaceutical companies or scientists from the CDC. If something were to happen to your child due to vaccination, none of them would be held responsible.

The subject of vaccination is very emotional. For some reason, it is very difficult for many people to rationally research this topic, or even read up on it. However, in order to understand it, one needs to set emotions aside. One needs to allow the possibility that the anti-vaccination arguments might be true (at least some of them), and rationally evaluate the arguments for and against vaccination.

It is not right to ask yourself whether vaccines, in general, are good or not. Some "experts" begin to argue that smallpox or yellow fever vaccines saved millions of lives. Even if it were true, it would still be completely irrelevant. Parents do not need to decide whether to vaccinate against smallpox or yellow fever. They need to make decisions about completely different vaccines.

4

Each vaccine is unique. Each has its own safety and effectiveness. There are some vaccines that are quite effective, and some that are almost useless, and then there are also those with negative effectiveness. There are safer vaccines, and there are those that should never be used. Each vaccine needs to be examined separately. They work in very different ways biologically, and that is important. The measles vaccine is very different from the pertussis vaccine, and they are both very different from the pneumococcal vaccine.

Most developed countries vaccinate against the same set of diseases, but the number of vaccines and the immunization schedule differs a lot between the countries. Immunization schedules of most countries usually include some or all of the following 17 vaccines: hepatitis B, diphtheria, tetanus, pertussis, poliomyelitis, haemophilus influenzae B, measles, mumps, rubella, chickenpox, hepatitis A, rotavirus, pneumococcus, meningococcus, human papillomavirus, influenza, and tuberculosis. A separate decision should be made in regards to each vaccine, as all of the diseases mentioned above are different by their nature—some are more dangerous, some are less. All of the vaccines are different as well. There is also a big variation between the efficacy and side effects of vaccines of different manufacturers. There is even a difference between the vaccines against the same disease in different countries. For example, ethyl mercury, a vaccine preservative that has not been used in childhood vaccines for 25 years in Western countries, is still being used in most other countries.

In addition to the vaccines, it is necessary to understand the diseases in which they intend to protect. One needs to understand whether childhood diseases are indeed as dangerous as they are made out to be. One needs to figure out how many years the vaccine immunity lasts, and how many years the exposure to the disease gives immunity for. It is necessary to find out whether the disease is just harmful, or maybe, perhaps, it also has its advantages.

The decision of whether to get or refuse each vaccine should not be emotional but purely rational. If the probability of being exposed to the disease and getting complications is higher than the probability of complications from the vaccine, then one should vaccinate. If it is lower, then it is not worth it. It is an oversimplification, of course, as the complications can be more or less severe.

It should be remembered that in addition to the active ingredient, vaccines contain many additives: adjuvants, preservatives and stabilizers, antibiotics, fragments of cell cultures, fragments of human and animal DNA, and many other components. One needs to make sure that the concentration of all of these ingredients is really safe enough to inject into their healthy newborn baby.

Surprisingly, even those people who do read the medication inserts, do not read the vaccine inserts and show little interest in vaccine side effects, despite the fact that they give these vaccines to their healthy newborn children. Moreover, unlike medications that are taken orally and are filtered by the liver and gastrointestinal tract, all the components of the intramuscular vaccines are fully absorbed into the circulatory, lymphatic, or nervous systems.

There are thousands of studies published in peer-review journals, which prove that vaccines are both unsafe and ineffective. Well, perhaps the anti-vaxxers are doing cherry-picking? Do they base their decision on a thousand studies on the dangers of the vaccines and ignore a thousand other studies proving their safety? Could be. Thus, it is necessary to also read the studies that prove that vaccines are safe, to make sure that, in fact, they usually do not prove safety, and to see who really does cherry-picking.

It is very important to read these studies in full and not just read the abstract since it happens all too often that the results speak of one thing, but the conclusion says something completely different. It happens time and time again that instead of actually using an inert placebo, a neurotoxin or another vaccine is used as a placebo. It happens that the data is played around with in a way that makes it statistically insignificant. It happens that the observation period is only a few days, while the conclusions are drawn regarding chronic consequences.

> Paradoxically, the studies attempting to prove vaccine safety prove the opposite even more than the studies trying to prove their harm.

The opportunity to independently study the subject of vaccination only appeared a few years ago, thanks to a Kazakh student Alexandra Elbakyan, who established the Sci-Hub website in 2011. Until then, almost all scientific studies were inaccessible to the general public, and one had to pay tens of dollars to read most articles. Science was hidden from ordinary people. Now, thanks to Sci-Hub, it is possible to find almost any study for free in just a few seconds, and personally see how some scientists distort the facts and design the studies to achieve the desired result. Alexandra Elbakyan has certainly done more to popularize science than all the scientists and journalists combined.

All that is needed to prove that vaccines are safe and effective is a randomized, placebo-controlled study. One group of children should be vaccinated with all the vaccines, while the other group should not be vaccinated at all. There are no such studies since it is currently considered unethical not to vaccinate children. Therefore, almost all existing studies are observational studies, descriptions of clinical cases, hypotheses, expert opinions, animal studies, and so on. There are no studies that examine the entire immunization schedule. Never mind the whole schedule; there are no adequate studies testing the safety of any vaccine! Thus, when it is claimed that "vaccines are safe and effective,"—it is an *a priori* unproven statement. Until such a randomized study is conducted, the decision of whether to vaccinate or not is basically a choice in the face of uncertainty.

Serious side effects from vaccination are believed to be extremely rare. One in every hundred thousand or even a million.

This is a lie. Since there are no adequate vaccine studies, it is difficult to assess the real number of side effects, but even with the most optimistic estimates, serious side effects happen more often than once in every 50 cases (see chapter 4). According to a 2011 study, half (!) of the children in the USA have at least one chronic illness, and this number has constantly been increasing [1, 2]. Sure, not all diseases are associated with vaccines, but who knows how many actually are, if no one is studying this subject?

After thorough research into vaccine safety, I personally suppose that almost everyone has post-vaccination consequences. It is just that for the majority, these consequences are not obvious and delayed in time. And even if they are obvious, few people actually associate them with vaccination. For example, it is known that brain damage is one of the rare but possible consequences of vaccination. However, how many children will have some brain damage that will result in them only losing ten points off of their IQ, or have minor problems with memory, concentration, or social interactions? Could it be that the decline in the Flynn effect (a gradual decrease of the average IQ after 2000, which formerly was continuously increasing over the course of the 20th century) is the result of a sharp increase in the number of vaccines given over the past couple of decades?

No one has looked into this, even though it is a completely logical assumption.

If newborn babies, whose blood-brain barrier (a physiological barrier that protects the brain from harmful substances in the blood) has not fully formed yet, are injected with a vaccine containing neurotoxins such as mercury or aluminum, some of which will certainly reach the brain, would it not be logical to expect every child to be affected in one way or another? And if this procedure is repeated several dozen times during the first years of children's lives, would it not be logical to presume that the effect would be enhanced?

When you familiarize yourself with even a small part of the scientific research presented in this book, you will have no doubt left that the vaccines are much more dangerous than the diseases which they supposedly protect from, that the decision not to vaccinate children is much more scientifically sound than the decision to vaccinate, and that vaccination in its current form is one of the most terrifying medical inventions. Having thoroughly studied the subject, you will never voluntarily vaccinate your child.

Endnotes

1. Bethell CD et al. A national and state profile of leading health problems and health care quality for US children: key insurance disparities and across-state variations. *Acad Pediatr*. 2011;11(3):S22-33

2. AAP. Percentage of US children who have chronic health conditions on the rise. *ScienceDaily*. 2016 Apr 30

Chapter One

ANTI-VAXXERS

A minority may be right, and a majority is always wrong.
— **Henrik Ibsen**

Scientists usually receive very few grants to study the safety of vaccines and vaccine components. However, there is more than enough money to research the reasons why people refuse to vaccinate and to devise methods of forcing them to vaccinate their children. Hence, there are many studies that characterize the anti-vaccine parents.

There is an opinion that anti-vaxxers are usually uneducated, religious, and anti-scientific people. However, scientific research suggests the opposite. Most anti-vaxxers are wealthy and well-educated. In some private schools in Los Angeles, less than 20% of children are vaccinated [1]. How can it be that these rich and educated people do not vaccinate their children? Don't they know that vaccines are totally safe and protect from terrible diseases? Or maybe they know something about vaccines that other people don't? Here's what the research found.

According to a CDC study, unvaccinated children's mothers were married, over 30, had a college degree, and lived in a household with an annual income exceeding $75,000 [2]. Children of less-educated mothers and children in families with low income were more likely to have completed the vaccination series [3]. Parents who chose not to vaccinate their children placed a high value on scientific knowledge, knew where to look for and how to analyze information about vaccination, and at the same time expressed high levels of distrust in the medical community [4]. In the Netherlands, parents with a college degree were three times more likely to express a negative attitude towards vaccination. Health care workers were four times more likely to express a negative attitude towards vaccination, and atheists were 2.6 times more likely [5].

In California, the percentage of students with non-medical vaccination exemptions increased fourfold between 2001 and 2014. Personal belief exemptions were nearly twice as common in private schools as in public schools. Higher income, white ethnic background, and private schooling were associated with a greater number of vaccine exemptions [6]. The same phenomenon is observed in other states—exemption rates are significantly higher in private schools [7].

In Israel, university-educated parents were two times more likely to refuse vaccination. Jewish parents were four times more likely to refuse vaccination for their children compared to Muslim parents. The older the mother, the more likely is the refusal to vaccinate [8]. In the UK, mothers who don't vaccinate are older and more educated [9].

In Canada, parents with higher education were more likely to refuse the HPV (human papillomavirus) vaccine for their daughters [10]. A systematic review of 28 studies found that parents with lower levels of education reported higher HPV vaccine uptake [11].

British parents who are older, with a high level of education and higher income, were more likely to refuse the MMR (measles, mumps, and rubella) vaccine and choose a monovalent measles vaccine instead [12]. In California, parents with higher education were less likely to allow their daughters to get the HPV vaccine [13]. In Colorado, higher maternal education and income were associated with the refusal of the hepatitis B vaccine during the perinatal period [14].

According to a 2016 survey across 67 countries, vaccine safety-related sentiment was particularly negative in the European region. Countries with high levels of schooling and good access to health services showed the least confidence in vaccine safety [15].

After Australia passed a law obliging parents to vaccinate their children in order to receive child benefits ("no jab no pay"), immunization rates in the wealthiest suburbs of Melbourne markedly fell. Parents with higher levels of education, many with a background in science, have more concerns about the safety and the necessity of vaccines than parents with lower levels of education. Only 20% of those parents, who refused to vaccinate before this law was introduced, began to vaccinate because of it. Ten percent of Australian parents believe that vaccines are associated with autism [16, 17].

Almost all similar studies come to the same conclusions. Parents who do not vaccinate their children are older, more educated, and wealthier [18, 19].

> Contrary to the image habitually painted by the mass media, anti-vaxxers are far from being idiots.

In this chapter, I will also cite the results of several other important studies for which taxpayers' money was used.

According to a 2017 study conducted in the US, if a clinician declares, "Today you're gonna do flu vaccine," 72% of the parents agree. But if the clinician asks, "Are we gonna do the flu vaccine today?" only 17% agree. If a clinician recommends the influenza vaccine together with other vaccines, 83% of parents agree. And if a clinician offers the flu vaccine separately, only 33% agree [20].

Authors of another study analyzed YouTube, Google, Wikipedia, and PubMed, and concluded that online communities with greater freedom of speech lead to a dominance of anti-vaccine voices. On YouTube, the degree of freedom of speech is the greatest; on Google, it is lower; and on Wikipedia and PubMed, it is very low. This leads to the fact that on YouTube, 74% of the videos in search results link vaccination to autism; on Google, 41% of the search results do so; on Wikipedia—14%; and on PubMed, 17% of the top 100 articles link vaccines with autism. But the most awful thing, according to the authors, is that anti-vaccine activists use scientific arguments, certified physicians, celebrities, and personal stories to establish trust! They go on to say that the problem is that YouTube, unlike Google, does not prioritize institutional or scientific authority in its search results. Medical doctors participated in 36% of the anti-vaccine ads, and only in 28% of the pro-vaccine ads. The authors propose to moderate the Internet and urge medical institutions to step up their activity online [21].

11

Authors of a study published in 2016 analyzed the comments under Mark Zuckerberg's Facebook post, where he wrote about vaccinating his daughter. They concluded that the anti-vaccination comments were better structured logically and had a higher tendency to express ideas related to health, biology, research, and science, whereas the pro-vaccine comments demonstrated greater anxiety [22].

According to a 2002 study, in 43% of vaccine-related queries, the search engines showed anti-vaccination sites in the top ten. On Google, 100% of the sites in the top ten were anti-vaccination. More than half of those websites quote medical doctors who speak out against vaccination; 75% quote scientific sources. The authors conclude that there is a high probability that parents will be exposed to anti-vaccination materials on the Internet [23]. (As of 2020, the situation is reversed: Google, Facebook, and other social media websites don't return practically any anti-vaccination articles and groups in search results.)

A 2014 randomized study on effective messages in vaccine promotion showed that when parents are told about a child having nearly died from measles, it only strengthens their belief that the MMR vaccine leads to serious adverse effects. When parents are shown images of sick children, this only strengthens their belief that vaccines cause autism. When parents are told about the horrors of the diseases, this does not affect their intentions to vaccinate their children. When parents are told that MMR is not related to autism, they agree, but their intentions to vaccinate their children only decreases [24].

When people are told that the flu vaccine cannot cause the flu, they believe it, but their intention to get vaccinated only decreases [25]. When mothers are told that whooping cough is more dangerous than the vaccine, they believe it, but their intention to vaccinate their children only decreases [26].

Authors of a 2017 study found that parents who know someone, whose child has experienced a severe reaction to a vaccine, refused or postponed vaccines more often [27].

A British study found that many parents doubt physicians' recommendations because they are aware that general practitioners need to meet immunization targets and may partly be motivated by financial factors and not purely by the child's best interests [28].

There are quite a few studies that characterize anti-vaxxers and analyze methods of convincing them, and there are enough grants for all

these studies. However, there is no money for adequate vaccine safety studies, such that it would last longer than a few days or weeks and would use an inert placebo.

Endnotes

1. Shapiro N. With fewer vaccinations, is your child's school safe? *LA Times*. 2013 Aug 10

2. Smith PJ et al. Children who have received no vaccines: who are they and where do they live? *Pediatrics*. 2004;114(1):187-95

3. Kim SS et al. Effects of maternal and provider characteristics on up-to-date immunization status of children aged 19 to 35 months. *Am J Public Health*. 2007; 97(2):259-66

4. Gullion JS et al. Deciding to opt out of childhood vaccination mandates. *Public Health Nurs*. 2008;25(5):401-8

5. Hak E et al. Negative attitude of highly educated parents and health care workers towards future vaccinations in the Dutch childhood vaccination program. *Vaccine*. 2005;23(24):3103-7

6. Yang YT et al. Sociodemographic predictors of vaccination exemptions on the basis of personal belief in California. *Am J Public Health*. 2016;106(1):172-7

7. Shaw J et al. United States private schools have higher rates of exemptions to school immunization requirements than public schools. *J Pediatr*. 2014;165(1):129-33

8. Even D. More Israeli parents refusing to vaccinate their babies according to state regulations. *Haaretz*. 2013 Jun 4

9. Samad L et al. Differences in risk factors for partial and no immunisation in the first year of life: prospective cohort study. *BMJ*. 2006;332(7553):1312-3

10. Ogilvie G et al. A population-based evaluation of a publicly funded, school-based HPV vaccine program in British Columbia, Canada: parental factors associated with HPV vaccine receipt. *PLoS medicine*. 2010;7(5):e1000270

11. Brewer NT et al. Predictors of HPV vaccine acceptability: a theory-informed, systematic review. *Prev Med*. 2007;45(2-3):107-14

12. Pearce A et al. Factors associated with uptake of measles, mumps, and rubella vaccine (MMR) and use of single antigen vaccines in a contemporary UK cohort: prospective cohort study. *BMJ*. 2008;336(7647):754-7

13. Constantine NA et al. Acceptance of human papillomavirus vaccination among Californian parents of daughters: a representative statewide analysis. *J Adolesc Health*. 2007;40(2):108-15

14. O'Leary ST et al. Maternal characteristics and hospital policies as risk factors for nonreceipt of hepatitis B vaccine in the newborn nursery. *Pediatr Infect Dis J*. 2012; 31(1):1-4

15. Larson HJ et al. The state of vaccine confidence 2016: global insights through a 67-country survey. *EBioMedicine*. 2016;12:295-301

16. 9 News Melbourne. 2017 Jun 14

17. Fielding JE et al. Immunisation coverage and socioeconomic status - questioning inequity in the 'No Jab, No Pay' policy. *Aust N Z J Public Health*. 2017;41(5):455-7

18. Anello P et al. Socioeconomic factors influencing childhood vaccination in two northern Italian regions. *Vaccine*. 2017;35(36):4673-80

19. Feiring B et al. Do parental education and income matter? A nationwide register-based study on HPV vaccine uptake in the school-based immunisation programme in Norway. *BMJ open*. 2015;5(5):e006422

20. Hofstetter AM et al. Clinician-parent discussions about influenza vaccination of children and their association with vaccine acceptance. *Vaccine*. 2017;35(20):2709-15

21. Venkatraman A et al. Greater freedom of speech on Web 2.0 correlates with dominance of views linking vaccines to autism. *Vaccine*. 2015;33(12):1422-5

22. Faasse K et al. A comparison of language use in pro- and anti-vaccination comments in response to a high profile Facebook post. *Vaccine*. 2016;34(47):5808-14

23. Davies P et al. Antivaccination activists on the world wide web. *Arch Dis Child*. 2002; 87(1):22-5

24. Nyhan B et al. Effective messages in vaccine promotion: a randomized trial. *Pediatrics*. 2014;133(4):e835-42

25. Nyhan B et al. Does correcting myths about the flu vaccine work? An experimental evaluation of the effects of corrective information. *Vaccine*. 2015;33(3):459-64

26. Meszaros JR et al. Cognitive processes and the decisions of some parents to forego pertussis vaccination for their children. *J Clin Epidemiol*. 1996;49(6):697-703

27. Chung Y et al. Influences on immunization decision-making among US parents of young children. *Matern Child Health J*. 2017;21(12):2178-87

28. Evans M et al. Parents' perspectives on the MMR immunisation: a focus group study. *Br J Gen Pract*. 2001;51(472):904-10

Chapter Two

PHYSICIANS

Doctors are men who prescribe medicines of which they know little,
to cure diseases of which they know less,
in human beings of whom they know nothing.
— **Voltaire**

Argument 1: "If there were any problems with the vaccines, if they were unsafe or ineffective, doctors would have known about it. But there is an almost complete scientific consensus—that vaccines are safe and effective. After all, doctors with their long years of formal training have surely studied vaccines much more than what you could have read about them on the Internet."

My wife also used to believe that vaccines are safe and effective. It was what she was taught. I asked her how many hours of her education had been devoted to vaccines. It turned out that it was only a few hours. She studied the vaccination schedule for two hours, and another two hours were dedicated to a lecture on "how to respond to anti-vaccination arguments." By the way, after this lecture, almost all the students said that the lecturer's arguments did not convince them and that the anti-vaxxers' arguments made more sense. They, of course, didn't think that the anti-vaccine proponents were somehow right. They decided that the lecturer simply did not prepare well for this lecture.

In some countries, physicians have financial interest in vaccine promotion. The more vaccines they sell, the higher their bonuses are. For example, in the US, the insurance company Blue Cross Blue Shield pays pediatricians $400 for each fully vaccinated child, but only if the percentage of vaccinated children in their practice exceeds 63% [1]. This is the main reason why pediatricians in the United States refuse to treat unvaccinated children [2]. Indian doctors who order large quantities of vaccines receive presents from the pharmaceutical companies [3].

Argument 2: "But I have talked to several doctors and they all claim that vaccines are safe. Moreover, if they thought vaccines were unsafe, they would not vaccinate their own children."

Most people mistakenly believe that physicians can treat patients the way they see fit. That is far from being the case. For example, if a doctor has read several scientific articles and has come to the conclusion that a particular disease would be better treated in a certain way, they would have no right to put it into practice. Doctors must follow the approved treatment guidelines; otherwise, they risk losing their license or can get fired. If the doctor prescribes any unapproved medicine to the patient, such as treating pertussis with vitamin C instead of antibiotics, and something happens to the patient, the doctor might be taken to court. If the doctor does prescribe antibiotics (not particularly effective in the case of pertussis [4]) and something happens to the patient, the doctor will not bear any responsibility. So why would a doctor advise the patient anything not approved by the guidelines? Similarly, doctors do not really have a right to advise patients not to vaccinate. They can quickly lose their license, and even if they do not, their career will not go very far.

In Australia, for example, doctors who help parents to avoid vaccinating their children, or nurses and midwives who promote anti-vaccination messages via social media, face prosecution [5, 6]. In Canada, a former chiropractor who spoke out against vaccines on social media was ordered to pay a $100,000 fine [7]. A Spanish doctor was suspended for claiming vaccines are linked to autism [8]. The same happened in Poland [9]. And yet there are still many physicians who openly speak out against vaccines. Of course, these physicians usually have their own private practice. Here are some studies.

Despite the fact that 93% of Israeli doctors are aware of the Ministry of Health recommendation to vaccinate pregnant women against influenza and whooping cough, only 70% of them follow these recommendations. A third of the physicians hold the opinion that both vaccines are dangerous or controversial. Forty percent of the doctors, who believe that these vaccinations are dangerous, still recommend them to their patients [10].

In Switzerland, 5% of non-pediatricians did not vaccinate their children against measles, mumps, and rubella. They chose to avoid trivalent combined vaccines because of safety concerns and had a preference for infection-induced rather than vaccine-induced immunity. They were also convinced that homeopathic treatment helps with a benign outcome of measles, mumps, and rubella. Ten percent postponed the DTaP vaccination to a later date; 15 % postponed the MMR vaccination.

A third of pediatricians did not vaccinate their children against hepatitis B and Hib (haemophilus influenzae type *b*). Only 12% vaccinated against influenza and only 3% against chickenpox. Thirty-four percent of pediatricians did not vaccinate their children according to the vaccination schedule. The survey involved only subscribers to the InfoVac services, that is, physicians who are actively engaged in the topic of vaccination. This implies that the actual percent of physicians who do not vaccinate their children is probably higher [11].

In the US, 21% of sub-specialist pediatricians and 10% of generalist pediatricians will refuse at least one vaccine for their child. Nineteen percent of sub-specialist pediatricians and 5% of generalist pediatricians would delay MMR vaccination until after 18 months. Twelve percent of sub-specialist pediatricians will not give their child a rotavirus vaccine, 6% will not give them a hepatitis A vaccine [12].

A 2008 CDC study revealed that 11% of the physicians did not recommend parents to vaccinate children with all available vaccines. Family practitioners did not recommend all vaccines three times more often compared to pediatricians. It also turned out that physicians trust medical journals more than government health agencies, and that they trust the pharmaceutical companies less than the Internet [13].

In Italy, only 10.3% of the pediatricians had a very favorable attitude towards all recommended vaccinations for infants. Sixty percent of the pediatricians would like to know more about vaccines. Only 25% of the pediatricians administered "recommended" (as opposed to "mandatory") vaccines to their patients [14].

According to a 2013 French study, 27% of general practitioners were not vaccinated against hepatitis B, 36% were not vaccinated against whooping cough, and 23% were not vaccinated against influenza [15]. Thirteen percent of general practitioners consider measles a harmless disease. Twelve percent of general practitioners consider the second dose of MMR useless. Thirty-three percent of general practitioners do not believe that MMR vaccination should be mandatory for children under two years of age [16].

After a three-month-long campaign among the Israeli nurses to encourage them to immunize themselves against whooping cough, only 2% decided to do so. The nurses in question were employed by Mother and Child Centers, and their primary duty was to vaccinate children. Most of the nurses expressed a lack of trust in the health authorities and desperately resisted mandatory vaccinations. They were afraid of vaccines' adverse effects and assumed the danger of influenza and whooping cough to be less than that of the vaccines. They believed that the parents should have the choice whether or not to vaccinate their child, and they demanded the same respect for their own rights. The nurses distinguished between their work and personal lives. While those nurses' duty was to vaccinate other people's children, they considered their own vaccination status to be their private business and did not believe that informing the parents of their opinion about vaccinations or of their own vaccination status was necessary. The authors concluded that the nurses who administered vaccines were, in fact, anti-vaccinationists [17]. This is probably the most important study of all those presented herein. Practically in all the other studies, the data was collected from surveys. Physicians understand perfectly well that they are not supposed to refer to vaccinations in a negative way. Therefore, it is logical to assume that the real proportion of doctors who do not vaccinate their children is much higher. The data in this study, on the other hand, is not based on surveys but rather on factual immunization records. **Ninety-eight percent of nurses, whose main job was to vaccinate children, refused to be vaccinated themselves.**

Influenza Vaccination

Since most vaccines are administered in childhood, and physicians are usually not required to get new vaccines, there are practically no studies analyzing how willingly doctors submit themselves to this procedure. The

18

only exception is the influenza vaccine, which is recommended every year. So how do physicians and nurses react to flu vaccination campaigns?

According to a 2015 study, healthcare workers in Italy are refusing influenza vaccination despite ten years of efforts to increase vaccination coverage. Only 30% of physicians, 11% of nurses, and 9% of other clinical personnel received the influenza vaccine [18].

Forty-one percent of healthcare workers refused the vaccine against swine flu during the 2009 pandemic. The most common reasons for remaining unvaccinated were "side effects," "swine flu not severe," and "concerns about clinical effectiveness of the vaccine." Fifty-seven percent of healthcare workers refused the vaccine against seasonal influenza [19].

In China, only 13% of doctors and 21% of nurses were vaccinated against influenza. Thirty-five percent of healthcare workers believe that the flu vaccine can cause flu in some people [20].

Fifty percent of the healthcare workers in Madrid refused the influenza vaccine, and only 16% received the vaccine against swine flu during the 2009 pandemic. They had "doubts about vaccine efficacy" and "fear of adverse reactions" [21].

For more than 20 years, German healthcare workers have been encouraged to get the influenza vaccine, but only 39% of physicians and 17% of nurses are vaccinated. Their reasons included a low risk of infection, fear of side effects, the belief that the influenza vaccine might trigger the influenza virus infection, and skepticism about the effectiveness of the influenza vaccination [22].

In the US, 41% of nurses did not receive the influenza vaccine. They have a concern about adverse reactions, believe that the chance of contracting influenza is small, and they do not consider the flu vaccine to be effective enough [23].

Swiss nurses have skeptical attitudes towards infectious diseases and the influenza vaccine. They say that the outbreaks of diseases always turn out to be less dangerous than announced by public health authorities and by the media, decreasing public confidence in the reliability of expert sources of information. Conflicts of interest between public organizations and private corporations also reduce the level of trust in institutions responsible for fighting disease outbreaks [24].

This same story repeats itself all over the world. Physicians and nurses in all countries decline influenza vaccination [25, 26, 27].

According to a 2013 study in the US, the idea that the vaccines are the safest medical products and are getting better and safer is less supported by the recent medical graduates than by their older colleagues. Young medical specialists are more inclined to resist compulsory vaccination and are more convinced that vaccination causes more harm than good [28].

Regardless of how much physicians and nurses are being told that vaccines are safe and effective, not everyone believes it—far from it. Scientific evidence suggests that medical consensus on the safety and efficacy of vaccination is a myth.

Endnotes

1. Blue Cross Blue Shield 2016 performance recognition program
2. Haelle T. As more parents refuse vaccines, more doctors dismiss them - with AAP's blessing. *Forbes*. 2016 Aug 29
3. Iyer M. Pharma firms lure doctors with gold coins to push its vaccines. *The Economic Times*. 2017 Jan 21
4. Altunaiji S et al. Antibiotics for whooping cough (pertussis). *Cochrane Database Syst Rev*. 2005(1):CD004404
5. Percy K et al. Melbourne doctors investigated for allegedly helping parents avoid vaccinating children. *abc.net.au*. 2017 Aug 24
6. Davey M. Australian nurses who spread anti-vaccination messages face prosecution. *The Gardian*. 2016 Oct 20
7. Gorman M. Former chiropractor ordered to pay $100K related to anti-vaccine posts. *CBC News*. 2019 Jul 4
8. Güell O. Spanish doctor suspended for claiming vaccines cause autism. *El Pais*. 2019 Jun 21
9. Doctor who criticised vaccines banned from practising medicine for a year. *NotesFromPoland*. 2019 Nov 1
10. Gesser-Edelsburg A et al. Despite awareness of recommendations, why do health care workers not immunize pregnant women? *Am J Infect Control*. 2017;45(4):436-439
11. Posfay-Barbe KM et al. How do physicians immunize their own children? Differences among pediatricians and nonpediatricians. *Pediatrics*. 2005;116(5):e623-33
12. Martin M. Vaccination practices among physicians and their children. *OJPed*. 2012;2:228-35
13. Gust D et al. Physicians who do and do not recommend children get all vaccinations. *J Health Commun*. 2008;13(6):573-82
14. Anastasi D et al. Paediatricians knowledge, attitudes, and practices regarding immunizations for infants in Italy. *BMC Public Health*. 2009;9:463
15. Pulcini C et al. Factors associated with vaccination for hepatitis B, pertussis, seasonal and pandemic influenza among French general practitioners: a 2010 survey. *Vaccine*. 2013;31(37):3943-9
16. Pulcini C et al. Knowledge, attitudes, beliefs and practices of general practitioners towards measles and MMR vaccination in southeastern France in 2012. *Clin Microbiol Infect*. 2014;20(1):38-43

17. Baron-Epel O et al. What lies behind the low rates of vaccinations among nurses who treat infants? *Vaccine*. 2012;30(21):3151-4

18. Alicino C et al. Influenza vaccination among healthcare workers in Italy. *Hum Vaccin Immunother*. 2015;11(1):95-100

19. Head S et al. Vaccinating health care workers during an influenza pandemic. *Occup Med Lond*. 2012;62(8):651-4

20. Seale H et al. Influenza vaccination amongst hospital health care workers in Beijing. *Occup Med Lond*. 2010;60(5):335-9

21. Vírseda S et al. Seasonal and Pandemic A (H1N1) 2009 influenza vaccination coverage and attitudes among health-care workers in a Spanish University Hospital. *Vaccine*. 2010;28(30):4751-7

22. Wicker S et al. Influenza vaccination compliance among health care workers in a German university hospital. *Infection*. 2009;37(3):197-202

23. Clark SJ et al. Influenza vaccination attitudes and practices among US registered nurses. *Am J Infect Control*. 2009;37(7):551-6

24. Maridor M et al. Skepticism toward emerging infectious diseases and influenza vaccination intentions in nurses. *J Health Commun*. 2017;22(5):386-394

25. Hollmeyer HG et al. Influenza vaccination of health care workers in hospitals—a review of studies on attitudes and predictors. *Vaccine*. 2009;27(30):3935-44

26. Hofmann F et al. Influenza vaccination of healthcare workers: a literature review of attitudes and beliefs. *Infection*. 2006;34(3):142-7

27. Hulo S et al. Knowledge and attitudes towards influenza vaccination of health care workers in emergency services. *Vaccine*. 2017;35(2):205-7

28. Mergler MJ et al. Are recent medical graduates more skeptical of vaccines? *Vaccines*. 2013;1(2):154-66

Chapter Three

PLACEBO

*Those who could give up essential Liberty
to obtain a little temporary Safety
deserve neither Liberty nor Safety.*
— **Benjamin Franklin**

How should the safety of vaccines be determined? By conducting randomized, double-blind, placebo-controlled clinical trials, during which the data on adverse effects experienced by the vaccine recipients is collected and compared to the control group.

Clinical trials are very expensive: they cost tens of millions of dollars. Product development costs are estimated by hundreds of millions. However, those amounts aren't an issue for pharmaceutical companies. An FDA-approved vaccine very quickly becomes a part of the vaccination schedules in most countries and yields billions in profit on an annual basis. For example, sales of one of the recently licensed vaccines, Gardasil (against HPV), account for more than $3 billion per year [1].

Naturally, pharmaceutical companies want to lower the odds of failing in clinical trials. But do they have a legal opportunity to do so? It turns out that they do, and that it's quite easy to implement. Instead of a placebo, one simply needs to use a fairly toxic substance with adverse effects similar to those of the vaccine in question. One of the most toxic components in vaccines is aluminum (more details in chapter 6), which is used as an adjuvant (a substance that enhances the immune response) in most vaccines. If aluminum is added to the placebo, it is possible to increase the prevalence of adverse effects in the control group, making it comparable to the intervention group. This will allow the researchers to conclude that the new vaccine has no more adverse effects than the placebo, and therefore it is completely safe. It is also possible to add other toxic substances; for example, ethyl mercury, or simpler still—use another vaccine as the placebo. Based on such studies, the FDA and the CDC will also be able to conclude that the vaccine is safe, and so will the other countries around the world. Is this legal? Absolutely.

The thing is, you don't even have to bother with the choice of the placebo. It is by no means mandatory to use it in a randomized clinical vaccine study. Actually, the studies themselves don't even have to be either randomized or blind. In fact, you can simply give everyone the vaccine and observe what the adverse effects are. If the majority of the study participants remain alive, then the vaccine is completely safe.

According to a 2010 study, there are no inert substances and no regulations that guide placebo composition. The composition of the placebo does, of course, influence the trial outcomes. There is no requirement to disclose the contents of the placebo used in clinical trials, and medical journals do not require this information. The authors analyzed 167 clinical studies published in four of the most prestigious medical journals. Most clinical studies did not disclose the composition of the placebo. Studies of only 8% of pills and 26% of injections reported what was used as the placebo. For example, in the study of medication for cancer-acquired anorexia, it was found that the medication positively affects the gastrointestinal tract. However, lactose was used as a placebo. Cancer patients who are undergoing chemo and radiation therapy usually acquire lactose intolerance, and that is why the medication which does not contain lactose compares favorably with the "placebo." The authors conclude that failure to disclose placebo ingredients breaches scientific standards of rigor [2].

A 2009 study published in *Vaccine* journal reports that in 1930, in the town of Lübeck in Northern Germany, two physicians conducted a campaign to vaccinate newborn infants against tuberculosis. They used a BCG vaccine produced locally from a Parisian strain. The vaccine, although available since as early as 1921, was still not widely accepted at the time. In the next 12 months of this campaign, 208 children became ill with tuberculosis and 77 died. The two physicians were arrested and put on trial. The court eventually found them guilty of murder. This tragedy led to the first published discussion of medical research using human subjects.

In 2008, the US abandoned the Declaration of Helsinki (a set of ethical principles related to the research and experiments involving human subjects) for international clinical trials. Instead, the US uses Good Clinical Practice (GCP), which does not restrict pharmaceutical companies as much as the Declaration of Helsinki. Authors write that although the use of saline is allowed in the vaccine trials, the researchers frequently opt for other comparative agents. For example, a study of the pneumococcal conjugate vaccine used DTP-Hib (diphtheria-tetanus-pertussis-Hib) vaccine as a placebo. In another study on a pneumococcal vaccine (PCV23), vaccines for hepatitis A and B were used as placebos. In yet another study, a novel oral cholera vaccine was compared with a heat-killed E. coli vaccine, which has no therapeutic benefit. In a fourth study, aluminum hydroxide combined with thimerosal (a mercury-based preservative) was used as a placebo [3].

Unlike clinical trials of drugs, in which the placebo composition is often undisclosed, many vaccine manufacturers do not usually conceal the placebo composition. In order to find out this information, you simply need to read the vaccine insert. Here are only a few examples.

Daptacel (vaccine for diphtheria, tetanus, and whooping cough). Three vaccines were used as placebos: DTP, DT, and an experimental vaccine for whooping cough. This is not a mistake. An experimental vaccine was used as a placebo. Let that sink in [4].

Infanrix (another vaccine for diphtheria, tetanus, and whooping cough). Pediarix vaccine was used as the placebo. In addition, both groups received those vaccines alongside vaccinations for hepatitis B, pneumococcus, chickenpox, polio, Hib, measles, mumps, and rubella [5].

Pediarix (vaccine for diphtheria, tetanus, whooping cough, hepatitis B, and polio). This vaccine was tested together with a vaccine for Hib. The control group received the Infanrix vaccine, as well as a vaccine for polio and Hib [6].

In other words, Pediarix was used as the placebo in Infanrix trials, and Infanrix was used as the placebo in Pediarix trials. All of this was seasoned with a blend of several other vaccines in order to completely eradicate the possibility of distinguishing any adverse effects resulting from the vaccines being tested.

The first vaccines for diphtheria, tetanus, and whooping cough appeared long before anyone bothered with clinical trials or the use of placebos. Therefore, it can be argued that the use of a real placebo to test them (i.e., not vaccinating a part of the participating children) is unethical. But even the clinical trials of vaccines against diseases that weren't "vaccine-preventable" at the time of testing use other vaccines as the placebo.

Havrix (vaccine for hepatitis A). The clinical study included three groups. The first one received Havrix. The second one received Havrix + MMR (measles-mumps-rubella vaccine). The third one received MMR + chickenpox, and then Havrix 42 days after [7].

Prevnar (pneumococcal vaccine). The placebo was an experimental (!) meningococcal C vaccine [8]. The next version of this vaccine (Prevnar-13) used Prevnar as a placebo [9].

Cervarix (human papillomavirus vaccine). The placebo was a hepatitis A vaccine, as well as aluminum hydroxide [10].

Engerix-B (vaccine for hepatitis B). There was no control group [11].

Recombivax HB (vaccine for hepatitis B). There was no control group [12].

In order to license a new vaccine, it is sufficient to show the FDA that it is no more dangerous than some other vaccine, or even an experimental vaccine, or aluminum hydroxide, or any other substance the pharmaceutical company sees fit and has no obligation to publicly disclose.

> In vaccine clinical studies, a true, inert placebo is virtually never used.

So the next time someone claims that vaccines are completely safe, ask them: "Safe compared to what?" Vaccines are only completely safe when compared to extremely toxic substances or to other vaccines.

Endnotes

1. Keytruda and Gardasil will likely continue to drive Merck's earnings growth. *Forbes*. 2018 Oct 30
2. Golomb BA et al. What's in placebos: who knows? Analysis of randomized, controlled trials. *Ann Intern Med*. 2010;153(8):532-5
3. Jacobson RM et al. Testing vaccines in pediatric research subjects. *Vaccine*. 2009;27(25-26):3291-4
4. Daptacel vaccine package insert
5. Infanrix vaccine package insert

6. Pediarix vaccine package insert
7. Havrix vaccine package insert
8. Prevenar vaccine package insert
9. Prevenar-13 vaccine package insert
10. Cervarix vaccine package insert
11. Engerix-B vaccine package insert
12. Recombivax-HB vaccine package insert

Chapter Four

SAFETY

If you see fraud and do not say fraud, you are a fraud.
— **Nassim Taleb**

We have already seen that the safety of vaccines is tested without a real placebo, but instead in comparison with other vaccines, or in comparison with some other toxic compound. However, this is not all. There are a few more problems with testing vaccines' safety.

First of all, nearly all trials are done exclusively on healthy children, which does not stop physicians and FDA from recommending the vaccines to not-so-healthy children, preterm infants, children of a younger age, and not just to children.

Secondly, nearly all clinical trials of safety are looking only for short-term effects and last from several days to several weeks. Rare trials last several months. All the adverse effects that happen after this period a priori are considered to be unrelated to the vaccination.

Thirdly, even if there are serious adverse effects occurring during the trial, scientists can decide that those adverse effects, or even deaths, are not related to the vaccination and can be crossed out without being taken into account.

Fourthly, research is usually done on a relatively small group of children. For example, the hepatitis B vaccine was tested on 147 newborns

[1]. Usually, vaccines are tested on children from third-world countries, which halves the cost of clinical trials [2].

Here is an example of a clinical trial of Daptacel vaccine. To take part in the trial, a child should be absolutely healthy, be born after the 37th week, not be sensitive to any of the vaccine components, not have developmental delays, the family should not have a history of immune diseases, and so on. In addition, the child must receive a hepatitis B vaccine at least a month prior to the trial and remain absolutely healthy. This means that aluminum-sensitive children will not be part of the trial [3]. More or less, the same requirements are stated for all vaccine trials.

> That is, in contrast to medicines, which are usually tested on sick patients and then given to sick patients, vaccines are tested exclusively on healthy children and then given to both healthy, not-so-healthy, and even very sick children.

An article that reports the results of the aforementioned study states that safety was tested for 30 and 60 days after each dose. Serious adverse effects were registered in 5.2% of children from the test group and 5.2% of children from the control group (which received three other vaccines). The authors decided that these adverse effects were not related to vaccination. They did not report what these adverse effects were and why they were excluded [4].

Some additional examples.

In a clinical trial of Recombivax-HB (a vaccine against hepatitis B), safety was tested for 14 days. Seventy-seven percent of children had adverse events. Twenty-eight children (1.6%) had serious adverse events. One child died with a SIDS (sudden infant death syndrome) diagnosis. The authors report that his death was probably not related to the vaccination [5].

In clinical trials of Comvax (vaccine against Hib and hepatitis B), safety was tested for 14 days. Serious adverse events occurred in 17 infants (1.9%). Three children died with a SIDS diagnosis. The authors concluded that all serious adverse events, including deaths, were not related to the vaccine [6].

In clinical trials of the Infanrix Hexa vaccine, safety was tested for 30 days. Serious adverse events occurred in 79 infants (2.7%). Nearly all of them were not related to the vaccine, according to the researchers. One infant died with a SIDS diagnosis. It was not related to the vaccine [7].

In clinical trials of a pentavalent vaccine, safety was tested for 30 days. There were 8.5% of infants that had serious adverse events; almost all of them were reported as unrelated to the vaccine [8].

In clinical trials of a hexavalent vaccine, safety was tested for six months. Eighty-four infants (5.9%) had adverse events. Two died. No connection to the vaccine was found [9].

This is more or less how the majority of safety trials look. They rarely last longer than a few days or weeks. Most of them have serious adverse events occurring during this short period of time in absolutely healthy children, and it is almost never concluded that they are related to vaccination. They are deemed not related because, in the control group, which receives a different vaccine or the same vaccines without an antigen, the same adverse events are registered.

> In such short clinical trials, it is impossible to identify autoimmune, oncological, or neurological diseases, as well as many other diseases. These diseases might be triggered by vaccination, but it is impossible to diagnose them earlier than a few months or even years after vaccination. Moreover, vaccine inserts always state that "vaccine has not been evaluated for its carcinogenic potential, mutagenic potential, or potential for impairment of fertility."

A systematic review published in 2005 summarized how adverse events after vaccination are reported in clinical trials. Forty-five percent of the studies did not mention adverse events at all; 56% did not mention serious adverse events. Only 24% of the studies specified local and systemic adverse events. Twenty-eight percent of the articles did not mention the duration of the post-vaccination observation period. In 36% of the studies, the observation period was two days or less. Inconsistency of adverse events reporting between the sections "Methods" and "Results" was found in 24% of articles. The authors conclude that the information on adverse effects is provided inadequately. There are no guidelines for standardized collection, analysis, and publication of the adverse events. This is why it is very difficult or even impossible to do a meaningful comparison of safety data between different studies and surveillance systems [10].

Endnotes

1. Recombivax-HB vaccine package insert

2. Puliyel JM et al. Global access to vaccines: poor nations are being lured into a debt trap. *BMJ*. 2008;336(7651):974-5

3. Study of the safety, immunogenicity and lot comparability of Daptacel when administered with other recommended vaccine. clinicaltrials.gov/ct2/show/NCT00662870

4. Guerra FA et al. Safety and immunogenicity of a pentavalent vaccine compared with separate administration of licensed equivalent vaccines in US infants and toddlers and persistence of antibodies before a preschool booster dose: a randomized, clinical trial. *Pediatrics*. 2009;123(1):301-12

5. Vesikari T et al. Safety and immunogenicity of a modified process hepatitis B vaccine in healthy infants. *Pediatr Infect Dis J*. 2011;30(7):e109-13

6. West DJ et al. Safety and immunogenicity of a bivalent Haemophilus influenzae type b/hepatitis B vaccine in healthy infants. Hib-HB Vaccine Study Group. *Pediatr Infect Dis J*. 1997;16(6):593-9

7. Zepp F et al. Safety, reactogenicity and immunogenicity of a combined hexavalent tetanus, diphtheria, acellular pertussis, hepatitis B, inactivated poliovirus vaccine and Haemophilus influenzae type b conjugate vaccine, for primary immunization of infants. *Vaccine*. 2004;22(17-18):2226-33

8. Vesikari T et al. Randomized, controlled, multicenter study of the immunogenicity and safety of a fully liquid combination diphtheria-tetanus toxoid-five-component acellular pertussis (DTaP5), inactivated poliovirus (IPV), and haemophilus influenzae type b (Hib) vaccine compared with a DTaP3-IPV/Hib vaccine administered at 3, 5, and 12 months of age. *Clin Vaccine Immunol*. 2013;20(10):1647-53

9. Marshall GS et al. Immunogenicity, safety, and tolerability of a hexavalent vaccine in infants. *Pediatrics*. 2015;136(2):e323-32

10. Bonhoeffer J et al. Reporting of vaccine safety data in publications: systematic review. *Pharmacoepidemiol Drug Saf*. 2005;14(2):101-6

Chapter Five

THE UNVACCINATED

Never doubt that a small group of thoughtful,
committed citizens can change the world;
indeed, it's the only thing that ever has.

— **Margaret Mead**

Neither the CDC nor the FDA—and especially not the pharmaceutical companies—conduct studies comparing vaccinated and unvaccinated children. One of the directors from the CDC admitted to this fact after being cornered at the congressional hearing [1]. Nonetheless, there are some studies available comparing vaccinated and unvaccinated children. All of these studies are small and have flaws, but there is nothing better available at the moment. Only the studies comparing vaccinated and unvaccinated children can provide an adequate picture of the real benefits and harm of vaccination, and therefore despite all their shortcomings, these studies are the most important ones among all that exist.

A study published in 2017 compared 600 homeschooled children in four US states. Vaccinated children had chickenpox four times less often, whooping cough three times less often, and rubella ten times less often. On the other hand, vaccinated children had otitis media four times more often and pneumonia six times more often. Vaccinated children also had allergic rhinitis 30 times more often, allergies and ASD (autism spectrum disorder) four times more often, eczema three times more often, learning disabilities five times more often, neurodevelopmental disorders and ADHD (attention deficit hyperactivity disorder) four times more often, and they had some type of chronic illness 2.5 times more often. Vaccinated children used allergy medications 21 times more often, fever medications 4.5 times more often, ear-drainage tubes eight times more often, and antibiotics 2.5 times more often. They visited a doctor due to illness three times more often and were hospitalized 1.8 times more often [2]. Vaccination of preterm infants was associated with a 14-fold increase in the risk of neurodevelopmental disorders [3].

Children in Guinea-Bissau were vaccinated once in three months, which created a natural experiment. Some children have already been vaccinated by the age of three to five months, and some haven't. The risk of death in children vaccinated against diphtheria-tetanus-pertussis (with DTP vaccine) was ten times higher when compared to unvaccinated children. Children who were also vaccinated against poliomyelitis (with OPV vaccine) died only five times more often than unvaccinated children. After the introduction of these vaccines, the all-cause infant mortality rate after three months of age increased twofold. The authors of the study conclude: "*All currently available evidence suggests that DTP vaccine may kill more children from other causes than it saves from diphtheria, tetanus or pertussis*" [4].

> The authors can hardly be suspected of being anti-vaxxers. Peter Aaby, one of the study authors, created the Bandim Health Project in Guinea-Bissau, one of the main goals of which is to vaccinate children. He was also a pioneer of vaccination on the African continent.

According to a 1997 New Zealand study, 23% of vaccinated children had asthma, 22% received asthma consultations, and 30% had allergies. There wasn't a single case of asthma, asthma consultations, or allergies among unvaccinated children [5]. Also in New Zealand, a survey of parents of vaccinated and unvaccinated children revealed that vaccinated children had asthma five times more often, tonsillitis ten times more often, eczema two times more often, apnea four times more often, hyperactivity four times more often, ear infections four times more often, and they had an ear drainage tube inserted eight times more often. Five percent of vaccinated children had tonsils removed. There were no tonsil removals among unvaccinated children, and 1.7% of the vaccinated children had epilepsy. There were no cases of epilepsy among unvaccinated children [6].

A 2003 study compared vaccinated and undervaccinated children in the US. "Undervaccinated" are the children who have not received at least one vaccine or received at least one vaccine even a day later than the due date. Those who were undervaccinated by their parents' choice visited emergency departments 9% less often, visited doctors 5% less often, and had pharyngitis and upper respiratory illnesses 11% less often [7].

Rhesus macaques were given childhood vaccines according to the vaccination schedule in the US in 1999 and were compared with the unvaccinated macaques [8]. The vaccinated macaques had a much larger brain volume—a finding which is consistently observed in autistic children [9]. The amygdala (brain region responsible for emotions) was also much larger in the vaccinated macaques compared to the unvaccinated. This is also observed in autistic children [10].

In a 2011 study, the authors compared infant mortality in 30 countries and the number of vaccines given by the age of 12 months in those countries. There appears to be a linear correlation between the two. The more vaccinations there are in the country, the higher the infant mortality rate is [11].

> The more vaccinations there are in the country, the higher the infant mortality rate is.

In the US study, children vaccinated against tetanus or with the DTP vaccine had allergies 63% more often, asthma two times more often, and sinusitis 81% more often than the unvaccinated ones [12]. In Japan, among children vaccinated with the DTP vaccine, 56% had asthma, allergic rhinitis, or atopic dermatitis. Among the unvaccinated ones, only 9% had those diseases [13].

According to a 2020 study, vaccination before 24 months of age was associated with a threefold increase in the risk of developmental delays, a twofold increase in the risk of ear infections, and a sixfold increase in the risk of asthma [14].

In a study of 30,000 children in the UK, children vaccinated against diphtheria-tetanus-pertussis-polio had asthma 14 times more often and eczema nine times more often than unvaccinated children. Children vaccinated against measles-mumps-rubella had asthma 3.5 times more often and eczema 4.5 times more often. The numbers seem to speak for themselves, don't they? But these figures did not suit the authors, as they were looking to justify vaccinations, so they did two sleights of hand.

First, they determined that unvaccinated children visited doctors less. In their opinion, this does not mean that unvaccinated children got sick less often, but rather that their chance of being diagnosed was lower than of those vaccinated. Therefore, they made a correction. However, it turned out to be not enough, so they went further and divided all the children into four groups by the number of physician visits, and then analyzed each group separately. And, as if by a miracle, the statistical significance disappeared among those who visited the doctors often! But among those who went to see doctors less than three to six times, vaccinated children had asthma and eczema 10–15 times more often than the unvaccinated ones anyway. The authors concluded with a clear consciousness that vaccinations are not a risk factor for asthma or eczema [15]. Doctors, who only read the abstract (meaning almost everyone, since only a few people read these articles in full), see just the conclusion and, with a peace of mind, carry on vaccinating children. Such sleights of hand are often found in the studies that allegedly prove the safety of vaccinations.

Combination Of Vaccines

According to a 2012 study, the more vaccinations are given at the same time, the higher the likelihood of hospitalization and death. The mortality among those who received five to eight vaccinations was 1.5 times higher than among those who received one to four vaccinations [16].

Children from Guinea-Bissau, who received the DTP vaccine simultaneously with the measles vaccine, died two times more often than those who received only a measles vaccine. Authors cite several more studies with the same results in Gambia, Malawi, Congo, Ghana, and Senegal [17]. In another study in Guinea-Bissau, children who received a pentavalent vaccine (DTP-Hib-hepatitis B), in addition to measles and yellow fever vaccines, died 7.7 times more often than children who did not receive a pentavalent vaccine. The authors concluded that co-administration of live and inactivated vaccines is associated with increased mortality compared with the administration of live vaccines only [18].

In a study published by the CDC, the risk of hospital admission among children whose last vaccine was live was two times lower compared to those who received an inactive vaccine as their last one [19].

In New York, infants vaccinated with a combination vaccine (DTP-polio-hepatitis B) in addition to pneumococcal and Hib vaccines were two times more likely to visit the emergency department within three days of vaccination compared to infants vaccinated with each vaccine separately. They also had a sevenfold increased risk of receiving a full sepsis workup, a tenfold risk of receiving lumbar punctures, and a threefold increased risk of receiving antibiotics within seven days of vaccination [20]. In Israel, the number of newborns with unexplained fever doubled after the introduction of the hepatitis B vaccine [21].

In a 2016 study in Denmark, simultaneous administration of MMR with a pentavalent vaccine was found to be associated with a 27% increase in the risk of hospitalizations due to lower respiratory tract infections, compared to the administration of the MMR vaccine alone [22]. In Israel, adverse effects of vaccination were observed in 57% of children who received MMR and pentavalent vaccines simultaneously, but only in 40% among those who received these vaccines separately. The authors conclude that *"It may be necessary to reconsider the current vaccination policy regarding concomitant injections"* [23].

In 2011, India began to switch to pentavalent vaccines (DTP-Hib-hepatitis B) instead of trivalent ones (DTP). This made the comparison between post-vaccination mortality rates of both vaccines possible. The authors of a 2018 study have analyzed data on 45 million infants. The mortality rate within 72 hours after the pentavalent vaccine was twice as high as after the trivalent vaccine [24].

The CDC and other health agencies recommend using combined vaccines and administering several vaccines in one visit. Nonetheless, the above-mentioned scientific studies prove that such practice increases the risk of complications.

Endnotes

1. Posey questions CDC on autism research. *youtu.be/uNWTOmEi_6A*

2. Mawson A. Pilot comparative study on the health of vaccinated and unvaccinated 6- to 12- year old U.S. children. *JTS*. 2017;3(3):1-12

3. Mawson A. Preterm birth, vaccination and neurodevelopmental disorders: a cross-sectional study of 6- to 12-year-old vaccinated and unvaccinated children. *JTS*. 2017;3:1-8

4. Mogensen SW et al. The introduction of diphtheria-tetanus-pertussis and oral polio vaccine among young infants in an urban African community: a natural experiment. *EBioMedicine*. 2017;17:192-8

5. Kemp T et al. Is infant immunization a risk factor for childhood asthma or allergy? *Epidemiology*. 1997;8(6):678-80

6. Claridge S. Unvaccinated children are healthier. 2005

7. Glanz JM et al. A population-based cohort study of undervaccination in 8 managed care organizations across the United States. *JAMA Pediatr*. 2013;167(3):274-81

8. Hewitson L et al. Influence of pediatric vaccines on amygdala growth and opioid ligand binding in rhesus macaque infants: a pilot study. *Acta Neurobiol Exp Wars*. 2010;70(2):147-64

9. Hazlett HC et al. Early brain development in infants at high risk for autism spectrum disorder. *Nature*. 2017;542(7641):348-51

10. Schumann CM et al. The amygdala is enlarged in children but not adolescents with autism; the hippocampus is enlarged at all ages. *J Neurosci*. 2004;24(28):6392-401

11. Miller NZ et al. Infant mortality rates regressed against number of vaccine doses routinely given: is there a biochemical or synergistic toxicity? *Hum Exp Toxicol*. 2011;30(9):1420-8

12. McKeever TM et al. Vaccination and allergic disease: a birth cohort study. *Am J Public Health*. 2004;94(6):985-9

13. Hurwitz EL et al. Effects of diphtheria-tetanus-pertussis or tetanus vaccination on allergies and allergy-related respiratory symptoms among children and adolescents in the United States. *J Manipulative Physiol Ther*. 2000;23(2):81-90

14. Hooker B et al. Analysis of health outcomes in vaccinated and unvaccinated children: developmental delays, asthma, ear infections and gastrointestinal disorders. *SAGE Open Med*. 2020;8: 2050312120925344

15. Yoneyama H et al. The effect of DPT and BCG vaccinations on atopic disorders. *Arerugi*. 2000;49(7):585-92

16. Goldman GS et al. Relative trends in hospitalizations and mortality among infants by the number of vaccine doses and age, based on the Vaccine Adverse Event Reporting System (VAERS), 1990-2010. *Hum Exp Toxicol*. 2012;31(10):1012-21

17. Aaby P et al. DTP with or after measles vaccination is associated with increased in-hospital mortality in Guinea-Bissau. *Vaccine*. 2007;25(7):1265-9

18. Fisker AB et al. Co-administration of live measles and yellow fever vaccines and inactivated pentavalent vaccines is associated with increased mortality compared with measles and yellow fever vaccines only. An observational study from Guinea-Bissau. *Vaccine*. 2014;32(5):598-605

19. Bardenheier BH et al. Risk of nontargeted infectious disease hospitalizations among us children following inactivated and live vaccines, 2005-2014. *Clin Infect Dis.* 2017; 65(5):729-37

20. Thompson L et al. The impact of DTaP-IPV-HB vaccine on use of health services for young infants. *Pediatr Infect Dis J.* 2006;25(9):826-31

21. Linder N et al. Unexplained fever in neonates may be associated with hepatitis B vaccine. *Arch Dis Child Fetal Neonatal Ed.* 1999;81(3):F206-7

22. Sørup S et al. Simultaneous vaccination with MMR and DTaP-IPV-Hib and rate of hospital admissions with any infections: a nationwide register based cohort study. *Vaccine.* 2016;34(50):6172-80

23. Shneyer E et al. Reduced rate of side effects associated with separate administration of MMR and DTaP-Hib-IPV vaccinations. *Isr Med Assoc J.* 2009;11(12):735-8

24. Puliyel J et al. Deaths reported after pentavalent vaccine compared with death reported after diphtheria-tetanus-pertussis vaccine: an exploratory analysis. *Med J DY Patil Vidyapeeth.* 2018;11(2):99-105

Chapter Six

ALUMINUM

A foolish faith in authority is the worst enemy of truth.
— **Albert Einstein**

Most people assume that a vaccine is just a weakened or killed virus or bacteria. The immune system produces antibodies to the injected dead virus, and, if the person subsequently becomes infected, their immune system will be able to recognize the virus and quickly react to it. This description is simplified to such an extent that one might argue that it is completely false. If everything were that simple, then the vaccine would provide lifelong immunity, which is acquired after getting the actual disease. However, this is not what happens. Immunity obtained from a vaccine usually lasts for only a few years. The most effective vaccines give immunity for 10–20 years.

Our immune system is not stupid: it understands that a fragment of a dead virus or bacterium does not pose any real danger and thus produces antibodies against it very poorly [1]. How do the vaccine developers solve this problem? They add an **adjuvant** to the vaccine. An adjuvant is a molecule, which the immune system recognizes as a very toxic one and reacts to it strongly. At the same time, the immune system reacts to the virus as well and, to make things worse, it also reacts to all the other vaccine ingredients and not just to them. This, in turn, leads to allergies and various autoimmune diseases.

This is the reason why immunologists call aluminum the "immunologist's dirty little secret."

The second and probably even more important reason for using adjuvants is purely economic. Growing viruses is difficult, time-consuming, and expensive. Perhaps, if a significant amount of virus were injected, the immune system would respond to it appropriately and produce antibodies. It would, however, be a much more expensive vaccine. It is much cheaper to take a small amount of the virus, add some adjuvant, and get a strong immune reaction. When getting FDA approval, the vaccine's efficacy is much more important than its safety. Safety, as we have seen, is fairly easy to fake. Faking efficacy is much harder.

The two most common adjuvants are **aluminum hydroxide** and **aluminum phosphate**. Understanding just these two adjuvants is enough to exclude most vaccines. The topic of aluminum is worth understanding even unrelated to vaccination, just to grasp how corrupt science, WHO, the CDC, and the governments of different countries are. There are hundreds of studies proving that aluminum, even in minimal concentrations, is very toxic.

The authors of an article published in 2011 state that despite the fact that aluminum adjuvants have been used in vaccines for 90 years, it is still unknown why and how exactly aluminum causes such a strong immune response. High toxicity and danger of aluminum consumed orally have been known since 1911—when Dr. William Gies published the results of seven years of research on aluminum in baking powder, food preservation, and dye manufacturing. Gies concluded that "*The use in food of aluminum or any other aluminum compound is a dangerous practice.*" (Aluminum is still used in baking powder and food preservatives.) Aluminum affects memory, concentration, and behavior. Preterm infants that were given intravenous feeding solutions containing aluminum had reduced developmental attainment when compared to infants given feeding solutions without aluminum. Aluminum that is used in kidney dialysis leads to dementia, seizures, speech impairments, psychosis, and death. Aluminum is also associated with Alzheimer's disease, Parkinson's disease, ALS, multiple sclerosis, autism, and epilepsy. The authors conclude that "Newborns, infants and children up to 6 months of age in the U.S. and other developed countries receive 14.7 to 49 times more than the FDA safety limits for aluminum from parenteral sources from vaccines through mandatory immunization programs" [2].

A 2018 article states that the FDA approved amount of aluminum in vaccines was derived from the data, which demonstrated that this amount of aluminum enhanced the effectiveness of the vaccine, but did not include safety considerations. The conclusion about the safety of amounts of aluminum in vaccines was based solely on the studies of the dietary exposure of adult mice and rats. On day one of life, infants receive 17 times more aluminum than would be allowed if doses were adjusted for body weight [3].

According to a 2011 study, children from countries with the highest ASD prevalence appear to have the highest exposure to aluminum from vaccines. The increase in exposure to aluminum adjuvants strongly correlates with the increase in ASD prevalence in the United States observed over the last two decades. The authors use Hill's criteria (nine principles for establishing causality in epidemiological studies) and conclude that the correlation between aluminum in vaccines and autism may be causal [4].

In a 2009 Canadian study, mice were injected with aluminum in equivalent-to-human doses. Increased death of motor neurons, impairments of motor functions, diminished spatial memory capacity, and other effects, similar to the symptoms of dementia, Alzheimer's disease, and Gulf War syndrome were observed [5].

When pregnant rats were given subcutaneous injections of radioactive aluminum, it was observed that the aluminum reached the fetuses' brains in just a few days. After birth, the aluminum continued to accumulate in the brain, being passed on through the maternal milk [6]. A high level of aluminum in the mother's hair is associated with congenital heart defects in offspring [7]. Ninety-five percent of women who gave birth had aluminum found in the placenta, 81% had it in the placenta membranes, and 46% in the umbilical cord [8].

In some patients, the aluminum adjuvants do not dissolve after the vaccination, but instead remain at the injection site and form an aluminum granuloma. This diagnosis is called *macrophagic myofasciitis* (MMF). Accompanying symptoms are usually myalgia (muscle pains), chronic fatigue, cognitive dysfunction, as well as various autoimmune diseases [9].

A 2011 study reports that aluminum has no useful biological function. Despite the fact that aluminum is one of the most common metals on

Earth, in nature it is only found in the compounds with silicon and oxygen. Humans learned how to produce pure aluminum and create aluminum salts only in the late nineteenth century. Aluminum is a strong neurotoxin, which inhibits more than 200 biologically important functions and causes various adverse effects in plants, animals, and humans. Among other things, aluminum binds with ATP (which causes chronic fatigue), changes DNA, kills nerve cells, and destroys the homeostasis of useful minerals (such as magnesium, calcium, and iron) by mimicking them [10].

According to a 2014 study of patients with Alzheimer's disease, the closer the arteries to the brain are, the higher the concentration of aluminum in them is [11]. Patients with a familial form of Alzheimer's have been found to have incredibly high levels of aluminum in their brains [12].

A 2017 article states that even though the exact cause of Alzheimer's disease is still unknown, aluminum plays a major part in it [13].

Aluminum is accumulated in semen, and the more there is, the worse is the sperm quality [14]. Aluminum also damages the ovarian structure and inhibits the reproductive function of female rats [15].

A 2013 study reported that aluminum administered intramuscularly along with the vaccine gets into the brain, spleen, liver, and remains there for years. It is transported around the body by macrophages. Macrophages are the cells that engulf bacteria and other toxic substances. Macrophages swallow aluminum, but do not know how to dispose of it, and thus spread it throughout the body through the lymphatic system [16].

Where Does The Aluminum Go?

Although the aluminum adjuvants have been used since 1926, what exactly happens to them after they are injected into a muscle is still unknown to science. The authors of a 1997 study took several rabbits and injected two of them with radioactive aluminum hydroxide, and the other two with aluminum phosphate. Twenty-eight days later, the rabbits were sacrificed, and by that time, 94% of aluminum hydroxide and 78% of aluminum phosphate still remained in the rabbits' bodies. The authors examined several internal organs and concluded that small amounts of aluminum accumulated in each of them. However, it is unclear how exactly they determined that the amounts were small since there was no control group of rabbits in the experiment that were not injected with any kind of aluminum. The authors have not examined the rabbits' bones (because they damaged them), even though it is a known fact that aluminum accumulates in the bones. Neither did they examine the muscles that were injected with aluminum. It is known that aluminum stays in the body for years, but the study only lasted for 28 days. The authors concluded that the body successfully disposes of aluminum, regardless of the fact that most of the aluminum remained in the body, and it is completely unclear in which organs exactly [17].

In a 2013 study, 15 preterm infants were given several vaccines with 1,200 mcg of aluminum. This aluminum has not been found either in the blood or in the urine. Where it went remained unclear. The authors also found that vaccinated infants had a significant decline in serum levels of iron, zinc, selenium, and manganese [18].

In a 2017 review article, all the published studies of aluminum adjuvants' safety were analyzed. The authors state that the aforementioned study on rabbits is currently the only existing pharmacokinetic study on aluminum adjuvants. Moreover, the adjuvants tested in this study differ from the adjuvants actually used in vaccines. The FDA argues that aluminum in vaccines is safe based on two theoretical articles. The "safe dose" of aluminum for infants was extrapolated from the studies on mice that received aluminum orally. The authors conclude that comparing the toxicity of aluminum ions absorbed orally with the toxicity of aluminum salts administered intramuscularly is nonsense [19].

In another 2017 study, three groups of mice were injected with different doses of aluminum hydroxide. The experiment showed that aluminum granulomas only formed in the muscles of the mice that received high doses. The mice that got the low doses did not have granulomas, but the aluminum reached their brains, and they had behavioral disorders and decreased locomotor activity. The concentration of aluminum in the brains of the group that received the low dose was 50 times higher than that of the control group. The authors concluded that the simplified toxicity model, according to which the level of toxicity depends on the dose, does not work in the case of the aluminum hydroxide [20].

In a 2018 study, sheep were divided into three groups. The first group received 19 vaccines with aluminum in the course of 15 months. The second group received injections of aluminum adjuvant only. The third one was the control group and received a saline solution. One hundred percent of the vaccinated sheep and 92% of those injected with adjuvant had granulomas develop at the injection sites; the vaccinated sheep had significantly more granulomas. The aluminum particles in the granulomas of those vaccinated were much longer than in the granulomas of those injected with an adjuvant. The fact that the aluminum particles might increase in size in the presence of an antigen is known from other studies. **The concentration of aluminum in lymph nodes of the vaccinated sheep was 32 times higher than of those who only received an adjuvant and 86 times higher than that of the control group.** The authors conclude that the aluminum gets into the lymph nodes through macrophages. Degenerative changes were observed in macrophages of both groups [21].

Of children vaccinated with the Infanrix vaccine in a Swedish study, 0.83% had aluminum granulomas form at the injection site. Eighty-five percent of them became allergic to aluminum. Two vaccines with aluminum doubled the risk of granulomas. Fifty-seven percent of the children had itchy granulomas form two weeks to 13 months after the vaccination; they disappeared after 22 months on average. In another study, 0.98% of vaccinated children had granulomas form, and 95% of them became allergic to aluminum. The MMR vaccine, which does not contain aluminum, can become a trigger for the formation of granulomas [22].

A 2004 article analyzes different types of adjuvants. One of the adjuvants previously used in vaccines is calcium phosphate. It has properties similar to those of the aluminum adjuvants, but since it is a molecule natural to the body, it does not cause neurological reactions and does not lead to allergic reactions. Even though it is safer, no one is in a hurry to replace aluminum with calcium phosphate. The author concludes that it is likely that *"if aluminum hadn't been in use all these years and was first put forward to regulatory bodies for approval today, it would be refused registration on the basis of safety concerns"* [23].

A 2015 article states that aluminum salts induce cell death and inflammation, which could explain why granulomas might form at the injection site. In cats, dogs, and ferrets, aluminum adjuvants cause local chronic granulomatous lesions that can progress into malignant fibrosarcoma. It is unknown why such tumors do not develop in humans. It is also unknown how cumulative doses of aluminum adjuvants contribute to the development of chronic diseases, such as Alzheimer's or chronic bone diseases. Aluminum and other adjuvants cause serious adverse effects in animals. Even though its relevance to humans is unknown, this data is still ignored when determining the adjuvant safety for new vaccines. For example, it has been known for many years now that squalene (adjuvant used in some influenza vaccines) can lead to autoimmune conditions in genetically susceptible animals. *Hence, one might reasonably ask why these animal toxicity data do not predict the possibility of the adjuvant causing autoimmune disease in human subjects who are also genetically susceptible. There is currently no good answer to this question* [24].

Feline injection-site sarcomas were first described in the early 1990s. Despite the extensive research, the pathogenesis of these tumors has not been elucidated conclusively. Their appearance and the marked increase in their incidence have been mainly connected with the injection of vaccines, and it is assumed that a chronic inflammatory reaction at the injection site triggers subsequent malignant transformation. This is why vaccines began to be administered in the flank or hindlimb instead of the shoulder—that way, the tumor is easier to remove. The incidence of fibrosarcomas in cats in Switzerland had risen sharply since 1986 after the introduction of the adjuvanted vaccine against feline leukemia virus, which contained aluminum. In 2007, after the introduction of the vaccine without aluminum, the incidence of fibrosarcoma began to drop rapidly. The authors conclude that non-adjuvanted vaccines might be safer for administration to cats than the vaccines containing aluminum [25].

The question of the safety of the aluminum salts is one of the cornerstone questions in the topic of vaccination safety, and thus vaccine advocates have to answer it quite often. As an example, I will cite an article by the most famous vaccination advocate Paul Offit, in which he explains to parents that aluminum in vaccines should not be feared. His arguments are:

1) aluminum adjuvants are safe because they have been used in vaccines for over 70 years;

2) there's aluminum in breast milk, baby formula—and in general, it is one of the most common metals;

3) there were experiments done on mice: they were fed aluminum lactate, and nothing happened to them [26].

The first argument is so ridiculous and anti-scientific that it is difficult to respond to it. Seventy years ago, half of the children did not have chronic diseases. And given the abundance of scientific research on the dangers of aluminum, this argument is simply false.

The second argument is also very easy to refute. Firstly, even one single hepatitis B vaccine, which infants get on their first day of life, has five times more aluminum than they would get from six months of breastfeeding. Secondly, it is not possible to meaningfully compare intramuscular aluminum and aluminum in food (only 0.25% of which is absorbed). Thirdly, it is impossible to compare aluminum on its own and aluminum adjuvant bound to the antigen, which is much harder for the body to dispose of [27].

The third argument is answered by the aforementioned article [2]. Offit fails to mention that the motor activity of 20% of the mice from that experiment was significantly impaired. Not to mention that aluminum lactate cannot be compared with aluminum phosphate or aluminum hydroxide, as different aluminum salts have different toxicity. In addition, the harmful effects of aluminum on mice have been proven in other studies [5].

If there is so much evidence of aluminum toxicity, how can the FDA justify its safety in vaccines? Very easily. As a basis for their calculations, FDA scientists took the level of aluminum, which is considered safe. As mentioned above, the "safe" level was established based on an experiment on adult mice that received aluminum orally [3]. They compared this "safe" level to the theoretical level of aluminum that remains in infants' bodies after intramuscular vaccination with aluminum hydroxide or aluminum phosphate. **To calculate this level in their theoretical model, the authors based their calculations on the aforementioned rabbit study in addition to the study of one (!) adult (!) volunteer who received aluminum citrate (!) intravenously (!).** Furthermore, the authors took into account only 17% of the aluminum that entered the blood of the rabbits and ignored the rest of the aluminum, which remained in various organs [28]. It is, however, known that most intravenous aluminum is rapidly excreted by the kidneys, while intramuscular aluminum remains in the body for years.

Another attempt to justify aluminum in vaccines was made in a 2004 systematic review and meta-analysis. The authors identified eight studies of aluminum adjuvants in DTP vaccines. The safety studies lasted from 24 hours to six weeks. The adverse effects these studies were looking for were mostly persistent crying and screaming, drowsiness, pain, fever, convulsions, and erythema. The authors concluded that although these studies were of very poor quality, there is no substitute for aluminum in vaccines. And even if an alternative was found, all the vaccines would need to be tested again, which "would threaten immunisation programmes worldwide." Then comes the final shocking conclusion: "Despite a lack of good-quality evidence we do not recommend that any further research on this topic is undertaken" [29]. It was a systematic review of all the current literature on the safety of aluminum in DTP vaccines. Well, not exactly. It was not just an ordinary systematic review. It was a systematic review by Cochrane, the most respected medical science organization, whose systematic reviews are recognized as being of the highest quality in the world. One could only imagine what the ordinary, lower quality systematic reviews look like.

Aluminum Unrelated To Vaccination

Aluminum hydroxide is used to stimulate allergies in mice [30]. Intracerebral injections of aluminum hydroxide cause epilepsy in monkeys [31]. Aluminum hydroxide and aluminum phosphate are also used as antacids—drugs used to treat heartburn and some other gastrointestinal diseases, many of which are sold without prescription. This, in turn, leads to food allergies [32]. Thirty-eight percent of ingested aluminum accumulates in the intestinal mucosa. Even though the intestines absorb only a small amount of aluminum, 2% of aluminum that enters the blood is retained within the body and accumulates with age. Adults consume most of the aluminum with hot beverages (except coffee) and vegetables (except potato); children also consume it with pasta and pastries; infants get it from the formulas, which contain a hundred times more aluminum than cow milk. Other sources of aluminum are kitchenware, packaging, antacids, and analgesics [33].

Aluminum is found in large quantities in sunscreens. Since aluminum is an oxidant, it could be an extremely significant factor in melanoma development [34]. Aluminum is used in drinking water treatment systems, and some of it remains in the water [35].

There is a lot of aluminum in frozen pizzas, sausages, cheese, pancakes, baking powder, and cake mixes [36]. There is also a lot of aluminum in drinks sold in aluminum beverage cans [37]. Rats that were given drinks from aluminum cans had 69% more aluminum in their bones [38]. There is a lot of aluminum in toothpaste, as well as in tea [39]. Sixty percent of all the toothpaste on the market contain aluminum [40]. Toothpaste with aluminum may aggravate dermatitis (which is caused by vaccination) and lead to tooth decay [41, 42].

The topic of antiperspirants (deodorants containing aluminum) is quite controversial, as is any topic where a lot of money is involved. There is still no absolute proof that antiperspirants cause breast cancer. However, there is ample evidence suggesting that a link between antiperspirants and breast cancer is more than likely. Aluminum gets into the bloodstream after just one use of the deodorant. Aluminum is genotoxic; it is capable of causing both DNA alterations and epigenetic effects. The cause of 90% of cases of breast cancer is environmental, not genetic. Aluminum salts in antiperspirants block the sweat glands preventing them from releasing sweat, which is what makes them so effective. In 1926 only 31% of breast tumors were located in the upper outer quadrant of the breast. In 1994 this number increased to 61%. This proportion is growing linearly every year. Among breast cancer patients, those who used antiperspirants more often were diagnosed at a younger age [43]. A 2016 article states that six times more aluminum is absorbed through damaged skin, and since women often apply antiperspirant after shaving, it increases the aluminum absorption. The concentration of aluminum in the outer part of the breast is much higher than in the inner part. The level of aluminum in tumors is higher than in the adjacent unaffected tissue. The concentration of aluminum in breasts and breast milk is higher than in blood. Breast cysts are also more common in the outer part of the breast, and the concentration of aluminum in them is higher than in the blood. For some women, breast cysts disappear following the cessation of underarm cosmetic use [44]. According to a 2017 study, women who use underarm deodorant several times per day have a four times higher risk of breast cancer. The concentration of aluminum in the breast is much higher in cancer patients than in healthy ones [45].

Silicon-rich mineral water facilitates the removal of aluminum from the body. Twelve weeks of drinking this water led to cognitive improvements in some Alzheimer's patients [46]. Judging by experiments on rats, curcumin might protect from the inflammatory effects of aluminum, as might omega-3 fatty acids, moringa, melatonin, olive oil, folic acid, propolis, lecithin, selenium, taurine, vitamin E, and quercetin [46-56].

Endnotes

1. Gayed PM. Toward a modern synthesis of immunity: Charles A. Janeway Jr. and the immunologist's dirty little secret. *Yale J Biol Med.* 2011;84(2):131-8

2. Tomljenovic L et al. Aluminum vaccine adjuvants: are they safe? *Curr Med Chem.* 2011;18(17):2630-37

3. Lyons-Weiler J et al. Reconsideration of the immunotherapeutic pediatric safe dose levels of aluminum. *J Trace Elem Med Biol.* 2018;48:67-73

4. Tomljenovic L et al. Do aluminum vaccine adjuvants contribute to the rising prevalence of autism? *J Inorg Biochem.* 2011;105(11):1489-99

5. Shaw CA et al. Aluminum hydroxide injections lead to motor deficits and motor neuron degeneration. *J Inorg Biochem.* 2009;103(11):1555-62

6. Yumoto S et al. Aluminium incorporation into the brain of rat fetuses and sucklings. *Brain Res Bull.* 2001;55(2):229-34

7. Liu Z et al. Association between maternal aluminum exposure and the risk of congenital heart defects in offspring. *Birth Defects Res A Clin Mol Teratol.* 2016;106(2):95-103

8. Kruger PC et al. A study of the distribution of aluminium in human placental tissues based on alkaline solubilization with determination by electrothermal atomic absorption spectrometry. *Metallomics.* 2010;2(9):621-7

9. Gherardi RK et al. Macrophagic myofasciitis: characterization and pathophysiology. *Lupus.* 2012;21(2):184-9

10. Kawahara M et al. Link between aluminum and the pathogenesis of Alzheimer's disease: the integration of the aluminum and amyloid cascade hypotheses. *Int J Alzheimers Dis.* 2011;2011:276393

11. Bhattacharjee S et al. Selective accumulation of aluminum in cerebral arteries in Alzheimer's disease (AD). *J Inorg Biochem.* 2013;126:35-7

12. Mirza A et al. Aluminium in brain tissue in familial Alzheimer's disease. *J Trace Elem Med Biol.* 2017;40:30-6

13. Exley C. Aluminum Should Now Be Considered a Primary Etiological Factor in Alzheimer's Disease. *JAD reports.* 2017;1(1):23-5

14. Klein JP et al. Aluminum content of human semen: implications for semen quality. *Reprod Toxicol.* 2014;50:43-8

15. Fu Y et al. Effects of sub-chronic aluminum chloride exposure on rat ovaries. *Life Sci.* 2014;100(1):61-6

16. Khan Z et al. Slow CCL2-dependent translocation of biopersistent particles from muscle to brain. *BMC Med.* 2013;11:99

17. Flarend RE et al. In vivo absorption of aluminium-containing vaccine adjuvants using 26Al. *Vaccine.* 1997;15(12-13):1314-8

18. Movsas TZ et al. Effect of routine vaccination on aluminum and essential element levels in preterm infants. *JAMA Pediatr.* 2013;167(9):870-2

19. Masson JD et al. Critical analysis of reference studies on the toxicokinetics of aluminum-based adjuvants. *J Inorg Biochem.* 2018;181:87-95

20. Crépeaux G et al. Non-linear dose-response of aluminium hydroxide adjuvant particles: selective low dose neurotoxicity. *Toxicology.* 2017;375:48-57

21. Asín J et al. Granulomas following subcutaneous injection with aluminum adjuvant-containing products in sheep. *Vet Pathol.* 2019;56(3):418-28

22. Bergfors E et al. How common are long-lasting, intensely itching vaccination granulomas and contact allergy to aluminium induced by currently used pediatric vaccines? A prospective cohort study. *Eur J Pediatr.* 2014;173(10):1297-307

23. Petrovsky N et al. Vaccine adjuvants: current state and future trends. *Immunol Cell Biol.* 2004;82(5):488-96

24. Petrovsky N. Comparative safety of vaccine adjuvants: a summary of current evidence and future needs. *Drug Saf.* 2015;38(11):1059-74

25. Graf R et al. Feline injection site sarcomas: data from Switzerland 2009-2014. *J Comp Pathol*. 2018;163:1-5

26. Offit PA et al. Addressing parents' concerns: do vaccines contain harmful preservatives, adjuvants, additives, or residuals? *Pediatrics*. 2003;112(6 Pt 1):1394-7

27. Dórea JG et al. Infants' exposure to aluminum from vaccines and breast milk during the first 6 months. *J Expo Sci Environ Epidemiol*. 2010;20(7):598-601

28. Mitkus RJ et al. Updated aluminum pharmacokinetics following infant exposures through diet and vaccination. *Vaccine*. 2011;29(51):9538-43

29. Jefferson T et al. Adverse events after immunisation with aluminium-containing DTP vaccines: systematic review of the evidence. *Lancet Infect Dis*. 2004;4(2):84-90

30. Nials AT et al. Mouse models of allergic asthma: acute and chronic allergen challenge. *Dis Model Mech*. 2008;1(4-5):213-20

31. Chusid JG et al. Experimental epilepsy in the monkey following multiple intracerebral injections of alumina cream. *Bull N Y Acad Med*. 1953;29(11):898-904

32. Pali-Schöll I et al. Antacids and dietary supplements with an influence on the gastric pH increase the risk for food sensitization. *Clin Exp Allergy*. 2010;40(7):1091-8

33. Vignal C et al. Gut: an underestimated target organ for aluminum. *Morphologie*. 2016;100(329):75-84

34. Nicholson S et al. Aluminum: a potential pro-oxidant in sunscreens/sunblocks? *Free Radic Biol Med*. 2007;43(8):1216-7

35. Srinivasan P et al. Aluminium in drinking water: an overview. *Water SA*. 1999;25:47-55

36. Saiyed SM et al. Aluminium content of some foods and food products in the USA, with aluminium food additives. *Food Addit Contam*. 2005;22(3):234-44

37. Duggan JM et al. Aluminium beverage cans as a dietary source of aluminium. *Med J Aust*. 1992;156(9):604-5

38. Kandiah J et al. Aluminum concentrations in tissues of rats: effect of soft drink packaging. *Biometals*. 1994;7(1):57-60

39. Rajwanshi P et al. Studies on aluminium leaching from cookware in tea and coffee and estimation of aluminium content in toothpaste, baking powder and paan masala. *Sci Total Environ*. 1997;193(3):243-9

40. Verbeeck RM et al. Aluminium in tooth pastes and Alzheimer's disease. *Acta Stomatol Belg*. 1990;87(2):141-4

41. Veien NK et al. Systemically aggravated contact dermatitis caused by aluminium in toothpaste. *Contact dermatitis*. 1993;28(3):199-200

42. Heidmann J et al. Comparative three-year caries protection from an aluminum-containing and a fluoride-containing toothpaste. *Caries Res*. 1997;31(2):85-90

43. Darbre PD. Aluminium, antiperspirants and breast cancer. *J Inorg Biochem*. 2005; 99(9):1912-9

44. Darbre PD. Aluminium and the human breast. *Morphologie*. 2016;100(329):65-74

45. Linhart C et al. Use of underarm cosmetic products in relation to risk of breast cancer: a case-control study. *EBioMedicine*. 2017;21:79-85

46. Davenward S et al. Silicon-rich mineral water as a non-invasive test of the 'aluminum hypothesis' in Alzheimer's disease. *J Alzheimers Dis*. 2013;33(2):423-30

47. Oda SS. The Influence of omega3 fatty acids supplementation against aluminum-induced toxicity in male albino rats. *Environ Sci Pollut Res Int*. 2016;23(14):14354-61

48. Ekong MB et al. Neuroprotective effect of Moringa Oleifera leaf extract on aluminium-induced temporal cortical degeneration. *Metab Brain Dis.* 2017;32(5):1437-47

49. Allagui MS et al. Pleiotropic protective roles of melatonin against aluminium-induced toxicity in rats. *Gen Physiol Biophys.* 2015;34(4):415-24

50. Yassa HA at al. Folic acid improve developmental toxicity induced by aluminum sulphates. *Environ Toxicol Pharmacol.* 2017;50:32-36

51. Yousef MI at al. Propolis protection from reproductive toxicity caused by aluminium chloride in male rats. *Food Chem Toxicol.* 2009;47(6):1168-75.

52. Khafaga AF. Exogenous phosphatidylcholine supplementation retrieve aluminum-induced toxicity in male albino rats. *Environ Sci Pollut Res Int.* 2017;24(18):15589-98

53. Wenting L et al. Therapeutic effect of taurine against aluminum-induced impairment on learning, memory and brain neurotransmitters in rats. *Neurol Sci.* 2014;35(10):1579-84

54. Nedzvetsky VS et al. Effects of vitamin E against aluminum neurotoxicity in rats. *Biochemistry (Mosc).* 2006;71(3):239-44

55. Sharma DR et al. Quercetin protects against chronic aluminum-induced oxidative stress and ensuing biochemical, cholinergic, and neurobehavioral impairments in rats. *Neurotox Res.* 2013;23(4):336-57

56. Viezeliene D et al. Selective induction of IL-6 by aluminum-induced oxidative stress can be prevented by selenium. *J Trace Elem Med Biol.* 2013;27(3):226-9

Chapter Seven

HUMAN PAPILLOMAVIRUS

The world will not be destroyed by those who do evil,
but by those who watch them without doing anything.
— **Albert Einstein**

H uman Papillomavirus (HPV) is transmitted mainly through sexual contact, but it can also be caught from parents and friends [1]. Most people contract it at some point in their lives. In 90% of the cases, the virus passes on its own without any symptoms, and only in a tiny percentage of cases the virus may result in cervical cancer. There are over 170 strains of papillomavirus. Seventeen of them are potentially oncogenic; some only cause warts.

Three HPV vaccines are currently available. Gardasil (Merck) is a tetravalent vaccine (protects against types 6, 11, 16, 18) and Cervarix (GlaxoSmithKline) is bivalent (protects against types 16 and 18). Types 16 and 18 are oncogenic and are "responsible" for 70% of the cases of cervical cancer, while types 6 and 11 cause warts. Since 2014 there also exists a new, nine-valent vaccine—Gardasil-9.

This vaccine is usually given to children, both boys and girls, in three doses, starting at the age of nine. In 2016 the CDC recommended reducing the number of doses to two [2]. In 2018 discussions about reducing the number of doses to just one have begun [3]. The vaccines contain recombinant (genetically modified) virus-like particles. The HPV virus for

Cervarix is grown in caterpillar cells, and the virus for Gardasil is grown in yeast. Yeast is a known trigger of autoimmune reactions [4].

Does HPV Cause Cervical Cancer?

How is it usually determined that a certain virus (or other pathogens) is the cause of a specific disease? Theoretically, by using Koch's postulates[1]. However, the causal link between HPV and cervical cancer does not meet the requirements of Koch's postulates. In practice, this does not mean much, as even Koch himself understood the limitations of his postulates. In reality, there are currently no generally accepted criteria for establishing a causal relationship in medicine. Statistical methods are usually used, but statistics can be used to prove absolutely anything. In 1996, new Koch's postulates were proposed for the 21st century [5]. However, it is stated that these postulates are quite controversial, as according to them, HPV is not the cause of cervical cancer, even though everyone knows that it is.

> Thus, whether HPV is the cause of cervical cancer or is far from being settled science.

An article published in 2000 states that despite the fact that HPV-16 and 18 play a major role in the development of cervical cancer, HPV is neither a necessary nor a sufficient factor for causing cervical cancer. HPV is found in only 90% of the tumors, and therefore a causal relationship between them does not satisfy Koch's first postulate. In the 1970s, researchers believed that it was the herpes virus (HSV-2) that was responsible for this disease. HPV-infected women get cervical cancer 4.3 times more often than those who are not infected. However, women who

---

[1] Koch's postulates – four criteria designed to establish a causative relationship between a microbe and a disease:
1. The microorganism must be found in abundance in all organisms suffering from the disease, but should not be found in healthy organisms.
2. The microorganism must be isolated from a diseased organism and grown in pure culture.
3. The cultured microorganism should cause disease when introduced into a healthy organism.
4. The microorganism must be reisolated from the inoculated, diseased experimental host and identified as being identical to the original specific causative agent.

have both viruses (HPV and herpes) get cancer nine times more often. In other studies, HPV was found in 60–77% of cervical cancer cases [6, 7].

Smoking and vaginal douching significantly increase the risk of cervical cancer. Women who regularly douched with commercial douche products were 2.4 times as likely to develop invasive cervical cancer as opposed to women who never douched. Women who usually douched with water and vinegar showed no increase in risk. Commercial douching products contain tar. Tar is also found in cigarettes and is a known carcinogen. It is noteworthy that the rates of cervical cancer among African American women are about twice those of white American women, as are the rates of vaginal douching. Contraceptive pills increase the risk of cervical cancer by three times, and intrauterine devices by 1.6 times, while condoms and diaphragms decrease the risk. The authors conclude that the cause of cervical cancer is the interaction between viruses (especially HPV and HSV-2) and tar (smoking and douching) [7].

HPV and cervical cancer could be compared to aluminum and Alzheimer's disease. Despite the fact that many scientists think that aluminum plays a major role in the occurrence of Alzheimer's disease, admitting it would not benefit anyone. It would not benefit the aluminum industry, or the cosmetics industry, or the pharmaceutical industry, all of which will lose billion-dollar profits and will have to pay out huge compensations. Neither would it benefit the governments, whose countries' economies will suffer because of this, nor would it benefit the scientists, who will lose their scarce grants and who do not wish to become another Wakefield. It would not benefit even the Alzheimer's Association, which will lose its financing as soon as the cause of the disease is determined.

On the other hand, recognizing HPV as the sole factor in cervical cancer does benefit everyone: the pharmaceutical industry, the governments, and even scientists.

> The HPV vaccine created a new multi-billion-dollar market that has not existed before.

Effectiveness

Cervical cancer develops very slowly; it is a process that usually takes 20–40 years (although rapid development is also possible) [9, 10]. It is preceded by cervical dysplasia. Cervical dysplasia is the presence of atypical cells in the cervix. There are three types of dysplasia: CIN 1 (mild dysplasia), CIN 2 (moderate dysplasia), and CIN 3 (severe dysplasia).

Having dysplasia does not mean that cervical cancer is inevitable. Only 1% of CIN 1, 5% of CIN 2, and 12–32% of CIN 3 develop into cancer [8].

In a 2013 article, which analyzes clinical trials of HPV vaccines, it is reported that in the developed countries where the PAP smear (a test that determines whether or not one has dysplasia) is widely used, cervical cancer mortality rates are very low (1.4-1.7/100,000 women). Ninety percent of deaths from cervical cancer are recorded in third-world countries. The risk of the disease is also very low—7/100,000 women. Moreover, the mortality rates from cervical cancer continue to fall rapidly. In the 90s, these rates more than halved without any vaccinations [9].

Since the development of cervical cancer takes decades, and pharmaceutical companies do not want to wait that long, surrogate markers (i.e., dysplasia CIN 1–3, which develop faster) are used instead of cancer in vaccine clinical trials. But since the vast majority of these dysplasia resolves on their own, they are a pretty bad marker for cervical cancer. The test for dysplasia, especially CIN 2, is very imprecise, which also makes it a bad marker. Therefore, the efficacy of a vaccine, determined on the basis of dysplasia, is not an indication of its efficacy against cervical cancer.

According to the analysis of clinical trials, the capacity of Gardasil to prevent CIN 2–3, associated with any HPV type, was only 14–17%. (This is the actual efficacy of the vaccine. But even this number is too high, as dysplasia does not always develop into cancer.) Gardasil efficacy for those who have already been exposed to HPV types targeted by the vaccine was negative (from -33% to -44.6%). That is, for those already infected, vaccine increases the risk of dysplasia. These results were not mentioned in the article published by Merck. Nevertheless, the FDA does not require testing for the infection before vaccinating. The vaccine was found to be 100% effective against HPV-16/18 infections and CIN 1–3 lesions. However, the significance of these results is questionable at best for two major reasons. The first reason is the low number of cases and a correspondingly wide confidence interval. In other words, the vaccine prevented 1.3% and 2.7% of all CIN 1–3 lesions. However, reporting a combined efficacy against CIN 1–3 gives a highly misleading impression about the true clinical value of the vaccine since the vast majority of the lesions within this population comprised of CIN 1 lesions. CIN 1s are a completely inadequate surrogate endpoint for assessing long-term clinical benefits of any HPV vaccine due to their benign nature as well as high frequency of regression. The authors conclude that vaccination with Gardasil is unlikely to have any notable effect in reducing the global cervical cancer burden.

Similar results were observed in clinical trials of the Cervarix vaccine. The efficacy of Cervarix against CIN 2+ lesions seven years after vaccination was only 40%, with no statistical significance.

Further down in the same article, vaccine safety studies are analyzed. From 2006 to 2012, more than 20,000 cases of adverse reactions of this vaccine have been reported in the US, 8% of which (1592) were serious, including 73 deaths, 348 life-threatening adverse reactions, and 581 events which resulted in permanent disability. Since the Vaccine Adverse Event Reporting System (VAERS) is passive, it records only 1–10% of all cases, according to various estimates. Therefore, the real amount of adverse events is 10–100 times higher. Out of all vaccine-adverse events in girls and women aged 6–29 years, 65% of all serious adverse events were due to the HPV vaccines. Eighty-two percent of cases of permanent disability in females under 30 years of age were also attributed to the HPV vaccines. In Australia, the number of adverse events increased by 85% almost entirely due to the HPV vaccination. The same is also happening in other countries.

In a Cervarix study, which included 9,000 women, 8% reported a serious event, 32% reported a medically significant condition, 9% reported a spontaneous abortion, and 3% reported a newly onset chronic disease. The same adverse event rates were observed in the control group (which received the same vaccine, but without the antigen). In the UK, adverse events from Cervarix were observed eight times more often than from the MMR vaccine [9].

Negative efficacy for the HPV-infected population and low efficacy of Gardasil in the general population have been identified in other studies as well [11].

A 2012 article states that despite the fact that the HPV vaccine is positioned as a vaccine against cervical cancer, to this day, it has not prevented a single case of cancer, let alone a single case of cancer death. The long-term benefits of this vaccine are based on the theoretical assumptions, rather than on research.

The authors also note that "With regard to Gardasil, often in trials sponsored by the vaccine manufacturer, the assessment of the frequency of adverse events was limited to those trial cohorts which comprised of participants who did not receive the full three doses of the HPV vaccine. The result of such population sample bias is a lesser sensitivity for detecting serious adverse reactions, as such events may be expected to occur less frequently if fewer doses of the vaccine are administered" [12].

Vaccines' adverse effects include seizures, paralysis, Guillain-Barré syndrome, transverse myelitis, facial neuritis, anaphylactic shock, deep vein thrombosis, chronic fatigue syndrome, cervical cancer, and death. In developed countries, more people suffer from serious adverse effects of HPV vaccines than die of cervical cancer. Although this comparison is not entirely appropriate, it should be remembered that this vaccine is given to children; therefore, even if the vaccine was very effective and prevented all 70% of cases of cancer from HPV 16 and 18 strains, cervical cancer would develop only decades later [13]. Should the theoretical potential of getting cervical cancer at the age of 50 be exchanged for the practical risk of lifelong paralysis, autoimmune disease, or death at the age of nine?

Safety

In a study published in 2017, mice were injected with Gardasil in doses equivalent to humans and then compared to the control mice. Vaccinated mice showed signs of depression, as well as neuroinflammation and autoimmune reactions [14].

In a 2015 study, the authors analyzed the serious adverse events of Gardasil in the US. The vaccine was associated with an increase in the risk of gastroenteritis by four times, arthritis by 2.5 times, systemic lupus by five times, vasculitis by four times, alopecia by eight times, and CNS conditions by 1.8 times. Vasculitis (inflammation of the blood vessels) started, on average, six days after the vaccination, lupus 19 days later, and arthritis after 55 days [15]. Gardasil causes 2.6 times more fainting and eight times more seizures compared to other vaccines [16]. According to a 2017 VAERS analysis, for those vaccinated with Gardasil, the risk of gastroenteritis was increased by 4.6 times, rheumatoid arthritis by five times, thrombocytopenia by two times, systemic lupus erythematosus by 7.6 times, vasculitis by 3.4 times, alopecia by 8.9 times, fainting by five times, ovarian damage by 15 times, and irritable bowel syndrome by ten times [17].

Out of 195,000 Canadian girls who received Gardasil, 10% visited the emergency department within 42 days of vaccination. Nine hundred fifty-eight were hospitalized. The authors, nonetheless, concluded that the vaccine is safe. Ten percent of emergency department visits among the ten-year-old girls are, of course, quite normal and have nothing to do with the vaccination [18].

Nature abhors a vacuum. By preventing the infection from two or four strains of HPV, the vaccination leads to other strains taking their place. A study published in 2016 found that there is a decrease in the prevalence of the four strains of HPV in young girls, but there was no change in the prevalence of HPV if all HPV types are taken into account [19]. Oncogenic strains of HPV 16 and 18 have been replaced with other oncogenic strains [20]. Studies that were conducted in Italy, the Netherlands, and the US came to the same conclusions [21–23].

After the European Medicines Agency (EMA) published a report stating that the HPV vaccine is completely safe, the Nordic Cochrane Center filed a complaint with the EMA. In the 19-page letter, Cochrane provides evidence of the report being written by people with conflicts of interest, which they forgot to mention. The letter also says that they completely ignored testimonies, expert opinions, and evidence of this vaccine being unsafe [24].

Orthostatic intolerance is a decrease in pressure upon rising from a position of sitting or lying down. In a study published in 2015, Danish doctors analyzed the symptoms of 35 girls. All of them had orthostatic intolerance that started, on average, nine days after the vaccination, but they were diagnosed, on average, two years later. Most of them also had severe chronic headaches, nausea, reduced cognitive function, palpitations, fatigue, muscular weakness, intermittent tremor, sleep disturbances, skin changes, neuropathic pain, etc. Five girls could not move about without a wheelchair. Anyone who did not take oral contraceptives had irregular periods. All but one reported that their daily activities were seriously affected, and 21 of them quit school or work due to their symptoms. **Before the vaccination, all girls were professionally involved in sports. Half of them were competing at a national or international level.** The fact that exercise enhances response to vaccination was also established in other studies [25].

In another study, the same authors analyzed post-vaccination symptoms of 53 girls. Common symptoms included severe headache, orthostatic intolerance, fatigue, nausea, cognitive dysfunction, disordered sleep, blurred vision, abdominal pain, involuntary muscle activity, neuropathic pain, etc. The symptoms started, on average, 11 days after the vaccination. None of the girls had any chronic diseases before the vaccination, and all of them were professionally involved in sports. After the vaccination, 98% reported that their daily activities were seriously affected, and 75% had to quit school or work for more than two months due to their symptoms [26]. An Italian study describes 18 similar cases among active and athletic young girls. Because of these symptoms, at least ten of them developed a long-standing social impairment (school absence, sport suspension, and daily activity impairment) [27]. Similar studies were published in Japan and the US [28, 29].

A 2012 study reported on two girls that died after getting the Gardasil vaccine. The first girl died at the age of 19, six months after receiving the third dose. The second girl died at the age of 14, two weeks after receiving the second dose. Autopsies of either of them did not reveal any pathologies. The authors of the study analyzed the samples of the girls' brain tissue and discovered that they both had autoimmune cerebral vasculitis (inflammation of the blood vessels of the brain) caused by the HPV-16 antibodies. They also found virus-like vaccine particles HPV-16L1, adhering to the blood vessels of the brain. Accumulation of immune cells in brain tissues could happen in one of the three cases: 1) direct brain infection; 2) brain trauma; 3) excessive stimulation of the immune system, such as through vaccination. From the autopsy results and the medical history, only the latter applied in both cases. The brain is very sensitive to ischemia (reduction in blood supply); therefore, vasculitis of the nervous system, if left untreated, almost inevitably leads to permanent injury. Cerebral vasculitis is thought to be rare, but this is because its symptoms are unstable, and it is hard to diagnose. The symptoms include severe headaches, orthostatic dizziness, syncope, seizures, tremors, tingling, weakness, locomotor deficits, cognitive and language impairments. The vast majority of these symptoms were experienced by both girls [30].

Impact On Reproductive Health

A 2015 article describes cases of three girls (ages 13, 14, and 21) with primary ovarian failure (menopause) following the HPV vaccination. Specific auto-antibodies were detected (anti-ovarian and anti-thyroid), suggesting that the HPV vaccine triggered an autoimmune response. All of them experienced regular symptoms as well—nausea, headache, sleep disturbances, cognitive and psychiatric disorders [4]. A 2014 article describes three more girls with menopause after the HPV vaccination, all from the same Australian state. The authors state that the premature ovarian failure in early- to mid-adolescence used to be so rare before that it was practically unknown [31]. In addition, this study analyzes pre-clinical, clinical, and post-licensing studies of the vaccine in terms of its effect on fertility.

Preclinical toxicology studies are performed on rodents. Merck (the Gardasil manufacturer) refused to provide a toxicology report on female rats' reproductive tract or ovaries but did provide the report on male rats' reproductive system. After vaccination, female rats conceived only once before euthanasia. In preclinical fertility studies submitted for licensing, no rats were tested with the complete vaccination course with representative interval administration, prior to mating.

Clinical studies were not any better. Firstly, the safety study enrolled predominantly females aged 16 to 23 years. There were very few girls under 16 years of age, even though they are the ones the vaccine was intended for. Secondly, they were all required to use effective contraception for at least seven months, which meant that irregularities in the menstrual cycle were impossible to identify. If anything happened after the seven-month period, then, by definition, it could not have been related to the vaccination. And if anything happened during those seven months, but the experimenter did not think it was vaccine-related, then it wasn't. And yet, two girls had amenorrhea, but Merck did not publish this data. Thirdly, serious adverse events were solicited for only two weeks after each vaccination, which obviously limits the ability to detect diminishing menstrual cycles. Moreover, menstrual cycle disruption, oligomenorrhea, and amenorrhea are not considered serious adverse events by definition. Serious adverse events are defined as life-threatening, resulting in death, permanent disability, congenital anomaly, hospitalization, prolongation of hospitalization, or necessitating medical or surgical intervention to prevent one of these outcomes. Menopause at the age of 12 is not a serious condition. VAERS recorded 104 cases of amenorrhea following Gardasil in 2006–2013. Post-licensing studies are usually based on data from the emergency departments and hospitalizations, and therefore they have no capacity to evaluate ongoing ovarian health since it rarely requires hospitalization. The authors conclude that "Small numbers of young persons represented in research, hormonal usage in older females' studies, vaccine report card limitations, omission of a true placebo, inconsistent rodent toxicity studies, limitations of serious adverse events recording, subjective investigator decisions of likelihood and failure to record new conditions arising after month 7 as vaccine-related have weakened safety research" [31].

A study published in 2018 found that the birth rate in the US decreased by 11% since 2007, even though it has been rising since 1995. Married women at the ages of 25–29, who received the HPV vaccine, got pregnant three times less often than those who did not get vaccinated. Among all women, the ones that got one dose got pregnant 2.4 times less often, and those who got three doses got pregnant 3.2 times less often, as compared to the women unvaccinated against HPV [32][2]. In another study, a link between the HPV vaccine and infertility has not been found. However, this study compared young vaccinated women to older unvaccinated women and did not analyze the number of doses the women received [33].

Polysorbate 80

One of the components of Gardasil is **polysorbate 80 (Tween 80)**. It's an emulsifier (E433) that is often used in the food and cosmetic industry and is considered to be safe enough to be used in vaccines as well. Although, of course, no one has ever evaluated its safety in vaccines. In a study on rats, however, it turned out that when newborn rats were injected with polysorbate 80, their estrous cycle was disrupted (increased from 4.3 to 9–14 days). In addition, they had decreased in the relative weight of the ovaries, cytological changes in the uterus, enlarged uterus, and accelerated aging of the reproductive organs [34].

---

[2] This study was retracted by the publisher in December 2019 without a valid explanation.

Furthermore, polysorbate 80 can penetrate the blood-brain barrier. Moreover, because of this property, it is often added to drugs intended for the central nervous system [35, 36]. This, in addition to aluminum, also explains why most adverse effects of the vaccine are neurological and psychiatric disorders.

According to the toxicology report of the manufacturer, polysorbate 80 is a carcinogen and causes DNA mutations. Animal studies show that it causes cardiac changes, psychological changes, and weight loss. Whether or not it penetrates the skin is unclear, but that does not prevent it from being widely used in soaps, shampoos, and other cosmetic products.

In the early 1980s, preterm infants were injected with E-ferol (intravenous vitamin E). It was associated with pulmonary deterioration, hepatomegaly, cholestatic jaundice, ascites, splenomegaly, renal failure, azotemia, and thrombocytopenia. At least 38 infants died. It turned out that polysorbate 80, contained in E-ferol, was responsible for these adverse effects [37]. Polysorbate 80 is also found in some vaccines against diphtheria, tetanus, pertussis, polio, Hib, hepatitis A and B, influenza, pneumococcus, meningococcus, and rotavirus [38].

Clinical Trials

In clinical trials of both vaccines, aluminum was used instead of a placebo. Therefore, it is impossible to determine the real number of adverse effects from the results of these trials. According to the document Merck provided to the FDA for approval of Gardasil, 20,000 girls participated in the vaccine trials. Seventy-five percent of these young girls developed some kind of new disease during the three years of the trial [39]. Whether or not this is a significant number is for you to decide.

However, one small control group of the girls in the Gardasil trials received saline, not aluminum. Although this saline also contained other components of the vaccine, excluding aluminum [40]. The existence of this small group allows Merck to claim that not only aluminum was used as a placebo, but also saline. As for the other components of this saline solution, they usually stay modestly silent. However, the data on the adverse effects of this group compared to other groups is not available. Merck summarized the serious adverse effects of all control groups together.

In a 2017 analysis of clinical and post-marketing studies of the vaccine, it is reported that in the two largest clinical trials, the number of serious negative events was significantly higher in the group that received the vaccine. In the group that received Cervarix, for example, 14 deaths were recorded, while in the control group, there were only three deaths. In the group that received Gardasil-9, the number of serious negative events was significantly higher compared to the group that received the previous version of Gardasil (3.3% vs. 2.6%). To prevent one case of dysplasia that is not prevented by Gardasil, 1,757 girls need to be vaccinated with Gardasil-9. To cause an additional serious adverse event, 140 girls need to be vaccinated with Gardasil-9, meaning that the chance of Gardasil-9 causing harm is 12 times higher than the chance of it doing good, as compared to Gardasil. Almost all serious adverse events in clinical trials were deemed by the investigators as unrelated to the vaccine [41].

A study conducted in Valencia showed that ten times more adverse events are recorded for the HPV vaccines as compared to other vaccines. Thirty-two percent of the adverse events were classified as severe. The authors suggested that it might be due to the bad publicity of this vaccine [41]. Japan suspended vaccination in response to the adverse events, after which diseases associated with this vaccination, such as orthostatic intolerance, ceased to occur [42]. It is also worth noting that only 48% of the completed HPV vaccine clinical trials were published [43].

Adjuvants And Other Components

At first glance, it is hard to understand how the manufacturers managed to create such a dangerous vaccine. After all, unlike most vaccines that are given to small children with an undeveloped immune system, this vaccine is given to adolescents and adults. So why is it that the number of adverse effects of this particular vaccine is so overwhelming? Vaccination advocates have a simple answer to this question. According to them, this happens because adolescents and adults, unlike infants, can speak. Infants can only express themselves through crying, and crying could be attributed to anything. If a 16-year-old girl starts fainting, stops thinking clearly, and cannot continue her studies, it is impossible not to notice, and impossible to write off as due to genetic factors. And if an infant stops thinking clearly, it only becomes apparent years later, and it can be concluded that the child was born that way.

But there is another answer: new types of aluminum salts were used as adjuvants in these vaccines. **Aluminum hydroxide** ($Al(OH)_3$) and

aluminum phosphate (AlPO₄) were discussed in the previous chapter. But there are new, more potent aluminum adjuvants. **Amorphous Aluminum Hydroxyphosphate Sulfate** (AAHS) is used in Gardasil. (Gardasil-9 contains 2.2 times more of this adjuvant than the previous version of the vaccine.) **Adjuvant system 04** (AS04) was used in Cervarix. AS04 is aluminum hydroxide mixed with salmonella endotoxin. Of course, no one conducted any studies on the safety of these new adjuvants.

Despite numerous studies proving its toxicity, aluminum is considered by the FDA as GRAS (Generally Recognized As Safe). This means that its new compounds are also safe enough to be added to the vaccines. A 2007 study compared the immune response to these new adjuvants with the response to aluminum hydroxide in mice. The authors concluded that both of the new adjuvants induce an immune response three to eight times greater than that of the aluminum hydroxide. For some reason, they never mention that an eightfold increase in the immune response also means an eightfold increase in the risk of the autoimmune response [44].

A 2012 study reported that despite the manufacturer's claims that the vaccine is purified and does not contain papillomavirus DNA, all 16 of the tested vials, collected from around the world, had fragments of the virus's DNA in them. Since these fragments are bound with aluminum adjuvant, (which is engulfed and spread throughout the body by macrophages), these virus DNA fragments enter all organs and further enhance the autoimmune response. Moreover, because the virus is bound to aluminum and macrophages do not know what to do with this aluminum, DNA fragments become protected by the aluminum and are not disposed of. Gardasil's papillomavirus DNA fragments were also detected in the blood and spleen of the 16-year-old girl that died six months after vaccination [45]. In response to this study, the FDA rushed to declare that the presence of DNA fragments is not at all dangerous and was even expected [46]. Although, according to the documents submitted to the FDA by Merck, there should be no DNA fragments in the vaccines [47].

According to VAERS, in the period from 2006 to 2019, more than 15,000 people visited the ER after being vaccinated against HPV in the US, more than 6,000 were hospitalized, 3,000 became permanently disabled, 480 died, more than 300 developed cervical dysplasia, and more than 400 developed cervical cancer. As indicated above, this data includes approximately 1–10% of all cases.

63

Probiotics may help in the treatment of cervical dysplasia [48]. Vitamins C, A, E, vitamin D, vitamin B group, green tea extract, turmeric, and healthy vaginal flora significantly reduce the risk of dysplasia [49–54]. This means that if you do not smoke, do not take oral contraceptives, eat well, do not destroy vaginal microflora with douching chemicals, get pap-smears once in a while, the risk of cervical cancer, which is already very low, is reduced to almost zero without any vaccinations.

Conclusions

It's not a proven fact that HPV causes cervical cancer.

In most cases, HPV disappears by itself without any symptoms.

The risk of cervical cancer in developed countries is very low (7/100,000) and continues to decline rapidly.

The vaccine increases the risk of cervical dysplasia by 44% in those already infected with HPV.

The vaccine contains new and unsafe aluminum adjuvants. Gardasil also contains polysorbate 80, which leads to the rapid aging of reproductive organs.

There are safer and more effective methods of preventing cervical cancer.

Vaccination is especially dangerous for athletes.

Endnotes

1. Rintala MA et al. Transmission of high-risk human papillomavirus (HPV) between parents and infant: a prospective study of HPV in families in Finland. *J Clin Microbiol.* 2005;43(1):376-81

2. Meites E et al. Use of a 2-dose schedule for human papillomavirus vaccination - updated recommendations of the advisory committee on immunization practices. *MMWR.* 2016;65(49):1405-8

3. Margaret Stanley PD. Preventing cervical cancer: how much HPV vaccine do we need? *Vaccine.* 2018;36(32):4759-836

4. Colafrancesco S et al. Human papilloma virus vaccine and primary ovarian failure: another facet of the autoimmune/inflammatory syndrome induced by adjuvants. *Am J Reprod Immunol.* 2013;70(4):309-16

5. Fredericks DN et al. Sequence-based identification of microbial pathogens: a reconsideration of Koch's postulates. *Clin Microbiol Rev.* 1996;9(1):18–33

6. Daling JR et al. A population-based study of squamous cell vaginal cancer: HPV and cofactors. *Gynecol Oncol.* 2002;84(2):263-70

7. Haverkos H et al. The cause of invasive cervical cancer could be multifactorial. *Biomed Pharmacother.* 2000;54(1):54-9

8. Ostör AG. Natural history of cervical intraepithelial neoplasia: a critical review. *Int J Gynecol Pathol.* 1993;12(2):186-92

9. Tomljenovic L et al. Human papillomavirus (HPV) vaccines as an option for preventing cervical malignancies: (how) effective and safe? *Curr Pharm Des.* 2013;19(8):1466-87

10. Hildesheim A et al. Risk factors for rapid-onset cervical cancer. *Am J Obstet Gynecol.* 1999;180(3 Pt 1):571-7

11. Mahmud SM et al. Effectiveness of the quadrivalent human papillomavirus vaccine against cervical dysplasia in Manitoba, Canada. *J Clin Oncol.* 2014;32(5):438-43

12. Tomljenovic L et al. Too fast or not too fast: the FDA's approval of Merck's HPV vaccine Gardasil. *J Law Med Ethics.* 2012;40(3):673-81

13. Tomljenovic L et al. Human papillomavirus (HPV) vaccine policy and evidence-based medicine: are they at odds? *Ann Med.* 2013;45(2):182-93

14. Inbar R et al. Behavioral abnormalities in female mice following administration of aluminum adjuvants and the human papillomavirus (HPV) vaccine Gardasil. *Immunol Res.* 2017;65(1):136-49

15. Geier DA et al. A case-control study of quadrivalent human papillomavirus vaccine-associated autoimmune adverse events. *Clin Rheumatol.* 2015;34(7):1225-31

16. Rodríguez-Galán MA et al. Adverse reactions to human papillomavirus vaccine in the Valencian Community (2007-2011). *An Pediatr (Barc).* 2014;81(5):303-9

17. Geier DA et al. Quadrivalent human papillomavirus vaccine and autoimmune adverse events: a case-control assessment of the vaccine adverse event reporting system (VAERS) database. *Immunol Res.* 2017;65(1):46-54

18. Liu XC et al. Adverse events following HPV vaccination, Alberta 2006-2014. *Vaccine.* 2016;34(15):1800-5

19. Markowitz LE et al. Prevalence of HPV After Introduction of the Vaccination Program in the United States. *Pediatrics.* 2016;137(3):e20151968

20. Fischer S et al. Shift in prevalence of HPV types in cervical cytology specimens in the era of HPV vaccination. *Oncol Lett.* 2016;12(1):601-10

21. Giambi C et al. A cross-sectional study to estimate high-risk human papillomavirus prevalence and type distribution in Italian women aged 18-26 years. *BMC Infect Dis.* 2013;13:74

22. Mollers M et al. Population- and type-specific clustering of multiple HPV types across diverse risk populations in the Netherlands. *Am J Epidemiol.* 2014;179(10):1236-46

23. Guo F et al. Comparison of HPV prevalence between HPV-vaccinated and non-vaccinated young adult women (20-26 years). *Hum Vaccin Immunother.* 2015;11(10):2337-44

24. Peter C Gøtzsche. Complaint to the European Medicines Agency (EMA) over maladministration at the EMA. *Nordic Cochrane Centre*

25. Brinth LS et al. Orthostatic intolerance and postural tachycardia syndrome as suspected adverse effects of vaccination against human papilloma virus. *Vaccine.* 2015; 33(22):2602-5

26. Brinth L et al. Suspected side effects to the quadrivalent human papilloma vaccine. *Dan Med J.* 2015;62(4):A5064

27. Palmieri B et al. Severe somatoform and dysautonomic syndromes after HPV vaccination: case series and review of literature. *Immunol Res.* 2017;65(1):106-16

28. Kinoshita T et al. Peripheral sympathetic nerve dysfunction in adolescent Japanese girls following immunization with the human papillomavirus vaccine. *Intern Med.* 2014; 53(19):2185-200

29. Blitshteyn S. Postural tachycardia syndrome following human papillomavirus vaccination. *Eur J Neurol.* 2014;21(1):135-9

30. Shaw LTC. Death after quadrivalent human papillomavirus (HPV) vaccination: causal or coincidental? *Pharma Reg Affairs.* 2012:S12-001

31. Little DT et al. Adolescent premature ovarian insufficiency following human papillomavirus vaccination: a case series seen in general practice. *J Investig Med High Impact Case Rep.* 2014;2(4):2324709614556129

32. DeLong G. A lowered probability of pregnancy in females in the USA aged 25-29 who received a human papillomavirus vaccine injection. *J Toxicol Environ Health A.* 2018; 81(14):661-74

33. McInerney KA et al. the effect of vaccination against human papillomavirus on fecundability. *Paediatr Perinat Epidemiol.* 2017;31(6):531-6

34. Gajdová M et al. Delayed effects of neonatal exposure to Tween 80 on female reproductive organs in rats. *Food Chem Toxicol.* 1993;31(3):183-90

35. Azmin MN et al. The distribution and elimination of methotrexate in mouse blood and brain after concurrent administration of polysorbate 80. *Cancer Chemother Pharmacol.* 1985;14(3):238-42

36. Pardridge WM. The blood-brain barrier: bottleneck in brain drug development. *NeuroRx.* 2005;2(1):3-14

37. Alade SL et al. Polysorbate 80 and E-Ferol toxicity. *Pediatrics.* 1986;77(4):593-7

38. www.cdc.gov/vaccines/pubs/pinkbook/downloads/appendices/B/excipient-table-2.pdf

39. Clinical Review of Biologics License Application Supplement for Human Papillomavirus Quadrivalent (Types 6, 11, 16, 18) Vaccine, Recombinant (Gardasil®) to extend indication for prevention of vaginal and vulvar cancers related to HPV types 16 and 18. 2008

40. Reisinger KS et al. Safety and persistent immunogenicity of a quadrivalent human papillomavirus types 6,11,16,18 L1 virus-like particle vaccine in preadolescents and adolescents: a randomized controlled trial. *Pediatr Infect Dis J.* 2007;26(3):201-9

41. Martínez-Lavín M et al. Serious adverse events after HPV vaccination: a critical review of randomized trials and post-marketing case series. *Clin Rheumatol.* 2017;36(10):2169-78

42. Ozawa K et al. Suspected adverse effects after human papillomavirus vaccination: a temporal relationship between vaccine administration and the appearance of symptoms in Japan. *Drug Saf.* 2017;40(12):1219-29

43. Jørgensen L et al. Index of the human papillomavirus (HPV) vaccine industry clinical study programmes and non-industry funded studies: a necessary basis to address reporting bias in a systematic review. *Systematic reviews.* 2018;7(1):8

44. Caulfield MJ et al. Effect of alternative aluminum adjuvants on the absorption and immunogenicity of HPV16 L1 VLPs in mice. *Hum Vaccin.* 2007;3(4):139-45

45. Lee SH. Detection of human papillomavirus (HPV) L1 gene DNA possibly bound to particulate aluminum adjuvant in the HPV vaccine Gardasil. *J Inorg Biochem.* 2012;117:85-92

46. FDA Information on Gardasil – Presence of DNA Fragments Expected, No Safety Risk. 2011

47. GARDASIL (Human Papillomavirus [Types 6, 11, 16, 18] Recombinant Vaccine) Vaccines and Related Biological Products Advisory Committee (VRBPAC) Briefing Document Presented to VRBPAC on 18-May-2006

48. Verhoeven V et al. Probiotics enhance the clearance of human papillomavirus-related cervical lesions: a prospective controlled pilot study. *Eur J Cancer Prev.* 2013;22(1):46-51

49. Hwang JH et al. Dietary supplements reduce the risk of cervical intraepithelial neoplasia. *Int J Gynecol Cancer.* 2010;20(3):398-403

50. Özgü E et al. Could 25-OH vitamin D deficiency be a reason for HPV infection persistence in cervical premalignant lesions? *J Exp Ther Oncol.* 2016;11(3):177-80

51. Hernandez B et al. Diet and premalignant lesions of the cervix: evidence of a protective role for folate, riboflavin, thiamin, and vitamin B12. *Cancer Causes Control.* 2003;14(9):859-70

52. Ahn W-S et al. Protective effects of green tea extracts (polyphenon E and EGCG) on human cervical lesions. *Eur J Cancer Prev.* 2003;12(5):383-90

53. Basu P et al. Clearance of cervical human papillomavirus infection by topical application of curcumin and curcumin containing polyherbal cream: a phase II randomized controlled study. *Asian Pac J Cancer Prev.* 2013;14(10):5753-9

54. Mitra A et al. The vaginal microbiota, human papillomavirus infection and cervical intraepithelial neoplasia: what do we know and where are we going next? *Microbiome.* 2016;4(1):58

Chapter Eight

HEPATITIS B

First, do no harm.
— Hippocrates

S imilar to HPV, hepatitis B is a virus, which is most commonly spread through sexual contact or through the blood. If a mother is infected with hepatitis B, the virus can pass to the fetus through the placenta or during delivery. Hepatitis B does not pass through breast milk [1].

Eighty percent of infected adults show no or very mild symptoms, and they do not even know that they were infected. After having been infected, they get lifelong immunity. Of the remaining 20%, who get diagnosed with hepatitis B, 95% fully recover and get lifelong immunity. Of the remaining 5%, only 25% (that is 0.25% of all those infected) will develop cirrhosis or liver cancer in 20–30 years after the infection. This cirrhosis or cancer does not develop because of the virus itself, but rather because of the immune system's response to it. Seventy percent of patients with chronic hepatitis B are injection drug users, homosexuals, alcohol abusers, homeless people, and people with many sexual partners. Hepatitis B develops into cirrhosis or cancer mainly in alcohol abusers, smokers, patients with hepatitis C, obesity, and diabetes [2].

Why vaccinate a newborn child against an STD, which they have virtually no chance of contracting? Well, simply because the adult drug addicts and homosexuals refused to get vaccinated. Therefore, it was decided to vaccinate children immediately after birth, while they are not yet able to refuse [3]. Most family physicians and pediatricians did not support this venture [4].

This is the only vaccine that is given immediately after birth. It is not given to prevent the possibility of contracting the infection from the mother. In the USA and other countries, all women get tested for hepatitis B before childbirth. Children of infected mothers receive immunoglobulin together with the vaccine. In some countries, however, all children get vaccinated just because it is much cheaper than testing all the mothers [5].

Prior to the beginning of universal infant vaccination in 1990, only one out of 100,000 children under the age of 15 had a hepatitis B infection in the US. Currently, the risk of getting infected with hepatitis B at any age under 20 years old is 0.3 in one million [6]. In developed countries, hepatitis B is a rare disease. In Africa and Southeast Asia, it is much more common [7].

The first hepatitis B vaccine appeared in 1981 and contained a live virus. After its introduction, the number of people infected with hepatitis B increased rapidly [8]. A 1994 study showed that despite the existence of the vaccine, the number of patients with hepatitis B was not decreasing [9]. There are quite a few manufacturers of this vaccine, but in developed countries, Recombivax (Merck) and Engerix-B (GSK) are most commonly used, as well as combination vaccines.

The Engerix-B vaccine contains aluminum hydroxide as an adjuvant, and Recombivax contains Amorphous Aluminum Hydroxyphosphate Sulfate (AAHS, the same adjuvant as used in Gardasil). Previously, the Recombivax package insert indicated that it contains aluminum hydroxide. Now they put it this way: *"0.5 mg of aluminum provided as amorphous aluminum hydroxyphosphate sulfate, previously referred to as aluminum hydroxide"* [10]. This raises the question of how trustworthy the list of vaccine ingredients is.

> In most European countries, newborns are not vaccinated against hepatitis B. Instead, they are vaccinated two to three months after birth. In some countries (Finland, Iceland, Denmark, Hungary), children are not vaccinated against hepatitis B at all, and yet there are no epidemics there.

Effectiveness

According to a Cochrane systematic review, vaccine efficacy in preventing infection from the mother is 72%, the efficacy of immunoglobulin is 50%, and vaccine + immunoglobulin has 92% efficacy. No statistically significant difference was found between vaccination immediately after birth and vaccination at one month of age. A single dose of immunoglobulin was as effective as multiple doses [11].

According to a 2018 study, in India, where hepatitis B is quite common, there is no difference in vaccine efficacy, whether it is given at birth or six weeks after. The risk of developing chronic infection is 90% in children younger than one year, 30% if infected at the ages of one to five, and 2% for adults. The prevalence of hepatitis B in India is 2.4%, which should result in 250,000 deaths from hepatocellular carcinoma each year. However, only 5,000 cases of hepatocellular carcinoma per year are recorded in India, which is much less than expected. At the age of one year, 45% of the unvaccinated children were naturally immune to hepatitis B. By the ages of four to five, the number of antibodies in vaccinated children decreased and was only insignificantly higher compared to unvaccinated children. The authors believe that unvaccinated children are probably protected by the mother's antibodies, which disappear only years after birth, and not within nine months, as is commonly believed [12]. The incidence of hepatocellular carcinoma in the US began to rise rapidly in the early 90s, after the beginning of universal vaccination, and by 2007 it already increased more than twofold [13].

The hepatitis B vaccine was originally intended only for risk groups, so clinical trials in the 1980s were conducted only on them. Seven hundred seventy-three homosexuals were given hepatitis vaccination and observed for five years. Eighty-two percent of them developed a sufficient level of antibodies after the vaccination. By the end of the observation period, the antibodies disappeared in 15% of the recipients, and decreased below the protective level in 27%. Fifty-five contracted hepatitis, and five became chronic carriers. The risk of infection was directly related to the extent of sexual activity. Persons who became infected had an average of 29 nonsteady sexual partners, as compared to 11.5 partners among those who did not become infected [14].

In Israel, the percentage of people infected with hepatitis B in 2012 has not changed if compared with 1977 and 1991. Despite vaccination, 8.4% of children were infected by their mothers [15]. In Taiwan, 15-year-old adolescents, vaccinated in childhood, had their level of hepatitis B antibodies tested, and it turned out to be very low [16]. That is, the immunity from vaccination disappears before the beginning of sexual activity, which is when it would finally become useful. According to another study, antibodies disappear by the age of five [17].

Hepatitis C is a disease with transmission methods similar to those of hepatitis B. As can be seen from the graph below, increase and decrease in the incidence of both types of hepatitis occurred almost simultaneously. Vaccination is considered to be responsible for the decrease in the hepatitis B incidence, whereas in the case of hepatitis C the CDC says: *"The reasons for this decrease were unknown but probably reflected changes in the behavior and practices among injection-drug users"* [18].

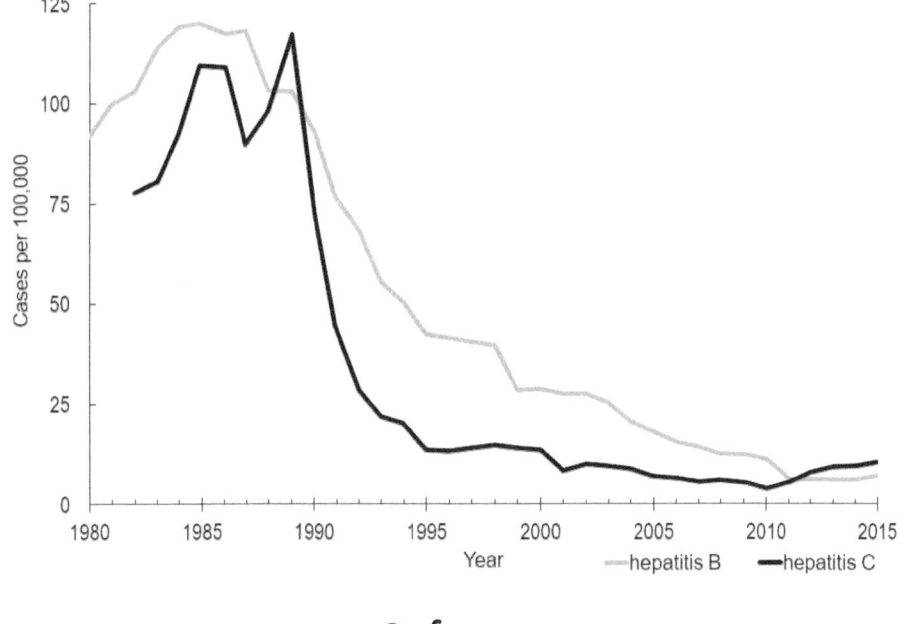

Incidence of hepatitis B and C in the US (1980-2015)

Safety

In a 2004 study, the hepatitis B vaccine was associated with a threefold risk of multiple sclerosis within three years after the vaccination. The authors also analyzed other studies, which did not find an increased risk of multiple sclerosis in the vaccinated. In these studies, the date of diagnosis was used, and not the date of onset of the first symptoms. Multiple sclerosis is usually diagnosed several years after the onset of symptoms [19].

In a 2009 French study, the Engerix-B vaccine was associated with a 2.8 times increase in the risk of multiple sclerosis, as compared to the other hepatitis B vaccines [20]. A 2014 study reported that after hepatitis B vaccination began in France, the number of multiple sclerosis cases increased by 65%. There is a high correlation between the number of doses of the vaccine received and the number of cases of multiple sclerosis within one to two years [21].

The hepatitis B virus antigen is similar in shape to the proteins found in myelin (insulating sheath of the nerve cells in the brain). After vaccination, 60% of people develop a cross-reactive response to myelin proteins, which weakens over time. This mechanism of molecular mimicry explains why multiple sclerosis can occur after the hepatitis B vaccination [22].

According to VAERS analysis, adults vaccinated against hepatitis B got multiple sclerosis five times more often than those vaccinated against tetanus. The risk of vasculitis in those vaccinated against hepatitis B was 2.6 times higher, alopecia seven times, lupus nine times, arthritis two times, rheumatoid arthritis 18 times, thrombocytopenia two times, and optic neuritis 14 times higher [23]. In another study, the hepatitis B vaccine was associated with a six times increase in the risk of arthritis, a 1.6 times increase in the risk of acute ear infections, and a 1.4 times increase in the risk of pharyngitis [24]. Also, the risk of liver problems was 1.5–2.3 times higher in those vaccinated against hepatitis B [25].

In a 2010 study, newborn macaques were given a hepatitis B vaccine with thimerosal and were compared to the unvaccinated ones. Vaccinated macaques acquired survival reflexes, as well as motor and sensory-motor reflexes, much later than the unvaccinated ones. Low birth weight and prematurity exacerbated the effect. Thimerosal (ethyl mercury) has not been added to childhood vaccines since 2003 in the US and Western Europe but is still used in vaccines in most other countries [26].

A 2008 article reported that after the introduction of vaccination, the number of children with type 1 diabetes increased by 61% in France, and by 48% in New Zealand. In Italy, those vaccinated against hepatitis B had type 1 diabetes 40% more often than those unvaccinated. The increase in the number of cases of type 1 diabetes occurs two to four years after the beginning of vaccination, which is consistent with the causal relationship [27].

According to a 2014 Israeli study, the hepatitis B vaccine is associated with chronic fatigue syndrome and fibromyalgia [28]. Autoimmune diseases such as Reiter's syndrome, arthritis, lupus, uveitis, myasthenia, erythema nodosum, thrombocytopenic purpura, Evans syndrome, and demyelinating diseases of the central nervous system are also associated with the hepatitis B vaccination [29].

Memory impairment, decreased blood cell count, and brain gliosis was observed in mice vaccinated with Engerix-B or aluminum hydroxide. Vaccination also increased the severity of kidney disease [30]. In another study, neurobehavioral impairments were observed in adult mice that were vaccinated against hepatitis B as newborns [31]. According to a 2012 study, the hepatitis B vaccine destroys mitochondria and kills liver cells in mice [32].

A 2015 Singapore study reported that the hepatitis B virus, passed from mother to child, might, contrary to popular belief, lead to better development of the immune system [33].

The authors of a Russian study published in 2009 write that 80% of the newborns in Russia have neonatal jaundice, which in recent years has been accompanied by the high levels of bilirubin and is taking longer to treat. Some doctors had concerns regarding vaccination of newborns, and this particular vaccine began to be regarded as a contributing factor to the increasing incidence of the prolonged conjugated jaundice in children. The study showed that the probability of development and prolonged treatment of neonatal jaundice is higher for those vaccinated against hepatitis B than for those unvaccinated [34].

VAERS recorded more than 1,300 deaths and more than 3,000 cases of permanent disability following the hepatitis B vaccination. Infants, of course, do not die from the hepatitis B itself.

Conclusions

Hepatitis B is a disease that is characteristic to risk groups such as drug users and homosexuals, people with multiple sexual partners, and to some extent, medical staff working with blood. The probability of contracting hepatitis B before the start of sexual activity is virtually zero.

It is often claimed that a child can get infected by using someone else's toothbrush or other household items. This way of contracting the infection is purely theoretical. There is not a single study proving that anyone has contracted hepatitis B this way.

Vaccines contain 250–550 mcg of aluminum. That is, three doses of this vaccine contain 15–30 times more aluminum than all the aluminum the child will get from breast milk in six months.

> By the way, the fact that infants get aluminum from mothers' milk does not mean that it is normal. It means that mothers are poisoned with aluminum, which they get from food and water, and are poisoning their infants with it.

The vaccine increases the risk of autoimmune diseases, such as multiple sclerosis, arthritis, type 1 diabetes, and others.

Endnotes

1. Chen X et al. Breastfeeding is not a risk factor for mother-to-child transmission of hepatitis B virus. *PloS One*. 2013;8(1):e55303

2. Elgouhari HM et al. Hepatitis B virus infection: understanding its epidemiology, course, and diagnosis. *Cleve Clin J Med*. 2008;75(12):881-9

3. Kolata G. U.S. panel urges that all children be vaccinated for hepatitis B. *New York Times*. 1991 Mar 1

4. Freed GL et al. Universal hepatitis B immunization of infants: reactions of pediatricians and family physicians over time. *Pediatrics*. 1994;93(5):747-51

5. Krahn M et al. Should Canada and the United States universally vaccinate infants against hepatitis B? A cost-effectiveness analysis. *Med Decis Making*. 1993;13(1):4-20

6. Viral Hepatitis Surveillance United States, 2013

7. Kim WR. Epidemiology of hepatitis B in the United States. *Hepatology*. 2009; 49(5):S28-34

8. Hepatitis B. *CDC Pink Book*

9. McQuillan GM et al. Prevalence of hepatitis B virus infection in the United States: the National Health and Nutrition Examination Surveys, 1976 through 1994. *Am J Public Health*. 1999;89(1):14-8

10. Recombivax HB vaccine package insert

11. Lee C et al. Hepatitis B immunisation for newborn infants of hepatitis B surface antigen-positive mothers. *Cochrane Database Syst Rev.* 2006(2):CD004790

12. Puliyel J et al. Evaluation of the protection provided by hepatitis B vaccination in India. *Indian J Pediatr.* 2018;85(7):510-6

13. El-Serag HB. Hepatocellular carcinoma. *N Engl J Med.* 2011;365(12):1118-27

14. Hadler SC et al. Long-term immunogenicity and efficacy of hepatitis B vaccine in homosexual men. *N Engl J Med.* 1986;315(4):209-14

15. Michaiel R et al. Vertical HBV transmission in Jerusalem in the vaccine era. *Harefuah.* 2012;151(12):671-4

16. Wu TW et al. Chronic hepatitis B infection in adolescents who received primary infantile vaccination. *Hepatology.* 2013;57(1):37-45

17. Petersen KM et al. Duration of hepatitis B immunity in low risk children receiving hepatitis B vaccinations from birth. *Pediatr Infect Dis J.* 2004;23(7):650-5

18. Daniels D et al. Surveillance for acute viral hepatitis - United States, 2007. *MMWR Surveill Summ.* 2009;58(3):1-27

19. Hernán MA et al. Recombinant hepatitis B vaccine and the risk of multiple sclerosis: a prospective study. *Neurology.* 2004;63(5):838-42

20. Mikaeloff Y et al. Hepatitis B vaccine and the risk of CNS inflammatory demyelination in childhood. *Neurology.* 2009;72(10):873-80

21. Le Houézec D. Evolution of multiple sclerosis in France since the beginning of hepatitis B vaccination. *Immunol Res.* 2014;60(2-3):219-25

22. Bogdanos DP et al. A study of molecular mimicry and immunological cross-reactivity between hepatitis B surface antigen and myelin mimics. *Clin Dev Immunol.* 2005; 12(3):217-24

23. Geier DA et al. A case-control study of serious autoimmune adverse events following hepatitis B immunization. *Autoimmunity.* 2005;38(4):295-301

24. Fisher MA et al. Adverse events associated with hepatitis B vaccine in U.S. children less than six years of age, 1993 and 1994. *Ann Epidemiol.* 2001;11(1):13-21

25. Fisher MA et al. Hepatitis B vaccine and liver problems in U.S. children less than 6 years old, 1993 and 1994. *Epidemiology.* 1999;10(3):337-9

26. Hewitson L et al. Delayed acquisition of neonatal reflexes in newborn primates receiving a thimerosal-containing hepatitis B vaccine: influence of gestational age and birth weight. *J Toxicol Environ Health A.* 2010;73(19):1298-313

27. Classen J. Clustering of Cases of IDDM 2 to 4 Years after Hepatitis B Immunization is Consistent with Clustering after Infections and Progression to IDDM in Autoantibody Positive Individuals. *Open Pediatr Med J.* 2008;2:1-6

28. Agmon-Levin N et al. Chronic fatigue syndrome and fibromyalgia following immunization with the hepatitis B vaccine: another angle of the 'autoimmune (auto-inflammatory) syndrome induced by adjuvants' (ASIA). *Immunol Res.* 2014;60(2-3):376-83

29. Cohen AD et al. Vaccine-induced autoimmunity. *J Autoimmun.* 1996;9(6):699-703

30. Agmon-Levin N. Immunization with hepatitis B vaccine accelerates SLE-like disease in a murine model. *J Autoimmun.* 2014;54:21-32

31. Yang J et al. Neonatal hepatitis B vaccination impaired the behavior and neurogenesis of mice transiently in early adulthood. *Psychoneuroendocrinology.* 2016;73:166-76

32. Hamza H et al. Hepatitis B vaccine induces apoptotic death in Hepa1-6 cells. *Apoptosis.* 2012;17(5):516-27

33. Hong M et al. Trained immunity in newborn infants of HBV-infected mothers. *Nature Comm.* 2015;6:6588

34. Shachova IV et al. Assessing the effect of hepatitis B vaccination on the development of protracted conjugated hyperbilirubinemia in children. *Pediatric pharmacology.* 2009 *cyberleninka.ru/article/n/otsenka-vliyaniya-vaktsinatsii-protiv-gepatita-v-na-razvitie-zatyazhnoy-konyugatsionnoy-zheltuhi-u-detey*

Chapter Nine

WHOOPING COUGH

Vaccination is nothing short of attempted murder.
— **George Bernard Shaw**

P ertussis (whooping cough) is caused by *Bordetella pertussis,* a bacterium that settles in the airways of the respiratory tract. While the bacterium itself is not dangerous, it secretes a toxin known as the pertussis toxin. This toxin irritates the respiratory tract and results in the release of mucus, ultimately leading to a severe cough with a characteristic sound (whoop). The cough can last for weeks, which is the reason why the Japanese and Chinese call it a "100-day cough." Although this disease can be quite unpleasant for both children and adults, it is generally not dangerous. However, for infants, especially those below the age of three months (who cannot really cough to remove mucus), whooping cough can be fatal. In infants up to four months old, about 1% of all the whooping cough cases have a fatal outcome [1].

> Pertussis is transmitted exclusively through airborne droplets. As such, you can only become infected if you come close enough to a sick person (within less than two to three meters). Outside of the human body, the bacterium very quickly dies.

Since the 1950s, a separate vaccine against pertussis is not manufactured. Instead, it is always administered as part of a combined vaccine that also includes diphtheria and tetanus. There are two types of pertussis vaccine.

DTP is a <u>whole-cell</u> pertussis vaccine (plus diphtheria and tetanus). This means that it contains the whole bacteria, which have been killed with formalin. While this vaccine has not been used in developed countries since 2001 because of its reactogenicity, it is still used throughout the rest of the world.

DTaP, on the other hand, is an <u>acellular</u> pertussis vaccine, meaning that rather than containing the whole bacteria, it only contains individual bacterial membrane proteins and the pertussis toxin. Nowadays, DTaP is rarely used as most countries have switched to five- and six-valent vaccines, which also intend to immunize the recipient against hepatitis B, polio-myelitis, and Hib.

All of the aforementioned pertussis vaccines contain aluminum. In addition, most of the pertussis vaccines also contain polysorbate 80.

Effectiveness

In 2014, the FDA conducted the most important pertussis vaccine study, which compared the vaccinated with the unvaccinated. However, it was not the study of people, but of baboons, who were divided into four groups. The first group received three doses of a whole-cell vaccine, the second group received three doses of an acellular vaccine, the third group was not vaccinated, and the fourth group consisted of baboons that were not vaccinated but had previously been infected with pertussis. A month after the administration of the last dose, all four groups were infected with pertussis, and the infection course was monitored. While the whole-cell, acellular, and unvaccinated groups remained infected for 18, 35, and 30 days respectively, the previously infected unvaccinated group resisted the infection altogether. Although the unvaccinated group had much more bacteria in the first two weeks compared to the two vaccinated groups, the acellular group remained infected for longer. This held true even though the acellular group had developed more antibodies against pertussis than the group that had previously been infected (we will come back to this point later on). **Thus, it appears that even three doses of either type of pertussis vaccine are not able to prevent pertussis infection.** The authors note that during vaccine trials, the participants were not screened for pertussis infection unless they presented with pertussis-like symptoms and a cough that lasted at least 7–21 days. Therefore, no experimental data exist on whether the vaccination prevents B. pertussis colonization or transmission in humans. The authors conclude that "The observation that acellular vaccine, which induces an immune response mismatched to that induced by natural infection, fails to prevent colonization or transmission provides a plausible explanation for the resurgence of pertussis and suggests that optimal control of pertussis will require the development of improved vaccines" [2].

A 2015 meta-analysis compared the efficacy of three and five doses of DTaP. The authors concluded that five doses of the vaccine are no more effective than three doses and that the average duration of the vaccine protection from DTaP is about three years. In fact, three years is a theoretical and overestimated period, since the authors *assume* the initial efficacy of 85%. According to other studies, the efficacy of the acellular vaccine is about 60% [3]. After the vaccination, the initial efficacy gradually decreases, and the risk of contracting pertussis increases by 33% each year. The authors conclude that very few children over the age of ten would be protected against pertussis, indicating the need for an earlier adolescent booster [4].

> Despite high vaccination coverage, more and more pertussis epidemics have been occurring worldwide since the beginning of the 21st century, and most cases turned out to be among the vaccinated population.

One example is a study of the 2013 pertussis epidemic in Spain (421 cases, mostly in children under the age of one year). The vast majority of the infected (90%) were fully vaccinated. Most primary cases were among fully vaccinated children aged five to nine. Only 8% of the 421 cases were hospitalized, and no one died. The authors state that the true incidence of pertussis was probably even higher because the study focused only on the cases confirmed by the laboratory tests or epidemiological relationship. They conclude that "Despite high levels of vaccination coverage, pertussis circulation cannot be controlled at all. The results question the efficacy of the present immunization programs" [5].

According to a 2014 Australian study, most infants six months of age and younger are infected with whooping cough by their fully vaccinated siblings, especially those who are two to three years old. Infants, who are not infected by their siblings, are often infected by their parents [6]. These results were confirmed in a CDC study [7].

In an article published in 2012 in *the BMJ* (British Medical Journal), a retired British general practitioner states that according to his long-term practice, whooping cough never went away. What went away was the ability of the doctors to recognize it, and in the absence of a practicable diagnostic test, the official figures fell [8]. Between the 1960s and 1970s, vaccination coverage against pertussis in England fell from 78% to 42%. The whooping cough-related death rate during the same period decreased threefold [9].

In light of this, it is no wonder that just 20% of adolescents and adults had antibodies against the pertussis toxin one month after the vaccination. Antibodies to the other vaccine antigens were found in only 39–68% of the subjects [10]. The ineffectiveness of the pertussis vaccine has also been noticed before. In 1978 it became clear that 84% of pertussis patients had been vaccinated with three doses of the vaccine. Based on this information, Sweden canceled the vaccination. Only when the acellular vaccine appeared in 1996 was vaccination reinstated.

Here I will give an example of an indicative case, which occurred in the year 2000 when a whole-cell (i.e., more effective) vaccine was administered to a two-month-old child in Israel. Despite the entire family (mother, aunt, and three siblings—two, five, and 11 years old) were fully vaccinated, the child died of whooping cough at the age of four months. Moreover, both younger brothers, who were at kindergarten, had also been fully vaccinated with four doses along with all the other kids who attended these kindergartens. The mother of the child had a three-month history of a persistent cough. The three other siblings had a paroxysmal cough, and an 18-year-old aunt, who took care of the infant and lived in the same house, reported a mild respiratory illness without paroxysmal cough. In the end, it turned out that the whole family—five people—was infected with pertussis. In addition, five children from both kindergartens (11%) were also infected, although only two of them fell under a "modified World Health Organization (WHO) case definition" of pertussis. The authors of this study concluded that vaccination does not fully protect children from whooping cough, that in some cases immunity does not persist even into early childhood, and that vaccinated children act as a "silent reservoir of infection in the transmission of pertussis in the community" [11].

What does a "modified WHO case definition" mean? Sometimes, when a new vaccine appears on the market, the definition of the disease changes. For example, before 1991, it was necessary for a person to have a paroxysmal cough and have pertussis antibodies or pertussis bacteria detected to diagnose pertussis. After 1991, when the clinical studies of the acellular vaccine began, these observations were no longer sufficient; it became necessary for the cough to last for at least three weeks. Without a paroxysmal three-week cough, whooping cough was now no longer diagnosed as whooping cough [12].

> This new definition obviously led to a sharp decrease in the number of patients diagnosed with whooping cough, and as a consequence, the apparent efficacy of the vaccine appeared to be high. Similarly, as soon as the polio vaccine came on the market, the definition of the disease immediately changed, which also resulted in fewer patients being diagnosed with polio. This led to a belief that the vaccine saved us from the polio epidemic, and not the new disease definition.

As the pertussis vaccine is extremely inefficient, and whooping cough is very dangerous primarily for the infants, scientists from the CDC decided that as soon as a new baby is born into the family, the entire family should be vaccinated. They recommended that mothers, fathers, siblings, grandparents, and everyone else who comes into contact with the child should be vaccinated in order to create a cocoon around the child. This is called "cocooning" and aims to prevent any pertussis bacterium from breaking through and reaching the child. Despite the fact that this strategy has been used since 2005, the number of cases of whooping cough has not decreased.

A 2015 study notes that in the last 20 years, the incidence of whooping cough in many countries has significantly increased. Three main hypotheses have been proposed to explain the resurgence: 1) waning of protective immunity from the vaccination or natural infection over time, 2) evolution of *B. pertussis* to escape protective immunity, and 3) low vaccine coverage. Recent studies have suggested a fourth mechanism: **asymptomatic transmission from those vaccinated** with the acellular *B.*

pertussis vaccines. The authors analyzed the incidence of whooping cough in the US and UK, conducted a genetic analysis of the bacterial strains, and concluded that asymptomatic transmission could account for the observed increase of pertussis, and that cocooning may be ineffective. According to their model, increased acellular vaccine coverage increases the incidence of the asymptomatic cases by a factor of 30, and the incidence of the symptomatic cases by a factor of 5–15 [13]. Nevertheless, cocooning has not been abolished and is still commonly used as a preventative technique along with the vaccination of pregnant women. Cocooning was also implemented in Australia, but it was found to be ineffective and was later abandoned.

How Does The Immune System Work?

In order to realize the absurdity of vaccination against pertussis, we need to understand a little about how the immune system works. Let's look at leprosy, a disease for which there is no vaccine and that we can study without bias. Roughly speaking, leprosy can either be tuberculoid or lepromatous. *Tuberculoid leprosy* is a relatively mild form of the disease during which only the skin is affected. It can often resolve without treatment. *Lepromatous leprosy*, on the other hand, is much more severe as all mucous membranes become affected, and the outcome is often fatal. Intermediate forms between these two kinds of diseases are also possible. What determines the type of leprosy an individual would develop? Solely the reaction of their immune system in response to the leprosy bacterium.

The immune system is divided into two subsystems: cellular immunity and humoral immunity.

Humoral immunity is immunity mediated by antibodies. B cells produce antibodies in response to antigens. The antibodies attach to pathogens and either neutralize them or notify other cells that the pathogen needs to be destroyed. T-helper cells of type 2 (**Th2**) are responsible for this system.

Cellular immunity is an immune response mediated by cells such as phagocytes, T-cells, and others. These cells recognize infected cells and either engulf or kill them. T-helper cells of type 1 (**Th1**) are responsible for this system. These systems suppress one another by producing signaling molecules called cytokines. In other words, the cytokines secreted by Th1 cells suppress Th2 cells and vice versa.

In the case of leprosy, if the immune response shifts towards cellular immunity, then the disease is more easily controlled, but if the immune response shifts towards humoral immunity, then the disease can take a heavy course. In this case, cellular immunity (Th1) is, therefore, much more effective at controlling the disease than humoral immunity (Th2), which interferes with the ability of cellular immunity to perform its task.

Immune response in leprosy

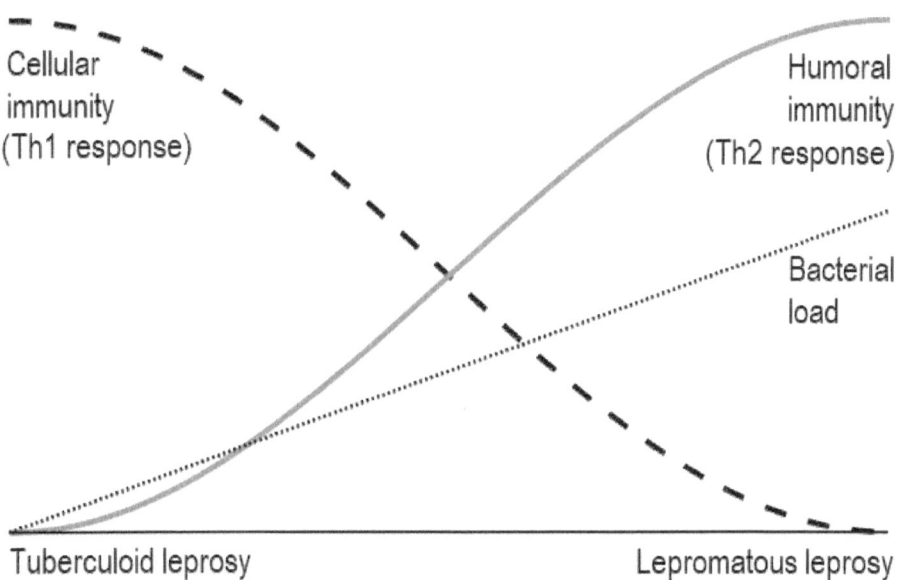

Let's now come back to whooping cough. While the acellular pertussis vaccine shifts the immune response towards humoral immunity (Th2), the whole-cell vaccine is associated more with cellular immunity (Th1), even though it shifts the immune response towards Th2 as well, just to a lesser extent. Despite containing far fewer antigens than the whole-cell vaccine, the acellular vaccine contributes to the production of a greater number of antibodies. The more doses of the acellular vaccine the person receives, the shorter the immunity from these doses is. This is because the additional doses shift the immune response further and further towards the humoral immunity (more antibodies are produced), making the immune response less and less efficient. In other words, the more vaccine doses a person receives, the more likely it is that they will get sick, and the longer they will remain infected [14].

How is vaccine efficacy measured during clinical trials? Scientists cannot simply infect vaccinated children and then see how many of them become ill. As such, the efficacy of the vaccines is measured by the number of antibodies that the immune system produces in response to the vaccination. In the case of whooping cough (and some other diseases), we see that the opposite is true: the more antibodies the immune system produces, the higher the probability of contracting the disease is. Therefore, one of the recommendations the authors of the previous article give is to reduce the amount of antigen in vaccines. Even the CDC states that "No level of antibody, presence of specific antibodies, or antibody profile has been accepted universally as a quantifiable serologic measure of protection... The cell-mediated immune responses to initial doses of pertussis vaccines are believed to correlate better with long-term immunity than antibody responses" [15].

That is, there is a big difference between the real effectiveness of the vaccine and its efficacy during clinical trials (immunogenicity). The more efficacious pertussis vaccine looks during clinical trials, the less effective it is, in reality, due to the stronger shift of immunity towards Th2.

Original Antigenic Sin

When the immune system meets a pathogen for the first time, it elicits an immune response. The second time the same or similar pathogen is encountered, the immune system produces the same immune response, even if another response would have been more effective. This phenomenon is called the "original antigenic sin."

In the case of whooping cough, pertussis bacterium secretes adenylate cyclase toxin (ACT) after settling in the airways. This toxin deceives the immune system, preventing it from recognizing pertussis as a pathogen. After two weeks, however, the immune system realizes that it has been deceived and begins to fight against the pertussis infection. The next time the immune system will come across the ACT, it will not be deceived and will immediately suppress the pathogen. This will prevent an individual from becoming infected for the second time. However, since there is no

ACT in the vaccine, the immune system of the vaccinated person does not know how to react to it, and that is why the vaccinated person can get infected with whooping cough. And as a consequence of the original antigenic sin, the immune system will never learn how to respond to pertussis effectively.

> Moreover, the more doses a person receives, the greater the effect of the original antigenic sin is. This is because each dose will make the immune system produce more and more specific B-cells. These cells end up competing with naive B-cells, which could have adapted and responded to a slightly altered pathogen more efficiently.

Consequently, since the vaccine pathogen and the natural pathogen differ from each other, the immune response to the real pertussis bacterium in an unvaccinated individual will be much more effective than the immune response in a vaccinated individual. In this way, an unvaccinated individual will suffer pertussis only once, while a vaccinated individual will have an ineffective response to the bacterium for the rest of his or her life [16, 17]. In a 2019 study, James Cherry, a leading pertussis researcher at the UCLA, states that "Because of the original antigenic sin, all children who were primed by DTaP vaccines will be more susceptible to pertussis throughout their lifetimes, and there is no easy way to decrease this increased lifetime susceptibility" [18].

Strain Replacement

Just as the excessive use of antibiotics can lead to mutations of bacteria and the emergence of antibiotic-resistant species, universal vaccination can lead to the rapid appearance of vaccine-resistant bacteria [19]. This led to the appearance of a new strain with a more virulent pertussis toxin among the vaccinated individuals, a strain that did not exist before the vaccination began. This strain leads to more hospitalizations and deaths than the original strain [20].

Sometimes, B. parapertussis (**parapertussis**) can take the place of the ordinary pertussis bacterium. Vaccination does not protect against B. parapertussis, which is already responsible for 16% of all disease cases [21]. According to another study, parapertussis is responsible for 36% of whooping cough cases [22]. According to research on mice, vaccination against pertussis increases the risk of parapertussis forty-fold [23].

Another component of the acellular pertussis vaccine is **pertactin**. Pertactin is a protein normally found in the membrane of the pertussis bacterium. In countries where the acellular vaccine is used, pertussis bacteria with pertactin are replaced by pertactin-free bacteria. In Australia, the strains without pertactin almost completely replaced strains with pertactin in just four years [24–27]. Genetic analysis of pertussis bacterial strains in the Netherlands concluded that the bacterium had mutated and adapted to the vaccine. Strains with different, mutated forms of pertactin and pertussis toxin became dominant. These strains did not exist before the beginning of vaccination against pertussis. The same trend was also observed in Finland, the US, and Italy [28].

Another bacterial strain that has been found to replace B. pertussis is B. holmesii. This strain causes the same symptoms, and its pathogenicity is not affected by the vaccine [29, 30].

Safety

In an analysis of 11,000 children in Canada who received a whole-cell vaccine, those who received the first dose of the vaccine two months later than normally developed asthma two times less often. Furthermore, those who received all three doses of the vaccine later in childhood had a 2.5-fold lower risk of developing asthma. This phenomenon happens due to the shift of the immune reaction towards Th2.

The exact cause of asthma is not yet known, but according to one of the prevailing theories, asthma is caused by increased hygiene. When children grow up in an extremely sterile environment, they do not come into contact with bacteria, which leads to the production of IgE antibodies. These IgE antibodies are responsible for asthma, allergies, dermatitis, and other problems that are much more common in vaccinated children. The reason for this is the shift of the immunity towards the antibody response (Th2), which happens directly (due to vaccine antigens), and indirectly (due to the protection against pertussis bacteria) [31].

In a study published in 2000, the odds of having a history of asthma were two times higher among vaccinated subjects than among unvaccinated subjects. The authors believe that "50% of diagnosed asthma cases (2.93 million) in US children and adolescents would be prevented if the DTP or tetanus vaccination was not administered. Similarly, 45% of sinusitis cases (4.9 million) and 54% of allergy-related episodes of nose and eye-related symptoms (10.5 million) in a 12-month period would be prevented after discontinuation of the vaccine" [32]. Similar results were obtained in other studies [33, 34]. Girls, who received the first dose of DTaP at least one month later than scheduled, developed allergies four times less frequently than those who were vaccinated on time. Both boys and girls developed eczema two times less often if they were vaccinated at least one month later [35].

A 2002 review reported that pertussis toxin, which is included in most pertussis vaccines, increases the permeability of the blood-brain barrier, allowing various other toxins and viruses to enter the brain. In an article from 1953, it was stated that virtually every child who receives pertussis immunization demonstrates some form of systemic toxicity, with often permanent CNS damage. In 1979, when four children in Tennessee died after being vaccinated with a vaccine from the same batch, the CDC concluded that the vaccine had a statistically significant link to these deaths. After the Tennessee incident, pertussis vaccine manufacturers arranged that entire batches would never again be sent to one area of the country. This small-batch plan meant that not one region of the country would have enough adverse reactions to a single batch of the whole-cell pertussis vaccine to alert the clinicians in that region to the fact that they were using a highly reactogenic batch [3].

The acellular vaccine is, of course, much less dangerous than the whole-cell vaccine. Nevertheless, according to VAERS, more than 1,300 people have died in the US since 2002 after receiving this vaccine; more than 1,000 became disabled, and more than 10,000 were hospitalized. At the same time, less than 200 people (including those vaccinated) died from whooping cough itself. In other words, the risk of dying from vaccination is at least six times higher than the risk of dying from whooping cough. Since VAERS figures should be multiplied by at least ten, the risk of dying after vaccination is 60–600 times higher than from the disease.

Treatment

A Cochrane systematic review of the antibiotic effects on whooping cough concluded that although antibiotics were effective in eliminating B. pertussis, they did not alter the subsequent clinical course of the illness.

There is no evidence that the preventive treatment of contacts with antibiotics is effective [36].

According to a 2003 study, children who received an antibiotic had a cough that lasted six to 11 days longer and a spasmodic cough that lasted four to 13 days longer than that of untreated patients [37].

In 1936, articles on the effectiveness of vitamin C against pertussis began to appear in the medical literature. The first study was by a Japanese physician, who administered the vitamin intravenously. Later, in 1937, an independent study by Canadian doctors reported on the use of vitamin C orally to treat pertussis [38, 39]. In 1938, vitamin C was successfully used, as reported in a US study [40]. The symptoms resolved in a matter of days. It was also reported that breastfed infants practically never get pertussis because of the high vitamin C level in their mother's milk. Also, in 1938, a controlled study found that vitamin C is not more effective than a control substance [41]. However, cod liver oil, belladonna, and bromide were used as control substances despite the fact that in an article published in the *Lancet* in 1871, it was shown that whooping cough could be successfully treated with cod liver oil [42]. Even back in those days, scientists knew how to choose a placebo well.

In the 1950s, several more articles were published on the treatment of pertussis with vitamin C. However, at that point, a vaccine has appeared, and vitamin C was completely forgotten. As a result, during the past 70 years, no one has made any further studies on the benefits of vitamin C against pertussis. Nonetheless, some doctors and parents successfully use it to treat and prevent whooping cough.

Statistics

The most frequent argument used to prove the pertussis vaccine's effectiveness is that when pertussis vaccination began in the 1950s, about 1,000 people in the US were dying from pertussis per year, whereas now this number is much lower. However, if the figures behind whooping cough-related mortality are looked at in more detail, then it becomes clear that the vaccine has nothing to do with this reduction at all: more than 90% of the decline in mortality occurred before vaccination began, even before antibiotics were introduced. Moreover, until the early 1990s, vaccination coverage did not exceed 70%.

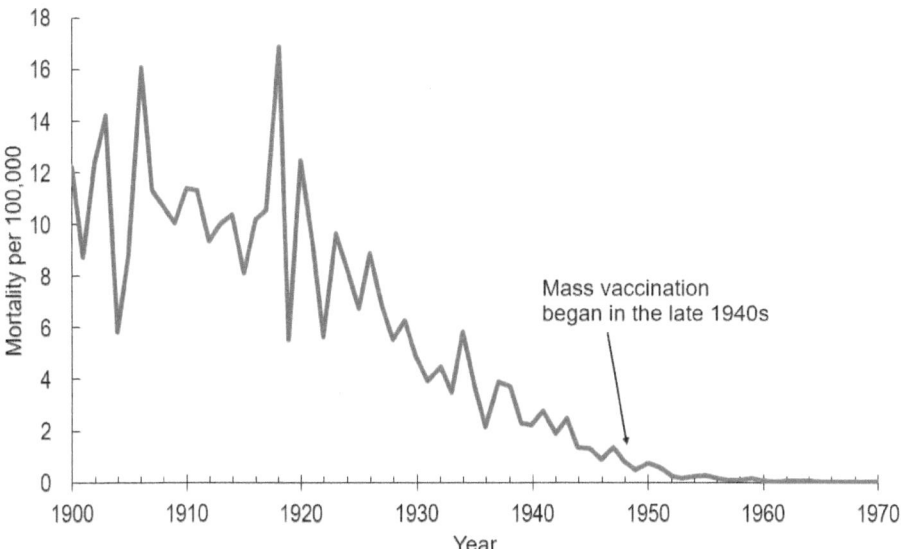

Pertussis mortality in the US (1900-1970)

Conclusions

Pertussis is only dangerous for infants, but since vaccination does not work for infants, both adults and children are vaccinated against whooping cough with the goal of creating herd immunity that will protect the infants. However, vaccination achieves the opposite effect. Instead of contracting pertussis once and forgetting about it for the rest of their life, vaccinated children and adults can become infected with pertussis time and time again. Furthermore, since the disease is often asymptomatic, they become a "silent reservoir" of infection, spreading the disease on their families and on infants. And the more vaccine doses they receive, the more they are susceptible to the infection. While before it was possible to isolate an infant from a sibling who has fallen ill with whooping cough, it is difficult to even diagnose the sibling now, because of the atypical course of the disease, altered disease definition, and simply because many doctors are unwilling to diagnose whooping cough in vaccinated patients.

The risk of dying after the vaccination, even with the DTaP, is much greater than the risk of dying from pertussis itself.

In recent years, the number of cases of whooping cough has been steadily increasing. This is not due to the appearance of anti-vaxxers, but rather because more people are being vaccinated against pertussis. We

vaccinate pregnant women, parents, grandparents, uncles, and aunts, and introduce booster vaccinations for children into the existing vaccination schedule. The more doses of this vaccine are received, the further immunity shifts towards Th2, and the more disease susceptible the person becomes.

Endnotes

1. Winter K et al. Risk factors associated with infant deaths from pertussis: a case-control study. *Clin Infect Dis.* 2015;61(7):1099-106

2. Warfel JM et al. Acellular pertussis vaccines protect against disease but fail to prevent infection and transmission in a nonhuman primate model. *PNAS.* 2014;111(2):787-92

3. Geier D et al. The true story of pertussis vaccination: a sordid legacy? *J Hist Med Allied Sci.* 2002;57(3):249-84

4. McGirr A et al. Duration of pertussis immunity after DTaP immunization: a meta-analysis. *Pediatrics.* 2015;135(2):331-43

5. Sala-Farré MR et al. Pertussis epidemic despite high levels of vaccination coverage with acellular pertussis vaccine. *Enferm Infecc Microbiol Clin.* 2015;33(1):27-31

6. Bertilone C et al. Finding the 'who' in whooping cough: vaccinated siblings are important pertussis sources in infants 6 months of age and under. *Commun Dis Intell Q Rep.* 2014;38(3):E195-200

7. Skoff TH et al. Sources of infant pertussis infection in the United States. *Pediatrics.* 2015;136(4):635-41

8. Jenkinson D. Increase in pertussis may be due to increased recognition and diagnosis. *BMJ.* 2012;345:e5463

9. Stewart GT. Re: "Whooping cough and whooping cough vaccine: the risks and benefits debate". *Am J Epidemiol.* 1984;119(1):135-9

10. Cherry JD et al. Prevalence of antibody to Bordetella pertussis antigens in serum specimens obtained from 1793 adolescents and adults. *Clin Infect Dis.* 2004;39(11):1715-8

11. Srugo I et al. Pertussis infection in fully vaccinated children in day-care centers, Israel. *Emerg Infect Dis.* 2000;6(5):526-9

12. WHO meeting on case definition of pertussis, Geneva, 10-11 January 1991

13. Althouse BM et al. Asymptomatic transmission and the resurgence of Bordetella pertussis. *BMC Med.* 2015;13:146

14. Diavatopoulos DA et al. What is wrong with pertussis vaccine immunity? Why immunological memory to pertussis is failing. *Cold Spring Harb Perspect Biol.* 2017;9(12)

15. Murphy TV et al. Prevention of pertussis, tetanus, and diphtheria among pregnant and postpartum women and their infants recommendations of the Advisory Committee on Immunization Practices (ACIP). *MMWR.* 2008;57(RR-4):1-51

16. Eberhardt CS et al. What is wrong with pertussis vaccine immunity? Inducing and recalling vaccine-specific immunity. *Cold Spring Harb Perspect Biol.* 2017;9(12)

17. Cherry JD et al. Determination of serum antibody to Bordetella pertussis adenylate cyclase toxin in vaccinated and unvaccinated children and in children and adults with pertussis. *Clin Infect Dis.* 2004;38(4):502-7

18. Cherry J. The 112-year odyssey of pertussis and pertussis vaccines-mistakes made and implications for the future. *J Pediatric Infect Dis Soc.* 2019:piz005

19. Bart MJ et al. Global population structure and evolution of Bordetella pertussis and their relationship with vaccination. *mBio.* 2014;5(2):e01074

20. Mooi FR et al. Bordetella pertussis strains with increased toxin production associated with pertussis resurgence. *Emerg Infect Dis.* 2009;15(8):1206-13

21. Cherry JD. Why do pertussis vaccines fail? *Pediatrics.* 2012;129(5):968-70

22. Liese JG et al. Clinical and epidemiological picture of B pertussis and B parapertussis infections after introduction of acellular pertussis vaccines. *Arch Dis Child.* 2003; 88(8):684-7

23. Long GH et al. Acellular pertussis vaccination facilitates Bordetella parapertussis infection in a rodent model of bordetellosis. *Proc Biol Sci.* 2010;277(1690):2017-25

24. Lam C et al. Rapid increase in pertactin-deficient Bordetella pertussis isolates, Australia. *Emerg Infect Dis.* 2014;20(4):626-33

25. Queenan AM et al. Bordetella pertussis variants lacking the vaccine antigen pertactin: first detection in the United States. *N Engl J Med.* 2013;368(6):583-4

26. Martin SW et al. Pertactin-negative Bordetella pertussis strains: evidence for a possible selective advantage. *Clin Infect Dis.* 2015;60(2):223-7

27. Barkoff A-M et al. Appearance of Bordetella pertussis strains not expressing the vaccine antigen pertactin in Finland. *Clin Vaccine Immunol.* 2012;19(10):1703-4

28. Mooi FR et al. Adaptation of Bordetella pertussis to vaccination: a cause for its reemergence? *Emerg Infect Dis.* 2001;7(3 Suppl):526-8

29. Pittet LF et al. Bordetella holmesii: an under-recognised Bordetella species. *Lancet Infect Dis.* 2014;14(6):510-9

30. Zhang X et al. Lack of cross-protection against Bordetella holmesii after pertussis vaccination. *Emerg Infect Dis.* 2012;18(11):1771-9

31. McDonald KL et al. Delay in diphtheria, pertussis, tetanus vaccination is associated with a reduced risk of childhood asthma. *J Allergy Clin Immunol.* 2008;121(3):626-31

32. Hurwitz EL et al. Effects of diphtheria-tetanus-pertussis or tetanus vaccination on allergies and allergy-related respiratory symptoms among children and adolescents in the United States. *J Manipulative Physiol Ther.* 2000;23(2):81-90

33. Bernsen RM et al. Reported pertussis infection and risk of atopy in 8- to 12-yr-old vaccinated and non-vaccinated children. *Pediatr Allergy Immunol.* 2008;19(1):46-52

34. Farooqi IS et al. Early childhood infection and atopic disorder. *Thorax.* 1998;53(11):927-32

35. Kiraly N et al. Timing of routine infant vaccinations and risk of food allergy and eczema at one year of age. *Allergy.* 2016;71(4):541-9

36. Altunaiji S et al. Antibiotics for whooping cough (pertussis). *Cochrane Database Syst Rev.* 2007(3):CD004404

37. Tozzi AE et al. Clinical presentation of pertussis in unvaccinated and vaccinated children in the first six years of life. *Pediatrics.* 2003;112(5):1069-75

38. Otani T. Concerning the vitamin C therapy of pertussis. *Klin Wochenschr.* 1936; 15(51):1884-5

39. Ormerod MJ et al. A further report on the ascorbic acid treatment of whooping cough. *Can Med Assoc J.* 1937;37(3):268-72

40. Vermillion E. A preliminary report on the use of cevitamic acid in the treatment of whooping cough. *J Kan Med Soc.* 1937;39(11):469

41. Gairdner D. Vitamin C in treatment of whooping-cough. *BMJ*. 1938;2(4057):742-4
42. Prestwich J. Cod liver oil in whooping cough. *Lancet*. 1871;98(2519):812

Chapter Ten

TETANUS

*As well consult a butcher on the value of vegetarianism
as a doctor on the worth of vaccination.*
— **George Bernard Shaw**

U nlike papilloma or whooping cough, tetanus is a dangerous
disease. Many parents, who refuse other vaccinations, still
consider it necessary to vaccinate against tetanus. But what is the
probability of contracting tetanus? Is it more dangerous than the vaccine?
Also, does the vaccine protect against tetanus?

Tetanus is caused by the bacteria *Clostridium tetani*. The spores of these
bacteria are everywhere. They are in the soil, inside human and animal
intestines (especially herbivores), in dust, on clothing, on the body, and
even in saliva. These bacteria do not multiply in an aerobic environment,
but once the bacteria get into the anaerobic environment, they come to life
and begin producing a very strong toxin (tetanospasmin). If this toxin gets
into the nervous system as a consequence of injury, it causes muscle spasms
and can lead to paralysis. In developed countries, about 11% of the disease
cases are fatal. Not all strains of the bacteria release the toxin [1].

Tetanus vaccine is almost always combined with diphtheria and
pertussis vaccine (DTaP/DTP), but it is also usually combined with
poliomyelitis, Hib, and sometimes also with hepatitis B. There is a vaccine
against tetanus and diphtheria, but without the whooping cough

component (DT for children and Td for adults). **All tetanus vaccines contain aluminum.** Theoretically, a tetanus vaccine without aluminum does exist and was used in France until 2008, but today it is not manufactured [2].

If tetanus toxin is treated with formalin, it gets converted into a *toxoid*, which is no longer toxic. This toxoid is what is used in a vaccine. In case of an injury, the vaccine is useless, since the process of antibody production happens in the period of several days to several weeks [3]. In this case, the immunoglobulin (i.e., the antibodies themselves) injections are given. Immunoglobulin (TIG) is isolated from the blood of repeatedly vaccinated horses or people. In developed countries, 70% of tetanus cases and 80% of deaths occur in those over 50 years old. Fatality from tetanus in people under 30 is almost zero, whereas among the elderly, the fatality rate is above 50% [4].

Natural Immunity

There is an absolute medical consensus on the fact that natural immunity against tetanus is impossible to attain, and only a vaccine can prevent the disease. However, in an Israeli study, the authors ran blood tests of two hundred randomly selected immigrants from Ethiopia to Israel and found tetanus antibodies in 98% of them. Thirty percent of them had the level of antibodies considered protective (above 0.01UI/ml). None of them have been vaccinated. The number of antibodies increased with age. The authors concluded that natural immunity is developed due to continuous contact with the bacteria [5]. In another study, researchers took blood samples of 120 randomly selected women living in Israeli kibbutzim. All of them had sufficient levels of antibodies against tetanus toxin, despite the fact that 12% of them had never been vaccinated [6].

The levels of tetanus antibodies of 57 tested inhabitants of the Galapagos Islands were above the protective level. None of them had been vaccinated. Two of them have had tetanus in the past. The authors also tested nine animals and all of them had sufficient levels of antibodies. They concluded that immunity is produced when bacterial spores that are swallowed multiply in the intestines, while skin wounds act like booster vaccines. Similar studies were also conducted in England, India, and Mali [7–10]. **All of those studies contradict the accepted dogma that the disease does not give immunity.**

In fact, the answer to the question of how natural immunity is produced was already given back in the 1920s. Tetanus bacteria were found in the intestines of 35% of men tested in Beijing, even though tetanus (excluding neonatal tetanus) was a very rare disease in China in the early 20th century. Researchers found tetanus bacteria in patients' stool even after they spent three months in the hospital on a practically sterile diet [11]. In the following study, the authors proved that tetanus bacteria multiply in the intestines. To test for the production of tetanus antibodies as a result of the ingestion of tetanus spores with food, one of the authors of the study swallowed a large number of bacterial spores (there were some proper scientists back in the day!). However, the experiment had to be stopped as he got constipation (it is unclear whether it was due to the ingestion of bacteria or not) [12].

In another study, guinea pigs that were fed tetanus bacteria developed antibodies within six months. Since there are many strains of tetanus bacteria, the antibodies were produced only to the strain, which was consumed. The immunity from other strains was not acquired. Those who were fed several different strains developed immunity to all of them.

In one of the experiments, the authors infected guinea pigs with tetanus, and all but two of them died. It turned out that those two guinea pigs were accidentally placed with a male and got pregnant. How did pregnancy save them from tetanus remains unclear. They gave birth to a healthy litter. In addition, the authors report that "It is well known spores alone will not produce an infection, but some irritating substance must be introduced at the same time in order that they may germinate." They used different materials as an irritant, including a glass capsule. A capsule filled with tetanus bacteria spores was inserted under the skin of guinea pigs and crushed after insertion. The fact that bacteria spores themselves are insufficient for infection also explains the fact that despite the prevalence of the bacteria, disease cases are extremely rare. The authors state that there is no correlation between the amount of antibodies in the blood and the immunity to tetanus. The authors conclude that antibodies to the toxin play only a small role in the tetanus immunity and that there is something else that protects against infection. They assume that proteins called agglutinins could play a role. Agglutinins are strain-specific: each bacterial strain will have its own agglutinin [13].

In a 1926 study, the researchers found agglutinins to several strains of tetanus bacteria in the blood of 80% of Californian residents, but they did not have antibodies. The authors believe that tetanus bacteria were in the intestines of these people in the past but did not survive there, and thus no antibodies were produced [14]. Tetanus agglutinins have not been studied ever since.

Does The Tetanus Vaccine Protect Against Tetanus?

A 1992 article reported on three men with severe tetanus. One of them died. All three of them were not only fully vaccinated but had very high levels of antibodies as well. One of them had the antibody level 2,500 times higher than the protective level. This patient was hyperimmunized for creating commercial immunoglobulin—that is, he was given the vaccine many times in order to create a lot of antibodies, which would then be isolated from his blood and sold as immunoglobulin. The other patient had an in vitro level of antibodies of 0.2 IU/ml, but when it was tested in vivo on mice, it turned out to be less than 0.01 IU/ml. The authors conclude that having immunity to toxoid is not at all equal to having immunity to toxin, and that "clinical diagnosis of tetanus should not be discarded solely on the basis of seemingly protective anti-tetanus titers or because of a history of complete tetanus immunizations" [15]. Cases of infection have also been described in people with an antibody level 16 times higher than protective, 100 and 278 times higher than the protective [16–18]. In a systematic review of cases of tetanus in vaccinated people, the authors analyzed 51 studies, which reported on 359 such cases [19].

The "protective" level of antibodies (0.01 IU/ml) was determined in 1937 on the basis of experiments on guinea pigs and was then extrapolated to humans. In recent years some countries started considering the level of antibodies 10–15 times higher as protective [20].

Neonatal Tetanus

One of the types of tetanus is neonatal tetanus, and it practically does not occur in developed countries. Its cause is the infection of the newborn through the umbilical cord, due to the non-sterile cord-cutting.

> Instead of raising the level of hygiene during childbirth, handing out hydrogen peroxide to pregnant women and teaching them not

to cut the umbilical cord with rusted scissors, WHO, of course, chose a different strategy—mass vaccination of pregnant women in third-world countries.

In a Nigerian study, 20 infants were admitted to the hospital with neonatal tetanus. The mothers of six of them had been vaccinated with at least two doses of the vaccine during pregnancy. All mothers and infants, including the unvaccinated ones, had the antibodies at a level much higher than the protective. The fatality rate among the unvaccinated was 43%. The fatality rate among the vaccinated was 50% [21]. However, there also exists a study proving that two to three vaccines during pregnancy significantly reduce the incidence of neonatal tetanus. On the other hand, the same study found that vaccination increased mortality from other causes by 18% [22].

In Tanzania, ten newborns with tetanus were studied. Mothers of all but one have been vaccinated during the last pregnancy. The level of antibodies of nine of them was above the protective level. The mother of the tenth newborn was vaccinated two weeks before giving birth. Two newborns had antibody levels 100 and 400 times higher than the protective level. The mother of one of them received 14 vaccine doses in five consecutive pregnancies; the other mother received six vaccine doses over a three-year period. The newborn, whose mother was not vaccinated, had the level of antibodies three times above the protective level. The authors concluded that there is no such thing as "protective level of antibodies" [23].

Ways Of Getting The Infection

One of the ways to get tetanus in the past was smallpox vaccination [24, 25]. Also, tetanus was caused by circumcision, medical bandages, sanitary pads, abortion, and hysterectomy (removal of the uterus). A case of tetanus infection due to the rapture of the foreskin during intercourse was reported, which means that tetanus bacteria probably live in the vagina as well.

The authors of a 1937 study analyzed 14 types of sanitary pads and found tetanus spores and *C. welchii* spores (more about them later) on all of them. Some of the pads were claimed by the manufacturer to be sterile. Tetanus spores were also found on sterile sets of hygienic bandages and pads intended for childbirth. The authors conclude that such non-sterile pads should not be used after childbirth and uterus removal since 3.5% of cases of tetanus are postpartum tetanus. They also state that "The sale of a tin of sardines is subject to more official control than a tin of accouchement dressings... The aboriginal, who uses no menstrual pad and no accouchement dressing tin, is safer from infection than her civilized sister" [26].

The above-mentioned *C. welchii*, which is nowadays called *C. perfringens*, is a bacterium from the same family as tetanus. It is also anaerobic, also lives in soil, in human and animal intestines, in dust, and is as common as the *C. tetani* bacteria. However, since there is no vaccine against this bacterium, you probably have not heard anything about it. **This is a bit strange since it causes a far more dangerous and more common disease—gas gangrene.**

Upon getting into an anaerobic environment through a deep wound, this bacterium begins to release a toxin, which quickly leads to tissue necrosis, leading to amputation at best. Unlike tetanus, for which anti-tetanus serum is effective in case of injury, gas gangrene serum does not work. One thousand people contract gas gangrene in the US every year. The fatality rate is 20–25%. How many people contract tetanus? Thirty per year [27]. Only three of them die. And while the nervous tissue of a person who survived tetanus is restored and they fully recover, the person who survived gas gangrene remains disabled at best.

C. difficile bacterium also belongs to the same family. You probably did not hear anything about it either, even though it is associated with almost 30,000 deaths per year in the US, meaning that it is ten thousand times more deadly than tetanus [28]. But maybe the incidence and mortality rates for tetanus are so low due to vaccination? In the 1950s, before the mass vaccination began, only 500 people a year contracted tetanus.

Who Gets Tetanus?

From 1987 through 2008, persons with diabetes accounted for 13% of all reported tetanus cases and 29% of all tetanus deaths. Diabetics are three times more likely to contract tetanus than nondiabetics, and the fatality rate among them is higher. Intravenous drug users accounted for 15% of cases [29]. Even if one were to assume that tetanus antibodies effectively neutralize the toxin, the antibodies would still need to get to the place of injury first. And if the injury occurs in a place with insufficient blood supply, antibodies are not able to get there. This is the reason why diabetics suffer from tetanus much more often.

Since 1955, 90% of tetanus cases in New York happen among heroin addicts [30]. A case of a brother and sister, who contracted tetanus from contaminated heroin, has been described. The brother had a severe form of tetanus, and the sister had a mild one. They both recovered—the brother within three weeks and the sister within two. Since the sister received a vaccine 15 years ago, the authors concluded that it was the reason why she got a mild form. They also concluded that the brother got severe tetanus because he probably was never vaccinated, although his antibody level was not tested, and whether he was ever vaccinated remains unclear [31].

Cases of tetanus among drug users, who injected morphine under their skin, were described even in the Victorian era. In Chicago, in the '50s, before the vaccination began, most tetanus cases were among heroin addicts. Of the 22 patients with tetanus, all of the 12 injection drug users died, compared to only four patients who died with other types of wounds [32]. The CDC reports that 55% of tetanus cases in California were among intravenous drug users [33].

Between 1984 and 1994, 40 deaths due to tetanus were detected in the Lazio region of Italy (population of 5.1 million). Sixty-three percent of tetanus deaths occurred in people over 60, and mostly intravenous drug users died among the younger people. Among people younger than 30, no deaths were recorded. Among those who were not drug users, only one person under the age of 40 died, and only two under the age of 50. The relative risk of death in retired people was 27 times higher, in farmers 167 times higher, and in drug users 186 times higher [34].

Until 2003, tetanus was a rare disease in Great Britain and mostly happened among the elderly. After 2003, drug users began to contract tetanus. In 2003 there were 35 cases of tetanus, and two patients died. The authors searched for common factors between these cases and found out that they all became infected through the contaminated heroin distributed from Liverpool [35].

Effectiveness

A randomized controlled study of tetanus vaccine effectiveness has never been conducted. So how was it determined that the vaccine is effective? Throughout the First World War, 70 cases of tetanus were observed among American soldiers (13.4 per 100,000 injuries). Throughout the Second World War, when all soldiers got vaccinated, 12 cases of tetanus were observed (0.44 per 100,000 injuries). In addition, 80 cases of tetanus were observed in German ground forces, who were not vaccinated. However, among the Luftwaffe (Air Force) soldiers, who were vaccinated, no cases of tetanus were reported. On the basis of this information, it was concluded that the vaccine is very effective, and since 1947 it has been given to the civilian population. **The fact that WWI was fought mainly on horses, while WWII was fought on tanks, did not seem to bother the researchers. Neither were they bothered by the fact that Luftwaffe fought in the air, while tetanus bacteria live mainly in the soil.**

Meanwhile, gas gangrene took the lives of 100,000 German soldiers during WWI (10–12% of all wounded). During WWII, less than 1.5% died from it, and during the Vietnam War, only 0.016% died. From the 1950s to the 1980s, the fatality rate of gas gangrene decreased from 70% to 41% [36]. **This happened without vaccination.**

Vaccines Against Pregnancy

Let's take a little break from tetanus. hCG (Human Chorionic Gonadotropin) is a hormone, which is released during pregnancy and is also the one on which the home pregnancy test is based. Since this hormone is absolutely necessary for the development of a pregnancy, scientists came up with a brilliant idea. They thought that if they could trigger an autoimmune reaction to this hormone, the immune system would begin to see it as a pathogen and destroy it. And thus, they would create a vaccine against pregnancy.

How does one trigger an immune response to a hormone? Simply by adding a tetanus toxoid and aluminum to it. The immune system will then produce antibodies to hCG, in addition to the tetanus antibodies. And so it was done. The work started back in the '70s but was not successful. However, in the early '90s, another adjuvant was added to the vaccine, along with the sheep lutropin (the hormone responsible for the ovulation) and diphtheria toxoid, and the vaccine started working! Unfortunately, the level of antibodies was constantly falling, so the vaccine had to be given once every few months. Hindu women, on whom the vaccine was tested, almost never got pregnant [37]. **However, some researchers accuse the** author of this experiment of skipping the preliminary animal testing and doing the testing straight on women. Maneka Gandhi, the former Minister of the Environment of India, claims that his contraceptive vaccine for male dogs killed too many of them [38]. Similar vaccines were also being developed by other research groups under the guidance of the WHO [39].

In the fall of 1994, the World Health Organization conducted a tetanus vaccination campaign in Mexico. For some reason, though, the vaccine was given exclusively to women of reproductive age. And despite the fact that one dose of tetanus vaccine gives protection for ten years, the women were vaccinated five times. A Catholic organization, Human Life International, found it strange and decided to test these vaccines for hCG, which was indeed found there. Similar hCG containing tetanus vaccines were found in the Philippines, where 3.4 million women were vaccinated, and in Nicaragua, where only women aged 12–49 were vaccinated [40].

In 2014, the WHO and UNICEF held a vaccination campaign for women of childbearing age (14–49 years old) in Kenya. Women received five doses of the vaccine. Vaccination in Kenya is usually carried out by the Church, but this time the WHO carried out the vaccinations itself. The Organization of Catholic Bishops in Kenya found it strange and decided to send the vaccine to four different labs for testing. According to the Bishops' statement, all labs found hCG in the tested vials. The WHO and UNICEF explained the vaccination of women of childbearing age by the fact that the vaccines were intended to prevent neonatal tetanus. However, according to the WHO's statistics, in five years prior to this campaign, only 19 cases of neonatal tetanus have been recorded in Kenya. The need for five doses of the vaccine instead of the regular one or two was never explained. One of the labs stated that they had no knowledge of what they were testing. If they had known that it was a vaccine, they certainly would not have found hCG there. Another lab's license was revoked after it refused to falsify the results.

A study published in 2017 reported the following:

1) WHO has been working on the development of vaccines against pregnancy since the 1970s, and on the issue of reducing birth rates in third-world countries since 1945. Since the 1970s the US government has been officially supporting the reduction in birth rates in third-world countries;

2) The vaccination protocol used in Kenya (five doses every six months) fully corresponded to the protocol of vaccination against

pregnancy, and did not correspond to the protocol of vaccination against tetanus;

3) Vaccines in Kenya were guarded by the police. Each vial had to be returned to the WHO under police supervision. All vaccines were kept in a hotel in Nairobi, and were only distributed from there;

4) Half of the vials provided by the WHO for testing contained hCG;

5) Women vaccinated against tetanus in the Philippines had hCG antibodies. The authors conclude that the WHO is responsible for the depopulation in Kenya [41].

Safety

The Institute of Medicine (IOM) report states that there is a causal relationship between tetanus/diphtheria vaccine and Guillain-Barré syndrome, anaphylactic shock, and brachial neuritis [42].

Tetanus booster vaccine temporarily lowers the level of T-lymphocytes in the blood to a level observed in AIDS patients [43]. Since tetanus vaccines are given at every opportunity, this leads to hyper-immunization (the antibody level above 5 IU/ml). In Italy, 11% of those born before 1968 and 17% of those born after 1968 were hyper-immunized [44, 45]. The level of antibodies of 53% of adults in Finland (over 50 years of age) was above 1 IU/ml [46]. A 2013 study found that 12- to 18-month-old children suffering from recurring infections had significantly higher levels of tetanus antibodies compared to healthy children [47].

According to VAERS, 24 deaths and 178 cases of permanent disability after tetanus vaccination (with no pertussis component) were recorded in the period from 2001 to 2008 in the US. These numbers should be multiplied by at least ten, and it should be remembered that these vaccines are quite rare—most children get a combined vaccine with pertussis. During these eight years, only 233 cases and 26 deaths from tetanus have been reported. Among those cases, 27% were vaccinated more than four times, and 40% were not vaccinated. Fifteen percent were intravenous drug users, 15% were diabetes patients, and 49% were over 50 years old. **Not a single tetanus case in children under the age of five was reported. No one under the age of 30 died from tetanus.**

Treatment

A 1966 German study found that rats, which received vitamin C injections, did not die from lethal doses of tetanus toxin [48]. In the early 1980s, a controlled study of the effects of vitamin C on tetanus was conducted in Bangladesh. One hundred seventeen patients were divided into two groups: the first group received 1g of vitamin C intravenously every day as well as the immunoglobulin, and the second group received the immunoglobulin only. Among children (one–12 years old) who did not receive the vitamin, the fatality rate was 74%, and no one died among those who got the vitamin. Among adults who did not receive the vitamin, the fatality was 68%. Among those who did, it was 37%. Since the vitamin C dose was the same for both groups despite the different weights of the patients, it is logical to assume that a higher dose of the vitamin in the adult group would further reduce mortality [49].

In 2013 Cochrane published a systematic review on the treatment of tetanus with vitamin C. In the entire medical literature, the authors of this review found only the aforementioned study on the effects of vitamin C on tetanus. They report the following among other things:

Infections and bacterial toxins deplete vitamin C in the adrenal glands. Several experiments proved that vitamin C improves the function of the immune system cells.

Dozens of animal experiments proved that vitamin C increases resistance to infections and bacterial toxins, including tetanus and other clostridium bacteria toxins.

One study reported that tetanus patients had lower plasma levels of vitamin C compared to healthy people and that tetanus patients who died had lower levels than those who survived. Furthermore, tetanus patients had elevated levels of dehydroascorbate (an oxidized form of vitamin C), which indicates that tetanus depletes vitamin C reserves.

Vitamin C is safe even in very large doses. One hundred grams administered intravenously did not cause adverse effects. When taken orally, large doses of vitamin C could cause diarrhea (more than 30 g/day for sick people, and more than 4–10 g/day for healthy people, which also indicates that infections deplete vitamin C reserves).

Since this Bangladeshi study was neither blinded nor randomized, the authors do not recommend using vitamin C in the treatment of tetanus, despite the complete absence of adverse effects. They recommend conducting additional clinical trials. Somehow, no one is in a rush to do that [50].

Statistics

As is the case with other vaccines, it is argued that tetanus vaccine is responsible for reducing the incidence of tetanus by 92% and the mortality rate by 99% [51]. However, since 1900, the tetanus mortality rate in the US decreased by more than 95% even before the vaccination began in the late '40s [52]. The tetanus mortality rate in Canada decreased by 80% from the 1920s to 1940s.

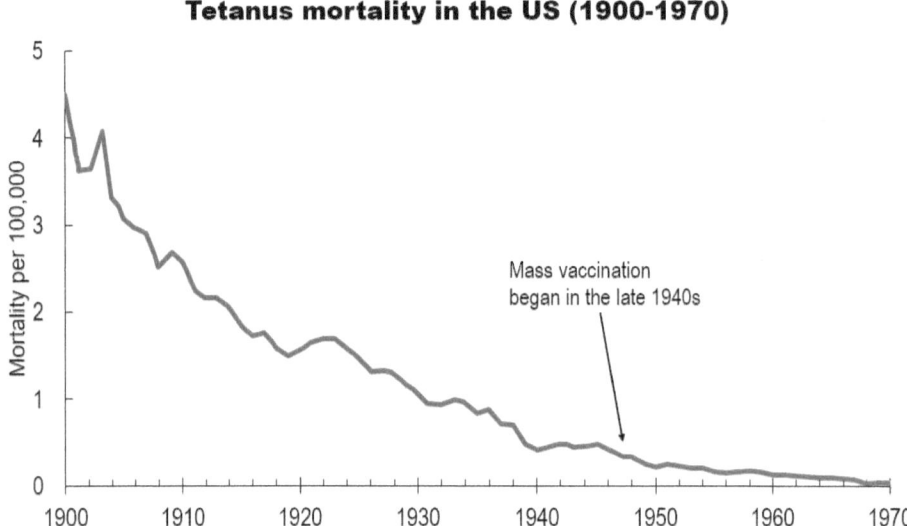

Tetanus mortality in the US (1900-1970)

Conclusions

Tetanus is an extremely rare disease, which is quite difficult to contract. It was extremely rare even during the First World War, despite countless wounds and lack of sanitation. Every year 50 people in the US die of a lightning strike, whereas only 30 people get tetanus; on average, three of them die, and most of them are intravenous drug users, diabetics, and the elderly. In developed countries, children do not die from tetanus, and barely ever contract it. It is far more logical to be afraid of gas gangrene, which is spread in the same way as tetanus, yet causes death 100 times more often, or lightning, which causes death 15 times more often.

The probability of death after vaccination is higher than the probability of death from tetanus, and the probability of permanent disability from vaccination is higher than the probability of contracting tetanus.

The efficacy of the tetanus vaccine has never been proved.

Endnotes

1. Tetanus. CDC Pink Book

2. Ullberg-Olsson K et al. Immunization aginast tetanus with aluminium free-versus aluminium contain triple vaccine. *Dev Biol Stand.* 1979;43:39-41

3. Porter JD et al. Lack of early antitoxin response to tetanus booster. *Vaccine.* 1992; 10(5):334-6

4. Cook TM et al. Tetanus: a review of the literature. *Br J Anaesth.* 2001;87(3):477-87

5. Matzkin H et al. Naturally acquired immunity to tetanus toxin in an isolated community. *Infect Immun.* 1985;48(1):267-8

6. Leshem Y et al. Tetanus immunity in kibbutz women. *Isr J Med Sci.* 1989;25(3):127-30

7. Veronesi R et al. New concepts on tetanus immunization: naturally acquired immunity. *J Hyg Epidemiol Microbiol Immunol.* 1975;19(1):126-34

8. Murphy NM et al. Objective verification of tetanus immune status in an apparently non-immune population. *Br J Clin Pract.* 1994;48(1):8-9

9. Dastur FD et al. Response to single dose of tetanus vaccine in subjects with naturally acquired tetanus antitoxin. *Lancet.* 1981;2(8240):219-22

10. Ehrengut W et al. Naturally acquired tetanus antitoxin in the serum of children and adults in Mali. *Immun Infekt.* 1983;11(6):229-32

11. Tenbroeck C et al. The tetanus bacillus as an intestinal saprophyte in man. *J Exp Med.* 1922;36(3):261-71

12. Tenbroeck C et al. Studies on the relation of tetanus bacilli in the digestive tract to tetanus antitoxin in the blood. *J Exp Med.* 1923;37(4):479-89

13. Tenbroeck C et al. The immunity produced by the growth of tetanus bacilli in the digestive tract. *J Exp Med.* 1926;43(3):361-77

14. Coleman G. Study of tetanus agglutinins and antitoxin in human serums. *J Infect Dis.* 1926;39(4):332-6

15. Crone NE et al. Severe tetanus in immunized patients with high anti-tetanus titers. *Neurology.* 1992;42(4):761-4

16. Livorsi DJ et al. Generalized tetanus despite prior vaccination and a protective level of anti-tetanus antibodies. *Am J Med Sci.* 2010;339(2):200-1

17. Pryor T et al. Elevated antitoxin titers in a man with generalized tetanus. *J Fam Pract.* 1997;44(3):299-303

18. Passen E. Clinical tetanus despite a 'protective' level of toxin-neutralizing antibody. *JAMA.* 1986;255(9):1171-3

19. Hopkins JP et al. A systematic review of tetanus in individuals with previous tetanus toxoid immunization. *Can Commun Dis Rep.* 2014;40(17):355-64

20. Sneath P. Tetanus immunity: the resistance of guinea pigs to lethal spore doses induced by active and passive immunization. *Am J Hyg*. 1937;25(3):464-76

21. de Moraes-Pinto MI et al. Neonatal tetanus despite immunization and protective antitoxin antibody. *J Infect Dis*. 1995;171(4):1076-7

22. Newell KW et al. The use of toxoid for the prevention of tetanus neonatorum. Final report of a double-blind controlled field trial. *Bull World Health Organ*. 1966;35(6):863-71

23. Maselle SY et al. Neonatal tetanus despite protective serum antitoxin concentration. *FEMS Microbiol Immunol*. 1991;3(3):171-5

24. Patel J. Tetanus following vaccination against small-pox. *Indian J Pediatr*. 1960;27:251-3

25. Tetanus following vaccination against smallpox, and its prevention: with special reference to the use of vaccination shields and dressings. *Public Health Rep*. 1927; 42(50):3061-71

26. Pulvertaft RJ. Post-hysterectomy and puerperal tetanus. *BMJ*. 1937;1(3973):441-4

27. Reported cases and deaths from vaccine preventable diseases, United States. *CDC*

28. Lessa F. Burden of Clostridium difficile infection in the United States. *N Engl J Med*. 2015;372(24):2369-70

29. Pascual B. Tetanus surveillance - US, 1998-2000. *MMWR*. 2003;52(SS03):1-8

30. Cherubin CE. Clinical severity of tetanus in narcotic addicts in New York City. *Arch Intern Med*. 1968;121(2):156-8

31. Berger SA et al. Tetanus despite preexisting antitetanus antibody. *JAMA*. 1978; 240(8):769-70

32. Beeching N. Tetanus in injecting drug users. *BMJ*. 2005;330(7485):208-9

33. Tetanus among injecting-drug users—California, 1997. *MMWR*. 1998;47(8):149-51

34. Sangalli M et al. Tetanus: a rare but preventable cause of mortality among drug users and the elderly. *Eur J Epidemiol*. 1996 Oct;12(5):539-40

35. Hahné SJ et al. Tetanus in injecting drug users, United Kingdom. *Emerg Infect Dis*. 2006; 12(4):709-10

36. Pailler JL et al. Gas gangrene: a military disease? *Acta Chir Belg*. 1986;86(2):63-71

37. Talwar GP et al. A vaccine that prevents pregnancy in women. *PNAS*. 1994;91(18):8532-6

38. Mukerjee M. Pushing the envelope for vaccines. *Sci Am*. 1996;275(1):38-40

39. Report of a meeting between women's health advocates and scientists to review the current status of the development of fertility regulating vaccines, Geneva, 17-18 August 1992

40. Tetanus vaccine may be laced with anti-fertility drug. International / developing countries. *Vaccine weekly*. 1995 May 29:9-10

41. Oller JW. HCG found in WHO tetanus vaccine in Kenya raises concern in the developing world. *OAlib*. 2017;4(e3937)

42. Stratton KR et al. Adverse events associated with childhood vaccines other than pertussis and rubella. Summary of a report from the Institute of Medicine. *JAMA*. 1994; 271(20):1602-5

43. Eibl MM et al. Abnormal T-lymphocyte subpopulations in healthy subjects after tetanus booster immunization. *N Engl J Med*. 1984;310(3):198-9

44. Wirz M et al. Prevalence of hyperimmunization against tetanus in a national sample of 18-26 year old immune subjects in Italy. *Vaccine*. 1987;5(3):211-4

45. Gentili G et al. Prevalence of hyperimmunization against tetanus in Italians born after the introduction of mandatory vaccination of children with tetanus toxoid in 1968. *Infection*. 1993;21(2):80-2

46. Olander RM et al. High tetanus and diphtheria antitoxin concentrations in Finnish adults - time for new booster recommendations? *Vaccine*. 2009;27(39):5295-8

47. Graziani S. Immune responses to tetanus vaccination in Italian healthy subjects and children with recurrent infections. *J Biol Regul Homeost Agents*. 2013;27(1):95-103

48. Dey PK. Efficacy of vitamin C in counteracting tetanus toxin toxicity. *Naturwissenschaften*. 1966;53(12):310

49. Jahan K et al. Effect of ascorbic acid in the treatment of tetanus. *Bangladesh Med Res Counc Bull*. 1984;10(1):24-8

50. Hemilä H et al. Vitamin C for preventing and treating tetanus. *Cochrane Database Syst Rev*. 2013(11):CD006665

51. Roush SW et al. Historical comparisons of morbidity and mortality for vaccine-preventable diseases in the United States. *JAMA*. 2007;298(18):2155-63

52. Fraser DW. Tetanus in the United States, 1900-1969. Analysis by cohorts. *Am J Epidemiol*. 1972;96(4):306-12

Chapter Eleven

DIPHTHERIA

The only safe vaccine is one that is never used.
— **Dr. James Shannon, Director of the NIH**

D iphtheria, like tetanus, is also a rather dangerous disease, but what is the probability of contracting diphtheria today, and how effective is the vaccine?

Diphtheria is caused by the bacterium called *Corynebacterium diphtheria*, which in itself is fairly harmless. However, if this bacterium is infected by a specific virus (bacteriophage), it begins to produce and secrete a strong toxin, which destroys the throat tissue and forms a pseudomembrane in it. This toxin is responsible for the severe symptoms of diphtheria, whereas without the toxin, this bacterium can only cause pharyngitis.

If this toxin enters the circulatory system, the complications could lead to myocarditis and temporary paralysis. The case-fatality rate is 5–10%. The disease is mostly transmitted through respiratory droplets, but it can also be transmitted through contaminated objects. Most people infected with diphtheria bacterium do not get sick, but simply become the bacteria reservoirs and carriers. During epidemics, most children happen to be carriers but do not get sick. The highest incidence of diphtheria is during winter and spring [1].

Diphtheria vaccine is not produced separately. It is always either combined with tetanus (DT, Td) or tetanus and pertussis (DTaP/DTP). Similar to the tetanus vaccine, this vaccine is made with a toxoid (i.e., formalin-inactivated toxin adjuvanted with aluminum). Antibiotics and diphtheria immunoglobulin are used as a treatment. Since diphtheria is an extremely rare disease, human immunoglobulin for it is not produced, and horse immunoglobulin is used instead, even in developed countries.

Among unvaccinated children in Afghanistan, Burma, and Nigeria, 40–78% acquire natural immunity by the age of five. In order to catch diphtheria, one needs to be within less than one meter of the infected person. If the distance is greater, the risk of infection is significantly reduced. Socioeconomic factors, such as overcrowding, poverty, alcohol abuse, and poor hygiene, contribute to the transmission of diphtheria [2].

In 1926, Alexander Glenny and his group experimented with the diphtheria vaccine and tried to improve its effectiveness. They accidentally discovered that adding aluminum to the vaccine triggers a stronger immune response. Since then, aluminum is added to most inactivated vaccines [3].

Who Used To Suffer From Diphtheria?

Diphtheria was always considered to be a childhood disease. However, the proportion of adult cases increased markedly in the 1960s. In 1960, 21% of the reported cases in the United States were in people over 15 years of age; by 1964, this figure was 36%, and in the 1970s it was already 48%. The fatality ratio has also changed. During the 1960s, 70% of deaths were in children, but during the 1970s, 73% of those who died were adults. **Since the 1960s, diphtheria was mainly observed in city districts with a low socioeconomic level, mostly among homeless people and alcoholics.** Since the 1980s, diphtheria has almost never been found in developed countries [4].

Not a single case of diphtheria has been recorded in Sweden from the late 1950s until the autumn of 1984. Three outbreaks were observed in 1984. Almost all patients were alcohol abusers. The protective level of antibodies of diphtheria is considered to be between 0.01 and 0.1 IU/ml. A more precise value cannot be established. In 48% of the ten-year-olds who received three doses of the vaccine as infants, titers fell below 0.01 IU/ml. It is possible that the low level of antibodies observed in people in Sweden could be due to the fact that the pertussis component had been excluded from the vaccine in 1972. Since the pertussis toxin acts as an adjuvant, its removal probably makes the diphtheria vaccine less effective. The authors report that the level of antibodies falls by 20–30% annually. A more rapid decrease was found in five-year-old children [5]. A low level of diphtheria antibodies was found in other studies as well. In another Swedish study, more than 70% of adult women and 50% of adult men lacked immunity [6]. About 80% of women in Minnesota had a diphtheria antibody level below 0.01 IU/ml [7]. In another study, 40% of Americans lacked immunity to diphtheria [8]. The authors of a study published in 1988 state that **the decline in the number of cases in the 1970s occurred despite the low immunity of adults, and that recent diphtheria outbreaks occurred only among alcoholics and the homeless [9].**

A 1985 article published in the *Lancet* states that "Recommendations to give adults diphtheria and tetanus toxoid every ten years have been based on serological surveys that have shown lower antibody levels in older populations. The purpose of an immunization program, however, is to prevent disease and not merely to produce antibodies. In Canada, although an immunization program against diphtheria has been in operation for nearly sixty years, age-specific morbidity and mortality rates for diphtheria do not show an increase with age. Similarly, age-specific death rates from tetanus do not show any increase." The authors conclude that the benefits of tetanus and diphtheria booster doses do not justify risks or costs [10].

In a study in Belgium, adults got revaccinated against diphtheria. In 24% of them, the antibodies produced did not go above the "protective" level. Among those whose antibody level was initially low, it remained insufficient in 42% of the cases [11].

The authors of a 2020 study analyzed more than 11 billion person-years in 31 countries and concluded that there is no benefit in booster vaccination against tetanus and diphtheria. They estimate that removing the recommendation of decennial adult booster vaccination would save more than $1 billion in the United States alone. The WHO has not recommended adult booster vaccination since 2017 [12].

Effectiveness

Since diphtheria almost never occurred in developed countries in recent decades, the effectiveness of the vaccine can only be judged from the historical data. Eighteen cases were registered in a 1946 outbreak in an English school. All except three children were vaccinated. Among the 23 unvaccinated children, 13% got sick. Among the 300 vaccinated children, 5% got sick. One of the unvaccinated children was actually vaccinated, but more than ten years ago. If he is excluded, then the percentage of sick children among the unvaccinated goes down to 9%. Dividing the vaccinated children into two groups—those vaccinated within five years and those more than five years ago—it was found that the percentage of cases was approximately equal. Nonetheless, for those who were recently vaccinated, the disease was milder than for those vaccinated a long time ago or those unvaccinated. The authors conclude that the vaccine is not very effective without the subsequent booster shots and urge to get booster vaccines every three years, in addition to being vaccinated in infancy [13].

In the early 1940s, there was a diphtheria epidemic in Canada (1,028 cases). Twenty-four percent of cases were vaccinated (or had antibodies). Five of them died, including one person who was vaccinated just six months before. Overall, those vaccinated had milder symptoms [14]. In the diphtheria outbreak in Halifax (Canada) in 1940, there were 66 cases, of which 30% were fully vaccinated [15]. Out of 103 cases in the diphtheria outbreak in Baltimore in 1943, 29% of patients were vaccinated, and another 14% claimed that they were vaccinated but had no formal proof. As a result of this, vaccination rates were increased in Baltimore. In the first half of 1944, 142 cases were recorded. Sixty-three percent of them have been vaccinated [16].

Diphtheria in Western countries is so rare that no one even remembers what it is like anymore. It is even hardly mentioned in medical school. However, in Russia and other former USSR countries, many still fear diphtheria because of the epidemic in the early '90s. But who got sick during this epidemic?

An article published by the CDC reports that prior to World War II diphtheria was rarely observed in Western European countries. During the war, an epidemic started in the Netherlands, Denmark, and Norway on the territories occupied by German troops. It was the last diphtheria epidemic in industrialized Western countries. The remaining isolated cases were observed mainly among the lower socioeconomic class.

In the early 90s in Russia, the incidence of diphtheria in the military was six times higher than that of the civilian population. In the epidemic in the former USSR countries in the 90s, most cases occurred in adults.

They were mainly among the homeless and patients of psychiatric hospitals, who lived in a crowded setting with poor hygiene. In a normal work setting, the cases were rare. Children rarely got sick, but they were disease carriers. The authors state that the economic crisis of the post-Soviet period may have worsened living conditions and contributed to the epidemic [17].

One thousand eight hundred sixty cases of diphtheria have been registered in the Botkin hospital in St. Petersburg. The fatality rate was 2.3%. **Sixty-nine percent of those who died were alcoholics.** Among those who suffered from the toxic form of the disease, the fatality rate was 26%. Six percent of vaccinated and 14% of unvaccinated patients suffered from the toxic form. However, only those who received the vaccine within the last five years were considered vaccinated. Overall, the diphtheria fatality rate was relatively low compared to previously known epidemics. If alcoholics were excluded, the fatality rate would come to about 1%. Most deaths occurred in patients admitted to the hospital late in the course of the disease. These patients were mainly alcoholics. The authors conclude that the diphtheria epidemic in developed countries is unlikely to have a high fatality rate in the future [18].

In a study of 218 cases of diphtheria in Georgia in the '90s, the fatality rate was 10%. Children whose mothers had only elementary-level education had a four times higher risk of diphtheria compared to those whose mothers had a university degree. Among adults, people with elementary-level education got sick with diphtheria five times more often than those who had a university degree. Chronic illnesses were associated with a three times increased risk of getting diphtheria. Unemployed got sick twice as often. Showering less than once a week was associated with a twofold risk of infection. Unvaccinated people got sick 19 times more often than vaccinated. However, only those who received all doses and boosters, and have been vaccinated within the last ten years, were considered vaccinated. The rest were considered unvaccinated. The authors write that, perhaps, the patients did not remember well whether they have been vaccinated or not.

> Among the 181 cases, just 9% were unvaccinated, 48% had a chronic health problem, and 21% showered less than once a week. The authors conclude that vaccination is the most important tool in the

control of diphtheria, but do not really emphasize that people should shower more than once a week.

Also, the authors state that diphtheria is not very contagious and that it takes prolonged contact with a patient to catch it. Visiting crowded places was not a risk factor. Compared to the previous epidemics in Europe and the US, which occurred mainly among alcoholics, the authors of this study did not find an increased risk for heavy drinkers. They conclude that low socioeconomic status, and not alcoholism per se, is likely to be a risk factor [2].

In the 90s, due to the opening of the borders, tourists flooded from Finland to Russia and from Russia to Finland. Four hundred thousand Finnish citizens visited Russia every year, and 200,000 Russians visited Finland. Despite the epidemic in Russia, only ten cases of diphtheria were registered in Finland. Almost all of them were middle-aged men; only three of them had severe form (described below), five had mild form, and two were solely carriers.

1. A 43-year-old resident of Finland visited St. Petersburg in 1993. During this trip, he "kissed his local girlfriend," and upon his arrival back to Finland, he was diagnosed with diphtheria. He was vaccinated against diphtheria 20 years ago and was considered as unvaccinated (antibody level 0.01 IU/ml). His Russian girlfriend did not get sick. Another diphtheria carrier who traveled in the same group was also identified. He also had intimate contact with the same woman in St. Petersburg. It was the first case of diphtheria in Finland in 30 years.

2. A 57-year-old male visited Russia for one day in 1993 and came back with diphtheria. He denied having had close contact with the locals, but his friends said that he had visited prostitutes. It is unknown whether or not he has been vaccinated (antibody level 0.06 IU/ml).

3. A 45-year-old male visited Russia for 22 hours and came back with diphtheria. His friends said that he also visited a prostitute. He had been vaccinated and even received a booster shot one year before the trip (antibody level 0.08 IU/ml). He was the only one fully vaccinated, and also the only one who died. All three consumed alcohol heavily during the trip, and at least two of them were regular heavy drinkers [19, 20].

According to the 2015 European CDC report, over the past few years, diphtheria became more common in Germany and France compared to the other developed countries (a few cases per year). The reason for this is the influx of migrants from the third-world countries [21].

In 2016, 25 years after diphtheria had been fully eradicated, a diphtheria outbreak began in Venezuela [22]. Since the vaccination coverage there was increasing every year, and also considering the humanitarian crisis, it is hard to blame the outbreak on the lack of vaccination [23]. However, the WHO wouldn't be the WHO if it would be side-tracked by the facts [24].

In November-December of 2017, diphtheria outbreaks began in Yemen and in a refugee camp in Bangladesh. This, of course, happened because of insufficient vaccination, and not because of the civil war in Yemen, and certainly not because the refugees in Bangladesh lived in tents, 30 people in each [25].

Treatment

Apart from humans and primates, guinea pigs are the only mammals that do not synthesize their own vitamin C. In a 1936 study, guinea pigs were injected with diphtheria toxin. Those who were on a low vitamin C diet lost more weight than those on a normal diet. Diphtheria toxin depleted vitamin C in the adrenal glands, pancreas, and kidneys [26]. According to a 1937 study, vitamin C deficiency is accompanied by a decreased resistance to injuries and infections resulting from bacterial toxins. The lowered resistance appears before the scurvy symptoms can be observed, and before there is a marked decline in the growth rate in young animals. Guinea pigs, who were injected with sublethal doses of diphtheria toxin and who were on a diet with severely restricted vitamin C, show more extensive tissue damage, greater weight loss, shorter life span, larger areas of necrosis, and poorer tooth development, than those who were not restricted in their vitamin C intake. It appears that a low level of vitamin C leads to a systemic disorder of the whole body, and particularly the entire endocrine system. The authors conclude that "The level of vitamin C intake for optimum in vivo detoxification of diphtheria toxin is considerably greater than that necessary to protect from scurvy or to show a favorable growth rate" [27].

A 1940 study found that when guinea pigs are injected with a sublethal dose of diphtheria toxin, a 30–50% decrease in the vitamin C level in tissues is observed within 24–48 hours. Children receiving small amounts of vitamin C were especially prone to the development of scurvy during periods of infection. Scurvy resolved spontaneously after the recovery from infection without an increase in vitamin C intake.

In another experiment, sublethal doses of diphtheria toxin were injected into guinea pigs. Among those who received 0.8 mg of vitamin C per day, tooth decay was observed. The teeth of those who received 5 mg of vitamin did not decay [28]. Similar results were obtained in other studies. After being injected with sublethal amounts of diphtheria toxin, guinea pigs kept on diets deficient in vitamin C developed arteriosclerosis in the lungs, liver, spleen, and kidneys [29]. Guinea pigs with low vitamin C levels died after the injection of diphtheria toxin faster than those on an adequate diet. Guinea pigs that received large doses of vitamin C survived after being injected even with multiple lethal doses of the toxin [30].

The effect of vitamin C on diphtheria has not been further studied since the '40s. In 1971, a case of a girl who was cured of diphtheria by intravenous injections of the vitamin was reported. Two other children did not receive the vitamin, and both died. All three received the antitoxin [31].

Statistics And Safety

As is the case with other diseases, the decline in the diphtheria mortality rate began long before the introduction of the vaccine. Since diphtheria vaccine is a toxoid, it cannot prevent the infection, but it is aimed to prevent disease complications. Therefore, it would be logical to expect the diphtheria fatality rate to decrease with the introduction of the vaccine. However, that did not happen. Despite the fact that the number of diphtheria cases was continuously decreasing, the fatality rate remained at approximately 10% in the period of the 1920s–1970s, regardless of the increasing vaccination coverage [4].

Diphtheria is an extremely rare disease nowadays. It is rarely found even in most third-world countries. Since 2000, only six cases of diphtheria have been reported in the US [32]. Only one of the patients died. He was 63 years old and was infected in Haiti [33]. This is such a rare disease that the CDC writes a separate report on almost every case. At the same time, more than 100 cases of bubonic plague were reported in the US since 2000. Twelve people died. Their deaths have not been widely reported because children are not vaccinated against the plague.

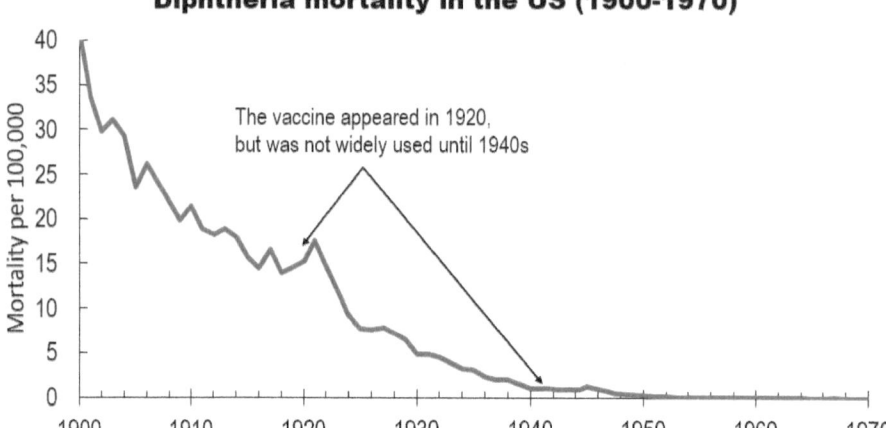

Since the diphtheria vaccine is always combined with tetanus/pertussis, its safety data is the same as was presented in the respective chapters. The vaccine (without the pertussis component) causes Guillain-Barré syndrome, anaphylactic shock, and brachial neuritis. It also lowers the level of lymphocytes and increases the risk of allergies.

From 2000 to 2018, VAERS has registered 36 deaths and more than 200 cases of permanent disability after the diphtheria vaccine without the pertussis component. During the same period, six people contracted diphtheria, and only one died. Considering that just 1–10% of all cases are registered with VAERS, the probability of dying from the vaccine is hundreds of times higher than the probability of contracting diphtheria. The probability of contracting diphtheria in developed countries is a maximum of 1 in 10 million, and usually even less. The probability of just the anaphylactic shock or brachial neuritis following vaccination is tens of times higher.

Conclusions

Since the diphtheria vaccine was developed back in the 1920s, there have been no clinical trials, let alone efficacy studies. Nonetheless, judging by the available data, it does provide certain immunity from diphtheria. It is clearly more effective than the tetanus vaccine, which makes sense: the diphtheria toxin is spread through the circulatory system, where antibodies are present, whereas tetanus is spread through the nervous system, where antibodies are not found. However, this immunity is very short-lived, which is why it is necessary to get vaccinated every three to five years to maintain a sufficient antibody level.

Diphtheria mainly affects alcoholics and homeless people, and even they suffer from it extremely rarely. It is virtually impossible to contract diphtheria nowadays.

The probability of dying after the vaccination is hundreds of times higher than the probability of contracting diphtheria.

Endnotes

1. Diphtheria. CDC Pink Book

2. Quick ML et al. Risk factors for diphtheria: a prospective case-control study in the Republic of Georgia, 1995-1996. *J Infect Dis*. 2000;181 Suppl 1:S121-9

3. Glenny A. Immunological notes. XVII–XXIV. *J Pathol*. 1926;29(1):31-40

4. Dixon JM. Diphtheria in North America. *J Hyg*. 1984;93(3):419-32

5. Mark A et al. Immunity and immunization of children against diphtheria in Sweden. *Eur J Clin Microbiol Infect Dis*. 1989;8(3):214-9

6. Christenson B et al. Serological immunity to diphtheria in Sweden in 1978 and 1984. *Scand J Infect Dis*. 1986;18(3):227-33

7. Crossley K et al. Tetanus and diphtheria immunity in urban Minnesota adults. *JAMA*. 1979;242(21):2298-300

8. McQuillan GM et al. Serologic immunity to diphtheria and tetanus in the United States. *Ann Intern Med*. 2002;136(9):660-6

9. Karzon DT et al. Diphtheria outbreaks in immunized populations. *N Engl J Med*. 1988;318(1):41-3

10. Mathias RG et al. Booster immunisation for diphtheria and tetanus: no evidence of need in adults. *Lancet*. 1985;1(8437):1089-91

11. Vellinga A et al. Response to diphtheria booster vaccination in healthy adults: vaccine trial. *BMJ*. 2000;320(7229):217

12. Slifka AM et al. Incidence of tetanus and diphtheria in relation to adult vaccination schedules. *Clin Infect Dis*. 2020;ciaa017

13. Fanning J. An outbreak of diphtheria in a highly immunized community. *BMJ*. 1947; 1(4498):371-3

14. Gibbard J. Some observations on diphtheria in the immunized. *Can J Public Health*. 1945;36(5):188-91

15. Morton AR. The diphtheria epidemic in Halifax. *Can Med Assoc J*. 1941;45(2):171-4

16. Eller C. An outbreak of diphtheria in Baltimore in 1944. *Am J Epidemiol*. 1945;42(2):179-88

17. Vitek CR et al. Diphtheria in the former Soviet Union: reemergence of a pandemic disease. *Emerg Infect Dis*. 1998;4(4):539-50

18. Rakhmanova AG et al. Diphtheria outbreak in St. Petersburg: clinical characteristics of 1860 adult patients. *Scand J Infect Dis*. 1996;28(1):37-40

19. Lumio J et al. Epidemiology of three cases of severe diphtheria in Finnish patients with low antitoxin antibody levels. *Eur J Clin Microbiol Infect Dis.* 2001;20(10):705-10

20. Lumio J. Diphtheria after visit to Russia. *Lancet.* 1993;342(8862):53-4

21. Cutaneous diphtheria among recently arrived refugees and asylum seekers in the EU. *ECDC.* 2015 Jul 30.

22. Venezuela: Diphtheria spreading as of early August. *garda.com.* 2017 Aug 5

23. WHO vaccine-preventable diseases: monitoring system. 2019 global summary

24. Nikolau L. Venezuela is ignoring another public health crisis: Diphtheria. *humanosphere.org.* 2016 Nov 1

25. Bichell R. Diphtheria: what exactly is it. And why is it back? *NPR.* 2017 Dec 8

26. Lyman C. The effect of diphtheria toxin on the vitamin C content of guinea pig tissues. *J Pharm Exp Ther.* 1936;56(2):209-15

27. Sigal A. The influence of vitamin C deficiency upon the resistance of guinea pigs to diphtheria toxin glucose tolerance. *J Pharmacol Exp Ther.* 1937;61(1):1-9

28. King CG et al. Effects of vitamin C intake upon the degree of tooth injury produced by diphtheria toxin. *Am J Public Health.* 1940;30(9):1068-72

29. King MMC. The influence of vitamin C level upon resistance to diphtheria toxin. *J Nutr.* 1935;10(2):129-55

30. Torrance C. The effect of diphtheria toxin upon vitamin C in vitro. *J Biol Chem.* 1937; 121:31-6

31. Klenner FR. Observations on the dose and administration of ascorbic acid when employed beyond the range of a vitamin in human pathology. *J App Nutr.* 1971;23:61-88

32. Reported cases and deaths from vaccine preventable diseases, United States. *CDC*

33. Fatal respiratory diphtheria in a U.S. traveler to Haiti—Pennsylvania, 2003. *MMWR.* 2004;52(53):1285-6

Chapter Twelve

MEASLES

> *Cancer was practically unknown until*
> *the cowpox vaccination began to be introduced.*
> *I have seen 200 cases of cancer,*
> *and never saw a case in an unvaccinated person.*
> — W.B. Clark, 1909

Today measles is undoubtedly the most frightening infectious disease. According to the media, measles is far more dangerous than Ebola [1]. Measles is indeed very dangerous in the case of malnutrition and vitamin A deficiency, which is why it was often fatal in the 19th and early 20th century and can still be fatal in third-world countries. **On the contrary, in developed countries, measles is far less dangerous than the flu. It is easy to recover from, gives lifelong immunity, and protects against much more dangerous diseases, as we will see later.**

In an article published in 1959 in *the BMJ*, several general practitioners explain that in England, measles has become a mild infection and passes with little or no complications. No treatment is required, no effort is made to prevent its spread, and disease cases are not registered anywhere. Moreover, they claim that it is better to catch measles between three and seven years old because, in adulthood, it often leads to complications. They go on to say that infants almost never get it, and if they do, the disease is very mild. They state that "Many mothers have remarked 'how much good the attack has done their children,' as they seem so much better after the measles" [2, 3].

Now, if measles was such a trivial disease, then why did people start being vaccinated against it in the first place? In his 1962 article, the CDC chief epidemiologist Alexander Langmuir claims that "This self-limiting infection of short duration, moderate severity and low fatality has maintained a remarkably stable biological balance over the centuries... To those who ask me, 'Why do you wish to eradicate measles?,' I reply with the same answer that Hillary used when asked why he wished to climb Mt. Everest. He said, 'Because it is there.' To this may be added, '... and it can be done'" [4].

In 1966 the plan was to completely eradicate measles within a year. It was considered that in order to achieve herd immunity, vaccination coverage of 55% was sufficient [5]. However, by 1980 it turned out that vaccination caused adults and adolescents to contract measles instead of children [6]. Later on, infants born to mothers who did not get measles during childhood because of the vaccine started to contract measles at ages younger than one year old, which was practically unheard of in the pre-vaccine era [7]. **In other words, pregnant women, infants, and adults, all of whom have a higher risk of complications, were now contracting measles instead of getting over it in childhood, when it is less dangerous [8].**

In 1978, the CDC set a goal to eliminate measles from the United States by 1982 [9]. However, it turned out that before 1980, the vaccine was unstable, and as a result, people vaccinated before 1980 may not be immune [10]. But even the 1980's version of the vaccine was not able to eradicate measles, so in 1989 the second MMR dose was introduced. It also turned out that measles outbreaks may very well occur in schools where 100% of children have a formal proof of vaccination. The CDC did not know how to explain this [11].

One of the world's leading vaccine proponents, Gregory Poland, published an article in 1994 analyzing 18 measles outbreaks in schools where almost all students were vaccinated. He concludes that it is impossible to completely eradicate measles even if 100% of the children are vaccinated because the vaccine is not 100% effective. So, as time goes on, measles will become a disease of the vaccinated, and since measles is highly contagious, herd immunity cannot be achieved, despite very high vaccination coverage (it's rather ironic that "herd immunity"—a term that gained popularity precisely in the context of measles, does not apply to measles) [12]. He also writes that vaccine given before 12 months of age is very ineffective, and even before 15 months of age, the vaccine's effectiveness is limited. Despite all this, in the United States as well as in many other countries, this vaccine is recommended at 12 months of age; meanwhile, the WHO recommends it routinely at nine months and at six months during epidemics [13].

Since 2000, measles has been considered eliminated in the United States. This does not mean people completely ceased to contract measles, because the definition of "elimination" itself had been revised. Today, elimination means that measles is transmitted from person to person for a time period of less than 12 consecutive months, and new cases are imported.

Nowadays measles vaccine is always given as part of the trivalent MMR vaccine (which includes rubella and mumps components) or the tetravalent MMRV vaccine (with rubella, mumps, and varicella). Monovalent measles vaccines are not manufactured in developed countries, but they are still available in Russia and some third-world countries.

In contrast to the inactivated vaccines, which we have examined so far, the measles vaccine is an attenuated vaccine containing a live virus. "Live"-attenuated vaccines are much more effective than inactivated ones, and therefore do not need aluminum adjuvants. The very first measles vaccine was inactivated, but after several years of common use, it turned out that it led to atypical measles, as well as to pneumonia and encephalopathy [14]. First attenuated vaccines were so potent that the immunoglobulin injection was also given with the vaccine. That is why, in 1965 and 1968, the vaccine was further attenuated [6].

What does the term "attenuated vaccine" mean? How exactly does one weaken a virus without killing it? For the virus to become attenuated, it is taken through a process of adaptation to living in non-human cells. As a result of this process, the virus mutates, becoming less adapted to humans.

A diagram of the mumps virus attenuation process is shown in the next figure [15].

The process starts with the isolation of a wild strain of the virus from an infected person. Next, the virus undergoes two serial passages through human embryonic kidney cells. Then it is transferred to green monkey kidney cells. Then it undergoes six serial passages through the egg amniotic cavity, then twice through the quail embryonic fibroblasts, and then again

Manufacturing processes of Urabe strain mumps vaccines

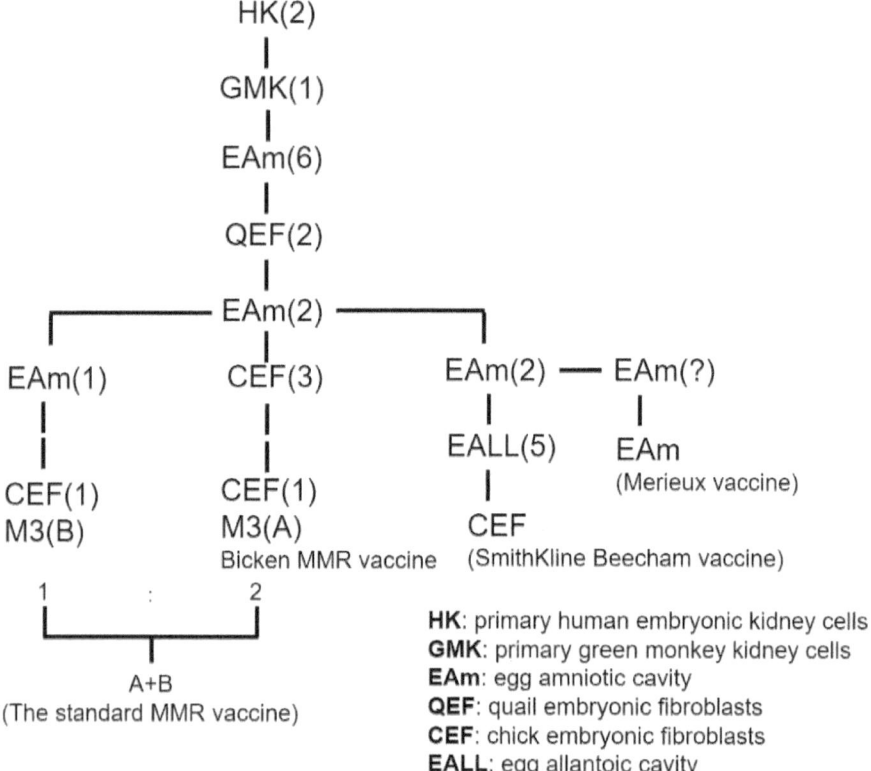

twice through the egg amniotic cavity. After this, several options are available. One may perform three serial passages through the chick embryonic fibroblasts, or two passages through the egg amniotic cavity and then another five through the egg allantoic cavity (embryonic respiratory organ), and then again through chick embryonic fibroblasts. This allows us to derive different vaccine strains, which can also be mixed with one another. Merck, for example, uses fetal lung cells (female WI-38 and male MRC-5) instead of kidney cells. In general, every vaccine manufacturer frolics to the best of their imagination.

Given that it is impossible to completely separate the virus from the cells where it multiplies, fragments of these cells are also part of the vaccine. Since the role of these cells is to multiply rapidly, they are often carcinogenic. Of course, scientists from the FDA are concerned about this, but not too much [16].

Moreover, these cells may contain other viruses that are not yet known to science. After all, in order to isolate a virus, one needs to know what to look for. And if the virus is not yet known, then it is impossible to isolate. But you shouldn't worry: the FDA scientists are working on new technologies to detect unknown viruses [17]. In 2010, a porcine virus was discovered in a rotavirus vaccine [18]. However, it was discovered by scientists from the University of California and not by the FDA. Later on, they decided to analyze the rotavirus vaccine by another manufacturer and found the DNA of two porcine viruses in it. But you shouldn't worry, as the FDA believes that these viruses are completely harmless to humans. At least their danger has not yet been proven, so it was decided to leave these porcine viruses in the vaccines. Indeed, why remake perfectly good vaccines because of something as insignificant as a couple of extra viruses?

Effectiveness

According to Cochrane's systematic review of MMR effectiveness and safety, the vaccine is 95% effective against measles and up to 88% effective against mumps. The vaccine increases the risk of aseptic meningitis by a factor of 14–22 (Urabe and Leningrad-Zagreb strains), the risk of febrile convulsions by a factor of 4–5, and the risk of thrombocytopenic purpura by a factor of 2–6. The authors conclude that "The design and reporting of safety outcomes in MMR vaccine studies, both pre- and post-marketing, are largely inadequate. The evidence of adverse events following immunization with the MMR vaccine cannot be separated from its role in preventing the target diseases." They recommend improving the design and reporting of clinical and post-marketing studies and standardize the definitions of adverse events. More evidence should be collected on whether the protective effect of MMR wanes with time [19].

The authors of an article published in 2014 wrote that it was previously believed that although those vaccinated against measles can still get measles, they are not able to infect others (the authors clearly did not read dozens of articles about measles outbreaks in fully vaccinated schools, in which the null patient was vaccinated [20]). But it turned out that it is possible. A 22-year-old girl, who was vaccinated twice, infected four people with measles, three of whom were healthcare workers. All four were either vaccinated with two doses or had measles antibodies [21].

> Although the vaccination coverage in China is greater than 99%, the incidence of measles, mumps, and rubella remains high.

Among 20- to 40-year-old women in Zhejiang Province, measles and rubella titers are much lower than in men of the same age category. This means that during pregnancy, when the protection against measles and rubella is of the biggest importance, many women do not have it due to the vaccination. Infants of seven months and younger have even lower titers (in China, measles vaccination is given at eight months). Most cases of measles are reported in the 20–29 age group. The same happens in other provinces. Rubella primarily occurs in the 15- to 39-year age group, and it is especially dangerous for pregnant women [22]. According to another Chinese study, despite the vaccination coverage of above 98.5%, the number of measles cases is growing, and adults contract it instead of children. The authors isolated 16 strains of measles virus from 14 vaccinated cases and two unvaccinated cases and concluded that the virus mutates, causing the vaccinated to contract the disease. The authors suggest that new vaccines should be developed to better control measles outbreaks [23].

In Korea, measles occurs mainly in infants younger than 12 months. Only 71% of the population have measles antibodies. Between 2010 and 2014, the average amount of titers decreased by 16% [24]. The same happened in Finland, Portugal, and the US [25–27]. Immunity after natural disease lasts longer than immunity after vaccination. In infants, maternal measles antibodies disappear by the age of eight months. Several studies of the early waning of maternal measles antibodies in infants have been published in recent years, and such waning may be related to low maternal measles titers. This is a limitation of a vaccine-induced immunity (compared with naturally developed immunity after wild measles virus infection) and the absence of natural boosters. According to a CDC study, infants of vaccinated mothers contracted measles 7.5 times more often than infants of unvaccinated mothers. Because of the vaccine, more and more infants are not protected against measles [7].

In a Japanese study, the vaccinated had nine times fewer antibodies than the unvaccinated. By the age of 20, their titers were significantly reduced. They increased again during their twenties, which implies a possible occurrence of natural infection in the vaccinated with low titers [28].

In the pre-vaccine era, 10.6% of the population was susceptible to measles, most of whom were children younger than ten. At the beginning of the measles vaccination program, from 1978 through 1981, the proportion of susceptible people in the population fell to 3.1%, but then began to rise by approximately 0.1% per year and is set to reach about 10.9% in the year 2050. According to a 2009 study, this will lead to large-scale epidemics [29, 30].

Immunoglobulins produced from donors' blood plasma are used for the treatment of measles in people with immune diseases. The authors of a 2017 study analyzed measles titers in donors' blood, and it turned out that those born after 1990 had seven times fewer antibodies than those born before 1962. Revaccination did not solve this problem, because it increased the antibody level only twofold, and only for a few months. The authors recommend that the FDA lowers the antibody level requirement for the immunoglobulin [31].

Agammaglobulinemia is a rare genetic disease, which manifests in the absence of humoral immunity, meaning that specific antibodies cannot be produced. This does not prevent people with this disease from recovering from measles. Therefore, antibodies and humoral immunity do not play a significant role in measles [32].

According to a 2009 Swedish study, children who were breastfed for more than three months had a 31% lower risk of clinical measles compared to those who were never breastfed, regardless of the vaccination status [33].

> As with some other diseases, the definition of measles has been revised and narrowed down. In the past, measles had been diagnosed only when a specific rash appeared (which was often confused with rubella [34]). Nowadays, a confirmed measles diagnosis requires either a laboratory analysis or a temperature above 38.3°C (101°F) with a rash and an epidemiological link to a confirmed measles case.

According to a 2017 study, approximately 5% of vaccine recipients develop symptoms that are indistinguishable from measles after measles vaccination. In the United States, 194 cases of measles were registered in 2015, of which **38% were caused by a vaccine strain** [35]. In a measles outbreak in Canada in 2015, 48% of the cases were caused by a vaccine strain. In a study in France, measles antibodies were found in 87% of the 133 unvaccinated children. However, only 42 of them (i.e., 41%) had clinical measles symptoms. This demonstrates that measles is asymptomatic in almost 60% of the cases. In a US study of the vaccinated patients who did not develop antibodies, measles was asymptomatic in only 17% [36, 37].

Vitamin A

In the 1920s, studies began to emerge proving that vitamin A protects against infections. Rats with vitamin A deficiency developed atrophies of the salivary glands and mucous membrane of the larynx and trachea. If vitamin A was withheld for a further period, a local bacterial invasion of these tissues followed, and the rats died from broncho-pneumonia. In 1931, it turned out that vitamin A protects against postpartum sepsis [38]. Back then, vitamin A was called "an anti-infective agent" [39].

The measles virus attacks epithelial cells. In the presence of vitamin A deficiency, these cells become atrophied, which allows generally harmless bacteria to attack them and invade the lungs, skin, middle ear, and gastrointestinal tract, causing complications.

In England, measles was dangerous mainly for children from the poorest families, whose diet lacked fats (and hence vitamins A and D). In a 1932 study, 600 children with measles admitted to a London hospital were randomly divided into two groups. One of the groups received vitamins A and D in the form of cod-liver oil, and the fatality rate in this group was 2.3 times lower than in the other group [40].

After this successful trial, the treatment of measles with vitamin A was simply forgotten.

Vitamin A was discovered again only 50 years later when it turned out that children with even mild vitamin A deficiency in Indonesia have a fourfold increase in mortality from all causes, and some age groups have an eight- to 12-fold increase. It also turned out that vitamin A supplementation decreases mortality by 34%, and that measles caused vitamin A levels in well-nourished children to fall to levels similar to those found in non-infected malnourished children [41, 42]. A 1968 WHO report states that "No nutritional deficiency is more consistently synergistic with infectious disease than that of vitamin A" [43].

In 1983 a randomized trial was conducted among children with measles in Tanzania. Among those who did not receive vitamin A, the fatality rate was 13%, and among those who received the vitamin, the fatality rate was 7%. Among children under two, vitamin A reduced mortality by 87%. The mortality of marasmic children was several times higher than that of better-nourished children, regardless of whether they had received vitamin A or not [44]. After this study, the WHO recommended the use of vitamin A for children with measles, but only in regions where case-fatality rates are over 1%.

Unlike in Tanzania, where children had an obvious vitamin A deficiency, clinically apparent vitamin A deficiency is rare in South Africa. Nevertheless, it turned out that in children with measles, the level of vitamin A was very low. In a randomized control trial, it was found that children who received vitamin A recovered from pneumonia and diarrhea two times faster, and also had less respiratory croup [45].

In the early '90s, researches studied vitamin A levels in 20 children with measles in California. To their surprise, half of them were vitamin A deficient, despite the fact that all the children were well-nourished. All uninfected children in the control group had normal levels of the vitamin. In the second control group, which included patients with other infectious diseases, 30% had low levels of vitamin A. The authors concluded that it is impossible to further assume that vitamin A levels during measles are not lower in well-nourished American children. They also suggest that vitamin A levels may decrease during other acute infections [46]. Similar results were obtained in studies in New York and Milwaukee [47, 48].

A Cochrane systematic review on treating measles with vitamin A, published in 2005, concluded that two doses of vitamin A (200,000 IU each) reduce measles fatality by 82% in children under the age of two. The risk of otitis media is reduced by 74%, the risk of croup by 47%. A single dose of vitamin A does not reduce mortality [49]. Could it be that three doses of vitamin A, or higher doses, will reduce mortality even more? For some reason, no one ever studied this hypothesis.

In a meta-analysis of the vitamin A impact on infant mortality, it turned out that vitamin A reduced measles-related mortality by 60%, and among infants by 90%. Pneumonia-related mortality decreased by 70% [50]. According to a Cochrane systematic review of the overall vitamin A impact on morbidity and mortality, vitamin A prophylactic supplementation in children reduces all-cause mortality by 12–24%. The risk of diarrhea is reduced by 15%; the risk of measles is reduced by 50% [51].

Similar to measles, the MMR vaccine also significantly depletes vitamin A levels [52, 53]. As opposed to vitamin A, there is not a single study proving that measles vaccination in developed countries reduces measles-related mortality.

The Benefits Of Measles And Other Infectious Diseases

According to a 2006 Italian study, measles was associated with a reduction in the risk of non-Hodgkin's lymphoma by 40% and Hodgkin's lymphoma by 70%. Chickenpox, mumps, and rubella were associated with a 50% lower risk of Hodgkin's lymphoma and an 80% lower risk of scarlet fever. Two childhood diseases were associated with a 50% reduction in the risk of non-Hodgkin's lymphoma and an 80% reduction in the risk of Hodgkin's lymphoma [54].

In a British study, measles was associated with a 47% reduction in the risk of Hodgkin's lymphoma, and two or more childhood illnesses were associated with a 55% decrease in the risk of lymphoma [55]. In a 2005 study, measles, mumps, or rubella in childhood were associated with a 70% reduction in the risk of Hodgkin's lymphoma associated with the Epstein-Barr virus in women. Those who had measles before the age of ten had a 96% lower risk of lymphoma than those who had measles after the age of ten [56]. According to the analysis of 17 studies published in 2012, measles and pertussis are associated with a 15% reduction in the risk of non-Hodgkin's lymphoma [57].

In a Swiss study, rubella in childhood was associated with a decrease in the risk of various types of cancer by 62%, and chickenpox by 38%. One or more childhood febrile illnesses were associated with a 73% reduction in the risk of cancer [58].

A study in Germany found that childhood diseases are associated with a reduced risk of melanoma (no statistical significance). Common colds or flu are associated with a 68% reduction in the risk of melanoma. An infected wound is associated with a 79% reduction and a chronic infectious disease, with a 68% reduction in the risk of melanoma [59]. In their next study, the authors concluded that almost all infectious diseases are associated with the reduction in melanoma risk: influenza is associated with a 35% risk reduction, pneumonia 55%, staphylococcus infection 46% [60].

A 2013 Italian study found that measles is associated with a 43% reduction in the risk of chronic lymphoid leukemia. The risk of lymphoid leukemia is inversely associated with a number of childhood diseases (mumps, chickenpox, rubella, whooping cough, etc.). One or two childhood diseases reduced the risk by 16%, three or more diseases by 53% [61]. A link between childhood infections and a reduced risk of leukemia has been identified in other studies [62, 63].

Since 1960, the incidence of Hodgkin's lymphoma in Israel has significantly increased. Some researchers believe that this is due to the fact that more people contract measles in adulthood after the introduction of measles vaccination [64, 65].

Measles is also associated with a 53% decrease in the risk of ovarian cancer, mumps decreases the risk by 39%, rubella by 38%, and chickenpox by 34% [66].

A 1971 article in the *Lancet* describes three children with confirmed Hodgkin's lymphoma in Poland who got measles. They all went into remission after recovery. Two of them had a minor relapse within two years [67]. A similar case was described in Portugal. A two-year-old child was diagnosed with Hodgkin's lymphoma. The child developed measles before radiotherapy was due to be started, and the tumor disappeared [68]. Similar cases were reported in Nigeria and Cuba [69]. In Uganda, a case of an eight-year-old boy was described, who suffered from an extremely swollen eye, and he no longer could see. He was diagnosed with Burkitt's lymphoma. Ten days after the diagnosis, he contracted measles, after which the tumor disappeared within two weeks, and he fully recovered [70]. In the Italian hospital in 1965, two out of four patients with lymphoblastic leukemia died, and two other contracted measles during the treatment and remained alive. In addition to measles, one girl also contracted rubella. The author believes that the rubella virus may also have a beneficial effect [71].

In 2014 a woman was cured of multiple myeloma using a huge dose of recombinant measles virus [72]. Currently, clinical trials are being conducted on the treatment of various oncological diseases with the measles virus [73]. The measles virus has also been used successfully to treat ovarian cancer and skin cancer [74–76]. The virus turned out to be much more effective than Avastin, a very toxic and very expensive cancer drug.

A study among 50,000 graduates of Harvard and the University of Pennsylvania found that those who had measles in childhood had a twofold lower risk of Parkinson's disease. Chickenpox and mumps also reduced the risk of Parkinson's disease [77]. Similar results were obtained in other studies [78]. A measles vaccine can, on the contrary, cause Parkinson's disease in children in rare cases [79].

A prospective study of more than 100,000 people in Japan, who were followed for 20 years, was published in 2015. Males who had measles in childhood had an 8% lower risk of death from cardiovascular diseases. Those who also had mumps had a 20% lower risk. Males who had mumps had a 48% lower risk of death from stroke. Women who had measles and mumps had a 17% lower risk of death from cardiovascular diseases [80].

According to a 2007 Swedish study, measles is associated with a 30% reduction in the risk of heart attack, chickenpox with a 33% reduction, scarlet fever with 31%, mumps with 25%, rubella with 9%, and mononucleosis with a 33% reduction. The more of these infectious diseases a person had in childhood, the lower was the likelihood of a heart attack. In those who had just one disease, the risk of heart attack was 35% lower. Two childhood diseases reduced the risk by 40%, three by 47%, four and five diseases by 54%, and all six of these diseases together reduced the risk of heart attack by 89% [81]. Several studies have found that those who had measles and other infectious diseases in early childhood have a lower occurrence of multiple sclerosis [82–84].

A 1947 article describes five patients with nephrotic syndrome, who contracted measles. In two of them, the syndrome had resolved after recovery from measles. Three others had a temporary improvement only. The authors analyzed the medical literature and found a few more cases of nephrotic syndrome resolution after measles and frequent cases of temporary improvement. The authors concluded that measles is the most effective treatment for nephrotic syndrome of all the methods they have used [85].

A 1978 article describes a severe case of nephrotic syndrome in a ten-year-old English boy in 1916. The child was sick for many months and was in critical condition. The doctors said that he would not survive, and his family had already bought mourning clothes. But suddenly, he got measles and recovered from nephrotic syndrome completely. For years after that, he had to wear his brothers' mourning costumes. When he grew up, this child became a famous pediatrician, a professor, and president of the national pediatric association [86].

According to a Danish study, those who did not have measles in childhood (or had atypical measles, without a rash), had an increased risk of oncological diseases, skin diseases, immunoreactive diseases, and degenerative diseases of the bone and cartilage in adulthood [87].

A 2002 study reports on a measles outbreak in a village in Senegal, during which some of the children had contracted measles, and some had not. They had been followed for four years after recovery. In children who had measles, the risk of death from other infectious diseases was 86% lower. Most patients were unvaccinated [88]. Similar results were observed in Guinea Bissau and in Bangladesh [89, 90].

A study published in the *Lancet* in 1996 reports that among children who had measles in Guinea-Bissau, allergies were three times less common than in vaccinated children who did not have measles. They also had dust mite allergy five times less often. This is explained by the fact that the measles virus stimulates cellular immunity, while humoral immunity is the one responsible for allergies [91]. In a British study, measles or whooping cough before the age of three years was associated with a reduced risk of asthma [92].

In a study of 15,000 children from five European countries, allergies were two times less common in those who had measles. Vaccination reduced the incidence of allergies as well, but not as much as measles. Amongst those who didn't have measles, the risk of rhinoconjunctivitis was 70% higher in vaccinated than in unvaccinated [93]. A lower risk of allergy in those who got measles and an increased risk of allergy in those who were vaccinated were also found in other studies [94–96].

Nodding syndrome is a new fatal seizure disorder found exclusively in some countries in Africa. Its incidence was sevenfold lower in children who had measles [97].

Safety

According to a Japanese study, the level of interferon-alpha (cytokine, responsible for the immunity from viral diseases) was reduced in children vaccinated against measles. This study lasted one year, and interferon levels did not recover during this period [98].

A 1992 Italian study found that MMR significantly reduces the function of polymorphonuclear neutrophils (i.e., increases susceptibility to infections). This is probably because attenuated strains of vaccine viruses do not replicate in lymphoid tissues as extensively as do wild-type strains [99]. MMR also leads to reduced lymphocyte function, which lasts one to five weeks after vaccination. The lymphocyte function is not restored until 10–12 weeks after vaccination. Other studies have shown similar results [100].

In a 2003 Italian study, measles vaccine was associated with a 92-fold increase in the risk of multiple sclerosis [101]. Cases of multiple sclerosis with onset almost immediately after vaccination with various vaccines have been reported [102]. A 2009 Swedish study found that in those who were vaccinated with MMR before the age of ten, the risk of multiple sclerosis was five times higher [103].

The risk of thrombocytopenic purpura increases 5.5 times following MMR vaccination [104]. This data was confirmed in a dozen studies. The risk of febrile seizures after MMR increases sixfold [105]. The risk of complex febrile seizures that last more than 30 minutes is also increased sixfold [106].

In 1993, a study of adverse effects of four different MMR vaccines was conducted in Japan. Thirty-eight thousand children were vaccinated. Aseptic meningitis (with a laboratory-confirmed vaccine strain of mumps in cerebrospinal fluid) was diagnosed in one in every 600 children vaccinated with the standard vaccine. One in every 350 vaccinated children had non-meningitis-related convulsions. However, one of the vaccines did not cause aseptic meningitis. It turned out that its manufacturer had something go wrong with the vaccine strains, but did not report it. **As a result of this study, the Japanese Ministry of Health suspended the use of MMR in 1993, and it remains suspended to this day [15].**

A 1996 article states that mortality rates of people vaccinated and non-vaccinated against measles have never been compared. However, several clinical trials in Guinea-Bissau, Senegal, and Gambia compared the mortality associated with different measles vaccines and found that girls who were given high-titer vaccines had an 86% higher mortality rate than girls who received a medium-titer vaccine [107].

132

> The WHO has been recommending the use of the high-titer vaccine from 1989 to the beginning of the 1990s, and who knows how many girls this vaccine has killed.

It is also unknown whether the mortality rate would have been further reduced if a low-titer vaccine had been used instead of a medium-titer vaccine, or if children had not been vaccinated against measles at all. An article published in *the BMJ* in 1993 claims that it was actually found by chance that a vaccine with high titers significantly increased the mortality rate since mortality happens a year, or even a few years, after the vaccination. Most studies do not last that long. The authors call for randomized studies and the use of mortality rather than surrogate markers, such as the level of antibodies, as a measure of vaccine efficacy [108]. The experiments with this vaccine were carried out not only in Africa but also on African Americans in Los Angeles, who were not informed that the vaccine was experimental because it was "overlooked" [109].

According to VAERS, between 2000 and 2018, 190 people died, and more than 950 became permanently disabled after being vaccinated with MMR or MMRV. During this time, four people died from measles. In 2015 the first case of measles death in the previous 12 years happened. It was a woman with chemotherapy-induced immune deficiency [110]. Prior to that, there were two deaths in the early 2000s: an immunocompromised child and a 75-year-old man [111]. **On the other hand, influenza reportedly causes thousands of deaths per year in the United States, but somehow almost no one is afraid of influenza, whereas measles causes full-blown horror.**

Measles Inclusion-Body Encephalitis And Subacute Sclerosis Panencephalitis

A healthy 12-month-old child was vaccinated with MMR, and within 8.5 months, he developed measles inclusion-body encephalitis (MIBE). A brain biopsy revealed that it was caused by a vaccine strain of measles. The child died after 1.5 months. A few more cases have been reported, but those usually occurred in immunocompromised people rather than in healthy ones [112]. It has been suggested that MIBE is fundamentally similar to Subacute Sclerosis Panencephalitis (SSPE—a rare measles complication that occurs several years after the disease), but the clinical symptoms appear earlier and progress more rapidly.

A Turkish study reported that out of nine cases of SSPE, three patients were vaccinated and two were not. The remaining patients' vaccination status was unknown [113]. According to another study, the proportion of vaccinated patients among SSPE cases is increasing, and it manifests faster in those vaccinated than in those previously exposed to measles [114]. Out of the 20 SSPE cases, in Bangladesh 70% were vaccinated, in England 45% were vaccinated, and in Pakistan 86% of patients were vaccinated. Several studies have found that panencephalitis mainly occurs in people with low income [115].

Measles-Induced Encephalitis

The authors of a 1997 Finnish study report that despite a decrease in cases of measles-induced encephalitis after the beginning of vaccination, the total number of encephalitis cases has not changed because the measles virus was replaced by other viruses [116].

Another study reports that the incidence of severe encephalitis cases in Finland has actually increased after the introduction of MMR [117]. In Vietnam, out of 15 cases of measles-induced encephalitis, 11 patients were vaccinated, two patients were not, and the status of the remaining two was unknown [118].

The CDC claims that the fatality rate of measles-induced encephalitis is 15%. However, before the introduction of the vaccine, this fatality rate was much lower. In 1961 there were 42 reported cases of measles-induced encephalitis with no fatalities. The risk of measles-induced encephalitis increases with age [119]. Essentially, the vaccine significantly increases the risk of measles-induced encephalitis by postponing the disease into adulthood.

A 2017 British study reported that although the number of cases of measles-induced and mumps-induced encephalitis decreased by 97–98% between 1979 and 2011, the overall incidence of encephalitis increased, mainly among infants [120].

The authors of a 1998 study published in *Pediatrics* journal described 48 children with encephalopathy after MMR. They conclude that a causal relationship between measles vaccine and encephalopathy may exist as a rare complication of measles immunization [121].

Statistics

Between the 1920s and 1960s, before vaccination against measles was introduced, measles mortality decreased by 99% even though the number of cases remained unchanged [4].

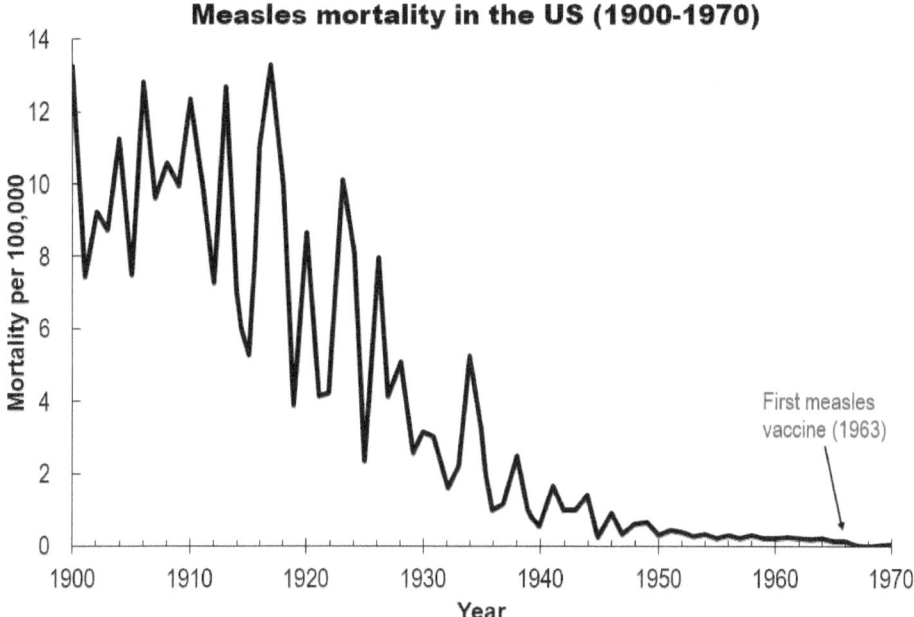

Measles mortality in the US (1900-1970)

During the American Civil War and World War I, measles was a significant cause of death among soldiers (0.2/100 person-years, fatality rate of 6%). On the other hand, during World War II, measles mortality was extremely low (0.0005/100 person-years, fatality less than 0.1%). The authors note that "The declines in measles-related mortality rates in military populations reflected the experiences in civilian populations; the declines preceded the availability of measles vaccine and antibiotics and were not attributable to any specific medical interventions" [122].

In the 1960s, measles mortality was one in 10,000 cases, or three per million people overall. Most of the measles-related deaths were among children with insufficient weight [123]. The same was revealed in a later study—children with low weight suffer from severe measles six times more often [124].

Conclusions

Measles is dangerous in cases of malnutrition and vitamin A deficiency.

Measles in childhood protects against cancer, neurological, cardiovascular, and atopic diseases in adulthood.

Measles vaccine is quite effective, but in the case of measles, it is more of a disadvantage. **Measles is a useful disease. It is preferable to contract it in childhood rather than not to have it at all, or to get sick when the vaccination no longer offers protection and measles is more dangerous: in adulthood or during pregnancy.**

Endnotes

1. Scared of Ebola? This measles outbreak is far more dangerous. *healthcareglobal.com.* 2015 Jan 30

2. Measles. Reports from general practitioners. *BMJ.* 1959;1(5118):380–3

3. Measles epidemic. *BMJ.* 1959;1(5118):351–4

4. Langmuir AD et al. The importance of measles as a health problem. *Am J Public Health Nations Health.* 1962;52(Suppl 2):1-4

5. Sencer DJ et al. Epidemiologic basis for eradication of measles in 1967. *Public Health Rep.* 1967;82(3):253-6

6. Cherry JD. The 'new' epidemiology of measles and rubella. *Hosp Pract.* 1980;15(7):49-57

7. Papania M et al. Increased susceptibility to measles in infants in the United States. *Pediatrics.* 1999;104(5):e59

8. Measles. CDC Pink Book

9. www.cdc.gov/measles/about/history.html

10. Belkin L. Measles, Not Yet a Thing of the Past, Reveals the Limits of an Old Vaccine. *NY Times.* 1989 Feb 26

11. Measles outbreak among vaccinated high school students—Illinois. *MMWR.* 1984; 33(24):349-51

12. Poland GA et al. Failure to reach the goal of measles elimination. Apparent paradox of measles infections in immunized persons. *Arch Intern Med.* 1994;154(16):1815-20

13. Biellik R et al. Strategies for minimizing nosocomial measles transmission. *Bull World Health Organ.* 1997;75(4):367–75

14. Fulginiti VA et al. Altered reactivity to measles virus. Atypical measles in children previously immunized with inactivated measles virus vaccines. *JAMA.* 1967;202(12):1075-80

15. Kimura M et al. Adverse events associated with MMR vaccines in Japan. *Acta Paediatr Jpn.* 1996;38(3):205-11

16. FDA briefing document. VRBPAC meeting Sep 19, 2012: Cell lines derived from human tumors for vaccine manufacture.

17. Khan A. Investigating viruses in cells used to make vaccines; and evaluating the potential threat posed by transmission of viruses to humans

18. Victoria JG et al. Viral nucleic acids in live-attenuated vaccines: detection of minority variants and an adventitious virus. *J Virol.* 2010;84(12):6033-40

19. Demicheli V et al. Vaccines for measles, mumps and rubella in children. *Cochrane Database Syst Rev.* 2012(2):CD004407

20. Nkowane BM et al. Measles outbreak in a vaccinated school population: epidemiology, chains of transmission and the role of vaccine failures. *Am J Public Health.* 1987; 77(4):434-8

21. Rosen JB et al. Outbreak of measles among persons with prior evidence of immunity, New York City, 2011. *Clin Infect Dis.* 2014;58(9):1205-10

22. Wang Z et al. Difficulties in eliminating measles and controlling rubella and mumps: a cross-sectional study of a first measles and rubella vaccination and a second measles, mumps, and rubella vaccination. *PloS One.* 2014;9(2):e89361

23. Shi J et al. Measles incidence rate and a phylogenetic study of contemporary genotype H1 measles strains in China: is an improved measles vaccine needed? *Virus Genes.* 2011; 43(3):319-26

24. Kang HJ et al. An increasing, potentially measles-susceptible population over time after vaccination in Korea. *Vaccine.* 2017;35(33):4126-32

25. Kontio M et al. Waning antibody levels and avidity: implications for MMR vaccine-induced protection. *J Infect Dis.* 2012;206(10):1542-8

26. Gonçalves G et al. Persistence of measles antibodies, following changes in the recommended age for the second dose of MMR-vaccine in Portugal. *Vaccine.* 2015; 33(39):5057-63

27. LeBaron CW et al. Persistence of measles antibodies after 2 doses of measles vaccine in a postelimination environment. *Arch Pediatr Adolesc Med.* 2007;161(3):294-301

28. Itoh M et al. Comparative analysis of titers of antibody against measles virus in sera of vaccinated and naturally infected Japanese individuals of different age groups. *J Clin Microbiol.* 2002;40(5):1733-8

29. Levy DL. The future of measles in highly immunized populations. A modeling approach. *Am J Epidemiol.* 1984;120(1):39-48

30. Heffernan JM et al. Implications of vaccination and waning immunity. *Proc Biol Sci.* 2009;276(1664):2071-80

31. Modrof J et al. Measles Virus Neutralizing Antibodies in Intravenous Immunoglobulins: Is an Increase by Revaccination of Plasma Donors Possible? *J Infect Dis.* 2017;216(8):977-80

32. Burnet FM. Measles as an index of immunological function. *Lancet.* 1968;2(7568):610-3

33. Silfverdal SA et al. Breast-feeding and a subsequent diagnosis of measles. *Acta Paediatr.* 2009;98(4):715-19

34. Stimson P. The Measles Rubella Confusion Continues. *JAMA.* 1965;193(5):403

35. Roy F et al. Rapid Identification of Measles Virus Vaccine Genotype by Real-Time PCR. *J Clin Microbiol.* 2017;55(3):735-43

36. Gendrel D et al. Underestimation of the incidence of measles in a population of French children. *Eur J Clin Microbiol Infect Dis.* 1992;11(12):1156-7

37. Gustafson T et al. Measles outbreak in a fully immunized secondary-school population. *N Engl J Med.* 1987;316(13):771-4

38. Green HN et al. Diet as a prophylactic agent against puerperal sepsis. *BMJ.* 1931;2(3691):595-8

39. Green HN et al. Vitamin A as an anti-infective agent. *BMJ.* 1928;2(3537):691-6

40. Ellison JB. Intensive vitamin therapy in measles. *BMJ.* 1932;2(3745):708-11

41. Sommer A et al. Increased mortality in children with mild vitamin A deficiency. *Lancet.* 1983;2(8350):585-8

42. Sommer A et al. Impact of vitamin A supplementation on childhood mortality. A randomised controlled community trial. *Lancet.* 1986;1(8491):1169-73

43. Scrimshaw N. Interactions of nutrition and infection; WHO. 1968

44. Barclay AJ et al. Vitamin A supplements and mortality related to measles: a randomised clinical trial. *BMJ.* 1987;294(6567):294-6

45. Hussey GD et al. A randomized, controlled trial of vitamin A in children with severe measles. *N Engl J Med.* 1990;323(3):160-4

46. Arrieta AC et al. Vitamin A levels in children with measles in Long Beach, California. *J Pediatr.* 1992;121(1):75-8

47. Frieden TR et al. Vitamin A levels and severity of measles. New York City. *Am J Dis Child.* 1992;146(2):182-6

48. Butler JC et al. Measles severity and serum retinol (vitamin A) concentration among children in the United States. *Pediatrics.* 1993;91(6):1176-81

49. Huiming Y et al. Vitamin A for treating measles in children. *Cochrane Database Syst Rev.* 2005(4):CD001479

50. Fawzi WW et al. Vitamin A supplementation and child mortality. A meta-analysis. *JAMA.* 1993;269(7):898-903

51. Imdad A et al. Vitamin A supplementation for preventing morbidity and mortality in children from six months to five years of age. *Cochrane Database Syst Rev.* 2017(12):CD008524

52. Yalçin SS et al. The effect of live measles vaccines on serum vitamin A levels in healthy children. *Acta Paediatr Jpn.* 1998;40(4):345-9

53. Yalçin SS et al. Sex-specific differences in serum vitamin A values after measles immunization. *Pediatr Infect Dis J.* 1999;18(8):747-8

54. Montella M et al. Do childhood diseases affect NHL and HL risk? A case-control study from northern and southern Italy. *Leuk Res.* 2006;30(8):917-22

55. Alexander FE et al. Risk factors for Hodgkin's disease by Epstein-Barr virus (EBV) status: prior infection by EBV and other agents. *Br J Cancer.* 2000;82(5):1117-21

56. Glaser SL et al. Exposure to childhood infections and risk of Epstein-Barr virus—defined Hodgkin's lymphoma in women. *Int J Cancer.* 2005;115(4):599-605

57. Becker N et al. Self-reported history of infections and the risk of non-Hodgkin lymphoma: an InterLymph pooled analysis. *Int J Cancer.* 2012;131(10):2342-8

58. Albonico HU et al. Febrile infectious childhood diseases in the history of cancer patients and matched controls. *Med Hypotheses.* 1998;51(4):315-20

59. Kölmel KF et al. Febrile infections and malignant melanoma: results of a case-control study. *Melanoma Res.* 1992;2(3):207-11

60. Kölmel KF et al. Infections and melanoma risk: results of a multicentre EORTC case-control study. European Organization for Research and Treatment of Cancer. *Melanoma Res.* 1999;9(5):511-9

61. Parodi S et al. Childhood infectious diseases and risk of leukaemia in an adult population. *Int J Cancer.* 2013;133(8):1892-9

62. van Steensel-Moll HA et al. Childhood leukemia and infectious diseases in the first year of life: a register-based case-control study. *Am J Epidemiol.* 1986;124(4):590-4

63. Ribeiro KB et al. Socioeconomic status and childhood acute lymphocytic leukemia incidence in São Paulo, Brazil. *Int J Cancer.* 2008;123(8):1907-12

64. Ariad S et al. A sharp rise in the incidence of Hodgkin's lymphoma in young adults in Israel. *Isr Med Assoc J.* 2009;11(8):453-5

65. Benharroch D et al. Does the measles virus contribute to carcinogenesis? - a review. *J Cancer.* 2014;5(2):98-102

66. Newhouse ML et al. A case control study of carcinoma of the ovary. *Br J Prev Soc Med.* 1977;31(3):148-53

67. Zygiert Z. Hodgkin's disease: remissions after measles. *Lancet.* 1971;1(7699):593

68. Mota HC. Infantile Hodgkin's disease: remission after measles. *BMJ.* 1973;2(5863):421

69. Taqi AM et al. Regression of Hodgkin's disease after measles. *Lancet.* 1981;1(8229):1112

70. Bluming AZ et al. Regression of Burkitt's lymphoma in association with measles infection. *Lancet.* 1971;2(7715):105-6

71. Pasquinucci G. Possible effect of measles on leukaemia. Lancet. 1971;1(7690):136

72. Russell SJ et al. Remission of disseminated cancer after systemic oncolytic virotherapy. *Mayo Clin Proc.* 2014;89(7):926-33

73. Russell SJ et al. Measles virus for cancer therapy. *Curr Top Microbiol Immunol.* 2009; 330:213-41

74. Heinzerling L et al. Oncolytic measles virus in cutaneous T-cell lymphomas mounts antitumor immune responses in vivo and targets interferon-resistant tumor cells. *Blood.* 2005;106(7):2287-94

75. Galanis E et al. Phase I trial of intraperitoneal administration of an oncolytic measles virus strain engineered to express carcinoembryonic antigen for recurrent ovarian cancer. *Cancer Res.* 2010;70(3):875-82

76. Galanis E et al. Oncolytic measles virus expressing the sodium iodide symporter to treat drug-resistant ovarian cancer. *Cancer Res.* 2015;75(1):22-30

77. Sasco AJ et al. Measles infection and Parkinson's disease. *Am J Epidemiol.* 1985; 122(6):1017-31

78. Kessler I. Epidemiologic studies of Parkinson's disease. III. A community-based survey. *Am J Epidemiol.* 1972;96(4):242-54

79. Alves RS et al. Postvaccinal parkinsonism. *Mov Disord.* 1992;7(2):178-80

80. Kubota Y et al. Association of measles and mumps with cardiovascular disease: the Japan Collaborative Cohort (JACC) study. *Atherosclerosis.* 2015;241(2):682-6

81. Pesonen E et al. Dual role of infections as risk factors for coronary heart disease. *Atherosclerosis.* 2007;192(2):370-5

82. Sullivan CB et al. Multiple sclerosis and age at exposure to childhood diseases and animals: cases and their friends. *Neurology.* 1984;34(9):1144-8

83. Alter M et al. Multiple sclerosis and childhood infections. *Neurology.* 1986;36(10):1386-9

84. Alter M et al. Does delay in acquiring childhood infection increase risk of multiple sclerosis? *Ital J Neurol Sci.* 1987;Suppl 6:11-6

85. Blumberg RW et al. Effect of measles on the nephrotic syndrome. *Am J Dis Child.* 1947; 73(2):151-66

To Vaccinate or not to Vaccinate: A Review of Scientific Literature on Vaccines

86. Gairdner D. A notable case of nephrosis. *Arch Dis Child.* 1978;53(5):363-5

87. Rønne T. Measles virus infection without rash in childhood is related to disease in adult life. *Lancet.* 1985;1(8419):1-5

88. Aaby P et al. Low mortality after mild measles infection compared to uninfected children in rural West Africa. *Vaccine.* 2002;21(1-2):120-6

89. Aaby P et al. No persistent T lymphocyte immunosuppression or increased mortality after measles infection: a community study from Guinea-Bissau. *Pediatr Infect Dis J.* 1996;15(1):39-44

90. Aaby P et al. No long-term excess mortality after measles infection: a community study from Senegal. *Am J Epidemiol.* 1996;143(10):1035-41

91. Shaheen SO et al. Measles and atopy in Guinea-Bissau. *Lancet.* 1996;347(9018):1792-6

92. Bodner C et al. Childhood exposure to infection and risk of adult onset wheeze and atopy. *Thorax.* 2000;55(5):383-7

93. Rosenlund H et al. Allergic disease and atopic sensitization in children in relation to measles vaccination and measles infection. *Pediatrics.* 2009;123(3):771-8

94. Kucukosmanoglu E et al. Frequency of allergic diseases following measles. *Allergol Immunopathol.* 2006;34(4):146-9

95. Flöistrup H et al. Allergic disease and sensitization in Steiner school children. *J Allergy Clin Immunol.* 2006;117(1):59-66

96. Alm JS et al. Atopy in children of families with an anthroposophic lifestyle. *Lancet.* 1999;353(9163):1485-8

97. Spencer PS et al. Nodding syndrome in Mundri county, South Sudan: environmental, nutritional and infectious factors. *Afr Health Sci.* 2013;13(2):183-204

98. Nakayama T et al. Long-term regulation of interferon production by lymphocytes from children inoculated with live measles virus vaccine. *J Infect Dis.* 1988;158(6):1386-90

99. Toraldo R et al. Effect of measles-mumps-rubella vaccination on polymorphonuclear neutrophil functions in children. *Acta Paediatr.* 1992;81(11):887-90

100. Munyer TP et al. Depressed lymphocyte function after measles-mumps-rubella vaccination. *J Infect Dis.* 1975;132(1):75-8

101. Zorzon M et al. Risk factors of multiple sclerosis: a case-control study. *Neurol Sci.* 2003;24(4):242-7

102. Miller H et al. Multiple sclerosis and vaccination. *BMJ.* 1967;2(5546):210-3

103. Ahlgren C et al. A population-based case-control study on viral infections and vaccinations and subsequent multiple sclerosis risk. *Eur J Epidemiol.* 2009;24(9):541-52

104. O'Leary ST et al. The risk of immune thrombocytopenic purpura after vaccination in children and adolescents. *Pediatrics.* 2012;129(2):248-55

105. Miller E et al. Risks of convulsion and aseptic meningitis following measles-mumps-rubella vaccination in the United Kingdom. *Am J Epidemiol.* 2007;165(6):704-9

106. Ward KN et al. Risk of serious neurologic disease after immunization of young children in Britain and Ireland. *Pediatrics.* 2007;120(2):314-21

107. Knudsen KM et al. Child mortality following standard, medium or high titre measles immunization in West Africa. *Int J Epidemiol.* 1996;25(3):665-73

108. Hall AJ et al. Lessons from measles vaccination in developing countries. *BMJ.* 1993; 307(6915):1294-5

109. Cimons M. CDC says it erred in measles study. *LA Times*. 1996 Jun 17

110. Szabo L. Measles kills first patient in 12 years. *USA Today*. 2015 Jul 3

111. Epidemiology of measles—United States, 2001-2003. *MMWR*. 2004;53(31):713-6

112. Bitnun A et al. Measles inclusion-body encephalitis caused by the vaccine strain of measles virus. *Clin Infect Dis*. 1999;29(4):855-61

113. Yilmaz D et al. Subacute sclerosing panencephalitis: is there something different in the younger children? *Brain Dev*. 2006;28(10):649-52

114. Dyken PR et al. Changing character of subacute sclerosing panencephalitis in the United States. *Pediatr Neurol*. 1989;5(6):339-41

115. Saha N et al. Clinical and investigation profile of subacute sclerosing panencephatitis (SSPE): an analysis of twenty cases. *J Dhaka Med Coll*. 2008;17(2):72-7

116. Koskiniemi M et al. Epidemiology of encephalitis in children. A prospective multicentre study. *Eur J Pediatr*. 1997;156(7):541-5

117. Koskiniemi M et al. Effect of measles, mumps, rubella vaccination on pattern of encephalitis in children. *Lancet*. 1989;1(8628):31-4

118. Fox A et al. Acute measles encephalitis in partially vaccinated adults. *PloS One*. 2013; 8(8):e71671

119. Ehrengut W. Measles encephalitis: age disposition and vaccination. *Arch Gesamte Virusforsch*. 1965;16:311-4

120. Iro M et al. 30-year trends in admission rates for encephalitis in children in England and effect of improved diagnostics and measles-mumps-rubella vaccination: a population-based observational study. *Lancet Infect Dis*. 2017;17(4):422-430

121. Weibel RE et al. Acute encephalopathy followed by permanent brain injury or death associated with further attenuated measles vaccines: a review of claims submitted to the National Vaccine Injury Compensation Program. *Pediatrics*. 1998;101(3 Pt 1):383-7

122. Shanks GD et al. Measles epidemics of variable lethality in the early 20th century. *Am J Epidemiol*. 2014;179(4):413-22

123. Barkin RM. Measles mortality: a retrospective look at the vaccine era. *Am J Epidemiol*. 1975;102(4):341-9

124. Capisonda R et al. Risk factors predictive of severe measles among patients admitted at MCU-hospital from 1988-1992. *Phil J Microbiol Infect Dis*. 1993;22:75-80

Chapter Thirteen

MUMPS

*Of all tyrannies, a tyranny sincerely exercised
for the good of its victims may be the most oppressive.*

— **C.S. Lewis**

M umps in children is usually such a mild disease that even the WHO does not scare anyone with it. In adults, however, they say that mumps can cause serious complications; hence, it is important to vaccinate infants [1].

According to the CDC, before the introduction of the mumps vaccine, 15% to 27% of infections were asymptomatic. It is difficult to estimate the number of asymptomatic infections in the post-vaccine era because it is unclear how vaccine modifies clinical presentation. Orchitis (testicular inflammation) is the most common complication of mumps, but it is only possible in post-pubertal males. Mumps orchitis is usually unilateral.

Sterility caused by mumps orchitis is quite rare, even in cases of bilateral orchitis.

Prior to the introduction of the vaccine, cases of mumps were not recorded. Monovalent mumps vaccine is virtually non-existent today, except for Japan, where MMR is still banned. Mumps vaccine in Japan is not sponsored by the state, and very few people are vaccinated against it [2].

A Bit Of History

A *BMJ* article published in 1967 states that mumps is a relatively benign disease in children, but it is a considerable nuisance since children have to miss school. Serious mumps complications are rare. The antibody levels after the mumps vaccine were considerably lower than after natural mumps. The authors conclude that despite the fact that recently released mumps vaccine looks promising, there is no obvious need for mass vaccination in the UK [3].

Thirteen years later, in 1980, *The British Medical Journal* wonders again whether the UK needs yet another vaccine for infants. Mumps is not notifiable, thus its incidence is unknown, especially since up to 40% of mumps cases are asymptomatic. Perhaps, authors ponder, a combination vaccine with measles might be the answer. This vaccine could be offered before school to those with no history of infection. Would the half of parents who currently accept measles vaccine also accept the combination vaccine? Only if the ill-founded but commonly held dread of sterility from mumps orchitis overcomes the British distrust of new vaccines. Otherwise, the acceptance rate would almost certainly be low. However, even low vaccination coverage can lead to an increase in the number of adults susceptible to mumps. It is already happening in the US. The authors conclude that "For the seronegative individual the vaccine might be a boon. For the general population it might be the reverse, since the pattern of natural infection resulting in a current 95% of immune adults would be altered. The disease, though painful, is rarely dangerous at present. To attempt its prevention on a mass scale might well increase its incidence in adults with all the troubles and risks which that implies" [4].

A 1974 article analyzes about 2,500 cases of mumps hospitalizations in 1958–1969 in 16 hospitals in England. They accounted for the majority of mumps cases in the country that required hospitalization. Half of the patients were 15 years old or older. Complications were recorded in 42% of all cases. Three patients died, but two of them had another serious underlying illness unrelated to mumps, and the third patient was probably misdiagnosed and did not even have mumps. The only complication, which may have been permanent, was deafness in five patients (four of them were adults). Meningitis in mumps is so frequent that some believe it should not even be regarded as a complication, but rather as an integral part of the disease. In any case, there is a consensus that mumps meningitis is benign and rarely has any consequences, which is confirmed by this study. Orchitis is what is usually feared the most. There is a general dread of sterility from orchitis, but its probability is overestimated. Even though it is impossible to exclude, a small retrospective study did not detect sterility as a consequence of orchitis. The authors conclude that there is little need for general vaccination against mumps. It might make sense to vaccinate postpubertal adolescents on admission to boarding schools or the military. Even then, however, it should be remembered that 90% of boys have already been infected with mumps by the age of 14. Consequently, the level of antibodies should be checked first, and only those who do not have the antibodies should be vaccinated [5].

If mumps can cause deafness in rare cases, maybe it does make sense to get vaccinated against it? The vaccine, however, can also cause deafness. A 1993 article describes nine cases of deafness after the MMR vaccine in four years following the vaccine introduction. The authors conclude that in three cases, deafness was unrelated to the vaccine (but they do not provide an explanation for this conclusion), and in six other cases, it may or may not have been related to the vaccine. Since unilateral deafness is hard to diagnose in children, and they are vaccinated at the age of 12 months, there may have been other cases that were missed. A 2008 article describes another 44 cases of deafness after MMR [6].

A 1957 article reports on 119 cases of meningoencephalitis caused by mumps in San Francisco in 12 years (1943-1955). Most cases were benign, without complications and without neurological consequences, lasted less than five days, and seldom required hospitalization. Death due to mumps meningoencephalitis is an extremely rare event, and in the entire medical literature, only three such cases have been described [7].

Effectiveness

Twenty years after the vaccine was developed and ten years after it became widely used, the first mumps outbreak occurred in the workplace (Chicago Futures Exchange). Total costs associated with the outbreak amounted to $120,000, whereas the vaccine costs only $4.47. The authors report that historically, mumps prevention has received less attention than other vaccine-preventable diseases because the illness was perceived as mild. However, $1,500 per case of mumps is too expensive. In the pre-vaccine era, mumps outbreaks were observed mainly in prisons, orphanages, and military barracks [8].

In the outbreak of mumps in London in the late 90s, 51% of cases were vaccinated. The effectiveness of one dose of the vaccine was 64% and of two doses, 88%. This effectiveness is much lower than it is stated in clinical trials since immunogenicity (i.e., the number of antibodies) is not an accurate biological marker of the vaccine's effectiveness [9]. In 2010, two weeks after the MMR vaccination of nursing students in Thailand, an outbreak of mumps occurred. The vaccine strain of the virus (Leningrad-Zagreb) was detected in those infected. This strain has repeatedly caused mumps outbreaks before [10]. **There are many more descriptions of outbreaks in schools and universities where almost all students have been vaccinated.**

In 2013, 15 mumps outbreaks were registered in France. Seventy-two percent of the cases had been vaccinated twice. Vaccine effectiveness was 49% for one dose and 55% for two doses. Among those who had been vaccinated once, the odds of mumps increased by 7% for every additional year since their last MMR dose. Among those who had been vaccinated twice, the odds of mumps increased by 10% for every additional year. Orchitis was observed in five men. One of them was unvaccinated, two were vaccinated with one dose, and another two were vaccinated with two doses. The authors note that in many other countries, mumps outbreaks are also observed among highly vaccinated young adults. The reason for this is waning vaccine-conferred immunity in the absence of natural boosters. The authors write that waning mumps vaccination-conferred immunity and the occurrence of outbreaks in highly vaccinated populations suggest the need for a third MMR dose. This kind of experiment was conducted in the US during the outbreaks in 2009 and 2010. Both times the outbreak subsided a few weeks after the administration of the vaccine. However, outbreaks always subside at some point, so it was unclear whether it had anything to do with the vaccination.

The introduction of a third regular dose into the national vaccination schedule has been considered in the Netherlands, but this idea was abandoned because mumps-associated morbidity was relatively low, and vaccine uptake of a third dose was unlikely to be satisfactory. This study and mumps outbreaks among the vaccinated led the French Public Health Council to recommend a third dose of MMR in outbreak settings. Even though it is unknown whether the vaccine is effective for those already infected with the virus, it is quite possible that the vaccine will shorten the virus shedding period. The Dutch study determined that two-thirds of cases during the outbreaks are asymptomatic. The role of asymptomatic patients in the transmission of the disease remains unknown [11].

In 2010 there was a mumps outbreak in Israel (over 5,000 cases). Seventy-eight percent had been fully vaccinated. Mostly adolescents and young adults had been affected.

> In other countries, mumps outbreaks are also observed among adolescents and college students, whereas in the countries where there is no vaccination against mumps, children aged five to nine are the ones most susceptible to mumps.

Despite the high vaccination coverage (90–97%), mumps antibodies were found in only 68% of the population. The authors report that recent mumps outbreaks have been caused by the genotype G virus, whereas the vaccine contains genotype A. However, they do not believe that genotype mismatch is a major factor in these outbreaks and suggest introducing a third dose of MMR [12].

A 2018 Dutch study reported that upon mumps infection, persistent polyfunctional memory T-cells are produced, but they are not produced upon vaccination. The authors speculate that this could explain why the vaccine gives temporary immunity only [13].

A 2018 Czech study found that among the 18–29 age group, only 19% of those vaccinated against mumps had antibodies. Among the unvaccinated of the same age group, 48% had antibodies. Among the unvaccinated in the 40 years and over age group, 63% had mumps immunity. The authors conclude that despite vaccination coverage of 98%, mumps outbreaks in the Czech Republic did not stop, but rather the incidence of mumps has shifted to adolescents and young adults [14].

In 2010, two virologists, who had previously worked for Merck, sued the company. They claimed that Merck manipulated the results of the mumps vaccine clinical trial, which allowed the company to remain the exclusive MMR manufacturer in the United States [15]. The lawsuit states that Merck organized a fictitious vaccine-testing program in the late 90s. The company obliged the scientists to participate in the program, promising them generous bonuses if the vaccine gets certified, and threatening with prison if they were to report this fraud to the FDA.

The effectiveness of the mumps vaccine is determined in the following way. A blood sample is taken from children before and after vaccination. After that, a virus is added to the blood, and as the cells get infected, the plaques are formed. The number of these plaques in the blood before and after vaccination determines the effectiveness of the vaccine. Instead of testing how well the wild strain of the virus is neutralized, Merck was testing the vaccine strain. However, this was still not enough to demonstrate the required 95% seroconversion. To overcome that, rabbit antibodies were added to the children's blood, bringing the seroconversion level to 100%. And it was not even everything that was done. Since adding animal antibodies showed pre-vaccine seroconversion of 80% (instead of 10%), the fraud was evident, and pre-vaccine samples had to be re-taken. They then tried to change the number of rabbit antibodies added, but it did not give the desired results. They then simply began to falsify the plaque counting and counted plaques that were actually not in the blood. Falsified data was entered into an Excel spreadsheet since changing paper forms proved too time-consuming, plus this tactic left no paper trail. Despite that, the virologists still contacted the FDA, and the FDA sent an agent to conduct a check. She asked questions for half an hour, got false answers, did not ask the virologists themselves any questions, did not check the lab, and wrote a one-page report, pointing out some minor issues with the process, but never mentioned neither the rabbit antibodies nor the falsified data. As a result, Merck has received the MMR and MMRV certification and is the sole licensed manufacturer of these vaccines in the United States. When the court asked Merck to provide evidence of the vaccine effectiveness, they provided data from 50 years ago. As of 2020, the case is still ongoing.

Because of the 2006 and 2009 outbreaks, the CDC has pushed back its target date for eradicating mumps from its original 2010 goal to no earlier than 2020 [16].

Safety

All MMR safety studies described in the section about measles are applicable to mumps as well. Here are some more.

In 1997, after the mass MMR vaccination campaign in Brazil with the Japanese strain of mumps (Urabe), an outbreak of aseptic meningitis began. The risk of the disease was increased by 14–30 times. The fact that Urabe strain is associated with aseptic meningitis was already known, but

Brazilian authorities decided to use this strain anyway, as it is cheaper and more effective than the Jeryl Lynn strain (which is used in the US), and because they thought the risk of meningitis was quite low.

In France, vaccination with the same strain did not cause a meningitis outbreak. The authors attribute this phenomenon to the fact that the outbreaks in Brazil were observed mainly in large cities, where people live close to hospitals. Moreover, a large number of children had been vaccinated in a very short time. These factors made it possible to identify the outbreak. The authors worry that reporting of adverse events could lead to a reduction in vaccination uptake. They state that public belief in the benefits of mass immunization campaigns is, perhaps, no longer enough by itself to prevent the increasing number of refusals of immunization and that it would be nice to also record adverse effects of the vaccination [17].

Urabe strain had been used in Great Britain from 1988 until 1992, when manufacturers declared that they were stopping its production. According to published documents, in 1987, authorities already knew about the dangers of this strain [18].

The following year, learning from their mistakes, the Brazilian authorities bought MMR with another strain of mumps (Leningrad-Zagreb) and vaccinated 845,000 children with it. Another outbreak of aseptic meningitis started, and this time the risk of disease increased 74-fold. It was, of course, known that this strain also increases the risk of meningitis, but since the vaccination campaign in the Bahamas did not cause a meningitis outbreak, they decided to see how it would turn out in Brazil. Moreover, a mumps outbreak also began. One out of every 300 doses of the vaccine resulted in mumps. The authors are wondering whether all the vaccination campaign funds should be used on vaccines, or maybe some of it should be allocated to surveil the adverse events? They write that this issue is controversial in the medical literature. Defenders of vaccination priority believe that the benefits of immunization campaigns are unquestionable and that there is no need to spend money on nonsense such as adverse effect surveillance. Defenders of improvements in surveillance argue that a lack of information scares people and leads to a lack of trust in vaccines [19]. The Leningrad-Zagreb strain was developed in Serbia based on the Leningrad-3 strain, which also caused meningitis, but is still used in Russia [20].

A 2016 Italian study found that in those vaccinated with MMR, the risk of Henoch-Schönlein purpura (hemorrhagic vasculitis) increased by 3.4

times. In children, this disease usually goes into complete remission in a few weeks, but less than 1% develop kidney failure [21]. Orchitis may well occur not only from mumps but also as a result of mumps vaccine [22].

A 2017 article reports a case of a 14-month-old boy who was given an MMR vaccine and then diagnosed with a severe combined immunodeficiency four months later. He then successfully underwent a bone marrow transplant, but developed chronic encephalitis and died at the age of five. A brain biopsy showed that he had the vaccine strain of mumps virus in his brain. This was the first case of panencephalitis caused by the mumps virus [23]. Since the mumps vaccine is a live one, mumps-vaccinated individuals might transmit the virus to close contacts [24].

The Benefits Of Mumps

Several studies, according to which childhood mumps is associated with a reduced risk of cancer, neurological, and cardiovascular diseases, among other things, were cited in the previous chapter. Here we will focus more on the link between mumps and ovarian cancer.

An article published in 1966 reported that unlike other types of cancer, the risk of which increases with age, the risk of ovarian cancer increases before the age of 70, and then declines. The author analyzed the relationship between ovarian cancer and 50 different factors and found that the only statistically significant factor associated with ovarian cancer was not having mumps in childhood (p=0.007). In fact, not having rubella as a child was also associated with ovarian cancer, but in this case, the p-value was equal to 0.02. Back then, scientists had slightly more self-respect, and p>0.01 was not considered statistically significant (today p<0.05 is considered a statistically significant result). It was also found that the risk of ovarian cancer in never-married women was significantly higher [25].

A 1979 article reported that clinical mumps in childhood is associated with a reduced risk of ovarian cancer. Moreover, it turned out that patients with ovarian cancer had fewer mumps antibodies. The authors believe that what influences the risk of ovarian cancer is not the actual mumps infection, but rather the subclinical course of the disease. In cases of the subclinical disease (without symptoms, like after vaccination), fewer antibodies are produced, which is what subsequently protects against cancer [26].

In addition to these two, seven more studies have been published on the association of mumps with the reduced risk of ovarian cancer. Nonetheless, the biological mechanism of this phenomenon has not been studied, and with the introduction of mumps vaccination, the association between mumps and ovarian cancer was rendered seemingly irrelevant and largely forgotten. All but two of the studies found the protective effect of mumps against ovarian cancer. The first of the two studies, which did not find the link, did not even find the known inverse correlation between pregnancies and ovarian cancer. The second study was conducted in 2008 and included many more vaccinated subjects than the previous studies, which makes it less relevant.

MUC1 is a membrane protein, which is associated with cancerous tumors. The authors of a Harvard University study found that women who have had a history of mumps parotitis had much more antibodies to this protein than those who did not have mumps. This biological mechanism is what explains the protective function of mumps. Mumps vaccination creates antibodies against the virus but does not create antibodies against MUC1. To create these antibodies, one needs to actually have mumps. Thus, it is possible to conclude that since symptomatic cases of mumps after the beginning of vaccinations are observed much less frequently, it will lead to an increase in the incidence of ovarian cancer. Indeed, the incidence of ovarian cancer has increased. The authors also conducted a meta-analysis of eight studies and concluded that the history of mumps is associated with a 19% decrease in the risk of ovarian cancer [27].

Ovarian cancer is the fourth biggest cancer killer among American women. It is estimated that 25,000 women are diagnosed each year, and 16,000 of them die from their disease. The authors from Mayo Clinic analyzed three viruses as a treatment for ovarian cancer in vitro and on mice: a recombinant measles virus and vaccine strains of mumps and measles. All three viruses successfully killed cancer cells. The authors note that since most people in Western countries are vaccinated against measles and mumps, the immune system can interfere with this type of therapy [28].

In a 1974 study, 90 patients with terminal cancer of various types received the mumps virus treatment (wild or almost wild strain). The virus was administered topically, intravenously, orally, rectally, by inhalation, or by local injection. Since the virus solution could not be obtained in a sufficient amount, most of the patients were given only a small quantity of it. Thirty-seven patients demonstrated very good results (the tumor disappeared completely or shrank by more than 50%), 42 patients had good results (the tumor shrank or stopped growing). Just a few days after the initiation of treatment, the patients experienced less pain and improved appetite, and within two weeks, the tumor disappeared completely in many patients. Adverse effects were minimal. Nineteen patients were cured completely [29].

In a 1978 study, 200 cancer patients received intravenous injections of mumps virus (Urabe strain). The only adverse clinical reaction was transient mild fever in about half of the patients. In 26 patients, tumor regression was observed. In most of the patients, the pain was alleviated. In 30 out of 35 patients, the bleeding decreased or stopped. In 30 out of 41 patients, ascites and swelling decreased or disappeared [30].

The two aforementioned studies were conducted in Japan, and the results were of no interest to anyone outside of the country. Then, in 2016, Mayo Clinic decided to take samples of this virus from Japan and test them in vitro and on mice. It turned out that the virus indeed has an anti-cancer effect [31].

Fetal Bovine Serum

One of the components of MMR and some other vaccines is fetal bovine serum. Cells, in which the virus is grown, need to multiply. In order to do so, they need a nutrient medium with hormones, growth factors, proteins, amino acids, vitamins, etc. Fetal bovine serum is commonly used as this medium. Since the serum should preferably be sterile, the blood of calves' fetuses is used instead of the grown cow's blood.

A 2002 article describes the process of fetal bovine serum manufacturing. A pregnant cow is slaughtered, and the uterus is removed. Then the calf is removed from the uterus, the umbilical cord is tied off, and the fetus is cleaned and disinfected. After that, the heart is punctured with a needle, and the blood is pumped out. Sometimes a vacuum pump is used for this, sometimes a massage. During the next step of the process, blood clots, platelets, and coagulation factors are separated from the blood by centrifugation. Fetal bovine serum is what remains as a result.

Apart from the necessary components, the serum can be contaminated with viruses, bacteria, mycoplasmas, yeast, fungi, immunoglobulins, endotoxins, and possibly prions. Many substances present in fetal bovine serum have not yet been identified. The function of many of the identified substances is unclear.

A bovine fetus of three months yields about 150 ml of raw fetal bovine serum, of six months 350 ml, and of nine months (near-term) 550 ml. At the beginning of the 2000s, the global production per year of raw fetal bovine serum was estimated to be around 500,000 liters, which requires approximately two million pregnant cows. Currently, the global serum market is at 700,000 liters.

The authors then go on to analyze the literature on the subject of whether the fetus suffers when its heart is punctured, and its blood is pumped out. Since the fetus experiences anoxia (an acute oxygen deficiency) when separated from the placenta, that perhaps prevents the pain signals from reaching the brain, and the fetus might not suffer. However, it turns out that unlike adult rabbits that die of anoxia within 1.5 minutes, preterm rabbits can survive without oxygen for 44 minutes. This happens because fetuses and newborns compensate for oxygen deficiency with anaerobic metabolism. Moreover, the fetal brain requires substantially less oxygen than the adult brain. Other species of animals show similar results, but calves specifically have never been studied.

Science has only recently raised the issue of whether a mammal's fetus or newborn feels pain. Just ten years before this article was published, it was still thought that human babies are less sensitive to pain; as a result, surgery was performed on premature and full-term babies without anesthesia. Today, it is considered that the human fetus can feel pain as early as the 24th week of pregnancy and has the ability to suffer starting from week 11 after conception. Moreover, fetuses and newborns are more sensitive to pain than adults since they have not yet developed a mechanism for suppressing physiological pain. Therefore, a fetus can feel pain even upon being touched. The authors conclude that the fetal calf can be expected to have normal brain function at the time of heart puncture, can experience pain and/or suffering at the moment of heart puncture for blood collection and possibly for a period after that, until it actually dies.

The authors then discuss whether it is possible to anesthetize the fetus so that it would not feel pain. Some believe that anoxia itself plays the role of anesthetic, but that is not the case. Mammal fetuses and neonates also

152

have a poor capacity to metabolize a variety of drugs, including anesthetics. It is also undesirable to have drugs in the serum, since it may increase batch-to-batch variations and contaminate the serum itself. Electrical stunning is not suitable either since it causes cardiac arrest. The authors believe that, perhaps, a bolt appropriately hammered into the brain would induce brain death. Some manufacturers claim that they kill the fetus before harvesting blood, but that is not true, since the blood coagulates immediately after death, so the fetus must be alive when it is collected. The authors conclude that the current practice of fetal blood harvest is inhumane [32].

According to a 1999 study, 20–50% of fetal bovine serum is infected with bovine viral diarrhea virus, as well as other viruses [33]. And these are only the viruses that are known to science, which constitute only a small fraction of the viruses that exist in nature [34]. A 2016 Harvard study found that fetal bovine serum contains extracellular RNA, which is impossible to separate from the serum. This RNA interacts with RNA of human cells, in which vaccine viruses are grown [35].

Japanese researchers examined five types of live vaccines and detected bovine viral diarrhea virus RNA in MMR vaccines of two different manufacturers, as well as in two monovalent vaccines against mumps and rubella, which most likely got there from fetal bovine serum. In infants, this virus might cause gastroenteritis, and in pregnant women, it might lead to the birth of children with microcephaly [36].

The fact that fetal bovine serum is infected with the bovine viral diarrhea virus was already known in 1977. It is also known that this virus passes through the placenta and can infect the calf fetus in the uterus. Sixty percent of serum samples in Australia were contaminated with the virus. Eight percent of the vaccines against bovine rhinotracheitis were contaminated as well. The virus was also found in bovine kidney cells, which are used in the production of the measles vaccine [37].

How can fetal bovine serum interact with other vaccine components? When mice were injected with pertussis toxin, none of them died, whereas, when they were injected with pertussis toxin together with bovine serum albumin (a fetal bovine serum component), most of them died from encephalopathy [38].

Conclusions

Mumps is a disease that is better to catch in childhood, rather than in adulthood. Vaccination causes a shift in the incidence towards adulthood, when the risk of complications, such as orchitis, is significantly higher.

Low vaccine effectiveness has been found in numerous studies.

Exposure to mumps in childhood decreases the risk of ovarian cancer and other diseases.

Endnotes

1. www.who.int/immunization/diseases/mumps/en/
2. Mumps. CDC Pink Book
3. Vaccine against mumps. *BMJ*. 1967;2(5555):779-80
4. Prevention of mumps. *BMJ*. 1980;281(6250):1231-2
5. A retrospective survey of the complications of mumps. *J R Coll Gen Pract*. 1974;24(145):552-6
6. Asatryan A et al. Live attenuated measles and mumps viral strain-containing vaccines and hearing loss: Vaccine Adverse Event Reporting System (VAERS), United States, 1990—2003. *Vaccine*. 2008;26(9):1166-72
7. Bruyn HB et al. Mumps meningoencephalitis; a clinical review of 119 cases with one death. *Calif Med*. 1957;86(3):153-60
8. Kaplan KM et al. Mumps in the workplace. Further evidence of the changing epidemiology of a childhood vaccine-preventable disease. *JAMA*. 1988;260(10):1434-8
9. Harling R et al. The effectiveness of the mumps component of the MMR vaccine: a case control study. *Vaccine*. 2005;23(31):4070-4
10. Gilliland SM et al. Vaccine-related mumps infections in Thailand and the identification of a novel mutation in the mumps fusion protein. *Biologicals*. 2013;41(2):84-7
11. Vygen S et al. Waning immunity against mumps in vaccinated young adults, France 2013. *Euro Surveill*. 2016;21(10):30156
12. Anis E et al. Mumps outbreak in Israel's highly vaccinated society: are two doses enough? *Epidemiol Infect*. 2012;140(3):439-46
13. de Wit J et al. Mumps infection but not childhood vaccination induces persistent polyfunctional CD8+ T-cell memory. *J Allergy Clin Immunol*. 2018;141(5):1908-11.e12
14. Smetana J et al. Serological survey of mumps antibodies in adults in the Czech Republic and the need for changes to the vaccination strategy. *Hum Vaccin Immunother*. 2018;14(4):887-93
15. Koleva G. Merck whistleblower suit a boon to vaccine foes even as it stresses importance of vaccines. *Forbes*. 2012 Jun 27
16. Pierson B. Merck accused of stonewalling in mumps vaccine antitrust lawsuit. *Reuters*. 2015 Jun 4

17. Dourado I et al. Outbreak of aseptic meningitis associated with mass vaccination with a urabe-containing measles-mumps-rubella vaccine: implications for immunization programs. *Am J Epidemiol.* 2000;151(5):524-30

18. Watts M. Vaccine officials knew about MMR risks. *The Telegraph.* 2007 Mar 5

19. da Cunha SS et al. Outbreak of aseptic meningitis and mumps after mass vaccination with MMR vaccine using the Leningrad-Zagreb mumps strain. *Vaccine.* 2002;20(7-8):1106-12

20. Cizman M et al. Aseptic meningitis after vaccination against measles and mumps. *Pediatr Infect Dis J.* 1989;8(5):302-8

21. Da Dalt L et al. Henoch-Schönlein purpura and drug and vaccine use in childhood: a case-control study. *Ital J Pediatr.* 2016;42(1):60

22. Clifford V et al. Mumps vaccine associated orchitis: evidence supporting a potential immune-mediated mechanism. *Vaccine.* 2010;28(14):2671-3

23. Morfopoulou S et al. Deep sequencing reveals persistence of cell-associated mumps vaccine virus in chronic encephalitis. *Acta Neuropathol.* 2017;133(1):139-47

24. Fanoy EB et al. Transmission of mumps virus from mumps-vaccinated individuals to close contacts. *Vaccine.* 2011;29(51):9551-6

25. West RO. Epidemiologic study of malignancies of the ovaries. *Cancer.* 1966;19(7):1001-7

26. Menczer J et al. Possible role of mumps virus in the etiology of ovarian cancer. *Cancer.* 1979;43(4):1375-9

27. Cramer DW et al. Mumps and ovarian cancer: modern interpretation of an historic association. *Cancer Causes Control.* 2010;21(8):1193-201

28. Myers R et al. Oncolytic activities of approved mumps and measles vaccines for therapy of ovarian cancer. *Cancer Gene Ther.* 2005;12(7):593-9

29. Asada T. Treatment of human cancer with mumps virus. *Cancer.* 1974;34(6):1907-28

30. Okuno Y et al. Studies on the use of mumps virus for treatment of human cancer. *Biken J.* 1978;21(2):37-49

31. Ammayappan A et al. Recombinant mumps virus as a cancer therapeutic agent. *Mol Ther Oncolytics.* 2016;3:16019

32. Jochems CE et al. The use of fetal bovine serum: ethical or scientific problem? *Altern Lab Anim.* 2002;30(2):219-27

33. Wessman SJ et al. Benefits and risks due to animal serum used in cell culture production. *Dev Biol Stand.* 1999;99:3-8

34. Cantalupo PG et al. Raw sewage harbors diverse viral populations. *mBio.* 2011;2(5)

35. Wei Z et al. Fetal Bovine Serum RNA Interferes with the Cell Culture derived Extracellular RNA. *Sci Rep.* 2016;6:31175

36. Harasawa R et al. Evidence of pestivirus RNA in human virus vaccines. *J Clin Microbiol.* 1994;32(6):1604-5

37. Nuttall PA et al. Viral contamination of bovine foetal serum and cell cultures. *Nature.* 1977;266(5605):835-7

38. Steinman L et al. Pertussis toxin is required for pertussis vaccine encephalopathy. *PNAS.* 1985;82(24):8733-6

Chapter Fourteen

RUBELLA

You medical people will have more lives to answer for in the other world than even we generals.

— **Napoleon Bonaparte**

R ubella in children is even milder than mumps, but it can be dangerous for pregnant women in their first trimester. In the case of pertussis, adults and children are vaccinated to protect infants, and in the case of rubella, infants are vaccinated to protect pregnant women. Or, to be more precise, infants are vaccinated to protect the unborn infants.

According to the CDC, rubella rarely results in any complications, and 50% of the cases are asymptomatic. Most rubella cases in adult women are accompanied by arthralgia (joint pain) and arthritis. Complications are more common in adults than in children. Rubella in the first trimester of pregnancy can cause birth defects and spontaneous abortion.

> Before the introduction of the rubella vaccine in 1969, mainly children of five to nine years of age were most susceptible to rubella infection. In the 1980s, 30% of rubella cases occurred in adults. Today, 60% of registered cases occur in the 20–49 age group.

Twenty-five percent of post-pubertal women develop acute arthralgia following rubella vaccination, and 10% develop acute arthritis. Although one dose of the vaccine is enough for rubella immunity, children receive two doses of MMR just because separate vaccines are no longer manufactured [1].

A 2004 review published in the *Lancet* reported that rubella is usually impossible to distinguish clinically from parvovirus B19, human herpesvirus 6, dengue fever, measles, and other viral diseases. **Therefore, laboratory confirmation is essential for the correct diagnosis.** Rubella can be contracted more than once. The probability of repeated infection after vaccination is higher than after naturally acquired infection [2].

The RA27/3 strain, which has been used since 1979 in almost all rubella vaccines, was first isolated in 1965 from an aborted fetus. RA means Rubella Abortus (i.e., fetus aborted due to rubella in mother); 27/3 means the third tissue (kidney) of the 27th fetus. In the previous 26 fetuses aborted due to rubella, the virus was not detected. The isolated virus was attenuated by 30 consecutive passages in aborted fetus lung cells. The vaccine was tested on orphans in Philadelphia. Five to ten times more antibodies are formed after natural infection than after vaccination [2–5].

A previous virus strain for rubella vaccine, HPV77.DK12, was attenuated by 77 serial passages in vervet monkey kidney cells and then by 12 passages in dog kidney cells. This vaccine was licensed in 1969 but was soon withdrawn due to a high incidence of adverse reactions (severe arthritis in children, lasting for up to three years).

The RA27/3 strain causes arthropathy (joint injury) lasting over 18 months in 5% of women, joint symptoms in 42%, and a rash in 25%. One study showed that joint pains were less likely to occur in those vaccinated six to 24 days after onset of menstruation, while another study showed that they were most likely to occur within seven days after onset of menstruation. The authors recommend vaccinating in the last seven days of the cycle.

Rubella revaccination is not particularly effective. Revaccinating people with a low level of antibodies resulted in only a transient antibody increase, and in 28%, there was no increase at all [5].

There are plenty of other viruses and bacteria, besides rubella, that increase the risk of birth defects and spontaneous abortion, if contracted during pregnancy. For example, herpes, varicella, cytomegalovirus, hepatitis, influenza, parvovirus B19, syphilis, listeria, toxoplasma,

chlamydia, trichomonas, etc. There is no vaccine against most of them, so they scare much fewer people [6].

Effectiveness

In a review article published by the WHO, it is reported that after the introduction of the MMR vaccine in Poland, Finland, and other countries, the incidence of rubella shifted from children to adolescents and adults. Mathematical models predict that if the vaccination coverage is less than 60–70%, the number of rubella-susceptible adults will increase, thus possibly increasing the incidence of congenital rubella syndrome [7].

Rubella vaccination in Greece began in 1975, but the vaccination coverage was below 50%. This led to a consistent increase in the number of pregnant women susceptible to rubella. As a result, there was a rubella epidemic in Greece in 1993, and in six to seven months, an epidemic of 25 cases of congenital rubella followed, the largest such epidemic in the country's history. Prior to this, congenital rubella syndrome was very rare in Greece. Before the vaccination began, the mean age of rubella cases was seven years, but in 1993 the mean age went up to 17 years. Although the number of recorded cases was smaller in 1993 than in 1983, the incidence of rubella in people aged 15 years or more was higher in 1993 than it was in the 1983 epidemic, which was the largest recorded in Greece [8].

Since both rubella and the congenital rubella syndrome are very difficult to diagnose, the true incidence could be 10–50 times higher. Authors of an article published in 2017 conducted a meta-analysis of 122 studies of rubella susceptibility among pregnant and childbearing-aged women. Eleven percent of women in Africa did not have rubella antibodies, 10% in America, 7% in Europe, 19% in Southeast Asia, and 9% in the Far East. Overall, 9% of pregnant women and women of childbearing age around the world did not have rubella antibodies, while the WHO's goal for rubella susceptibility is 5% or lower. At that time (in 2011), no country in Africa had a rubella immunization program, while in Europe, all the countries had two-dose routine immunization. It is also reported that in order to increase vaccination coverage among adolescents and adults, the US federal government spends $4 billion annually [9].

According to a British study, two to four years after receiving the first dose of MMR, the level of antibodies fell below the protective threshold for measles in 20% of children, for mumps in 23% of children, and for rubella in 5% of children. Similar results were documented in other studies. The second dose of the MMR vaccine causes an increase in the levels of measles and rubella antibodies, but within three years after vaccination, they decline back to the pre-vaccination levels. Similar results were recorded in other countries. The authors conclude that in highly vaccinated populations, the level of antibodies does not correlate well with the level of protection against the disease [10].

Between the 70s and 90s in Italy, the incidence of rubella decreased in children but significantly increased in adolescents and adults. The incidence of mumps significantly decreased in children under 14 years of age but remained almost the same among adults. It could be because Italy was using the Rubini strain, which turned out to be very ineffective and was replaced in 2001. The number of rubella cases among children increased in the 80s and then decreased again. Among adolescents and adults, the number of cases increased significantly in the 80s and then remained high in the following years. The incidence of rubella has not changed over the last decades, despite the fact that rubella vaccination for girls was introduced in Italy in the late 1970s. On the contrary, insufficient vaccination coverage, which does not eliminate the disease, as in the case of measles, causes a shift of the disease incidence into adulthood, which is much more dangerous in the case of rubella due to the risk of infection during pregnancy. The authors conclude that insufficient vaccination in Italy caused an increase in the number of adults susceptible to measles and rubella and had no effect on mumps [11].

In the 1990 outbreak of congenital rubella syndrome in California, 43% of mothers had been vaccinated. An Italian study showed that 10% of females caught rubella within five years of vaccination. In a study of 190 soldiers during an epidemic, 80% of those vaccinated caught it. Of those previously exposed to rubella, only 3.4% caught it again. Of those unvaccinated and never exposed, 100% caught it. Those who got infected for the second time showed no symptoms. Only a third of those infected for the first time showed symptoms [4].

A 2015 study reported that since childhood infections incidence shifted to adulthood due to vaccination, measles has become four times more dangerous, chickenpox two times more dangerous, and rubella five times more dangerous [12].

A Cochrane systematic review concluded that there is not a single study assessing the clinical effectiveness of the MMR vaccine against rubella [13].

Safety

The safety of the MMR vaccine was discussed in detail in the previous two chapters. Here are some more studies, focused more on rubella.

According to a 2008 British study, the risk of anaphylaxis due to vaccination is one in 5,300 cases for the measles vaccine and one in 4,400 cases for the rubella vaccine. The authors believe that these figures are underestimated since the exact number of administered vaccines is unknown and that the actual figures may be three to five times higher. Nevertheless, in 2004 the risk of anaphylaxis due to MMR vaccine was estimated as 1.4 in 100,000 cases, and the risk of anaphylaxis due to all the vaccines was estimated as 0.6 in a million [14].

A vaccine with the RA27/3 strain was introduced in 1979. A new disease appeared in the medical literature within three years—chronic fatigue syndrome, which was first attributed to the Epstein-Barr virus. The majority of the people suffering from chronic fatigue syndrome were adult women who started showing symptoms after receiving the rubella vaccine. Patients with this syndrome have elevated levels of antibodies for multiple common viruses. **The more rubella antibodies were found in a patient, the more severe the chronic fatigue symptoms were [15].**

A special committee of the Institute of Medicine, which spent 20 months reviewing a wide range of information sources, concluded that the RA27/3 strain causes chronic arthritis in adult women [16]. According to VAERS analysis, the rubella vaccine is associated with a 32–59 times increase in the risk of chronic arthritis compared to other adult vaccines [17].

Over 69% of women vaccinated against rubella after childbirth shed the virus in their breast milk. Fifty-six percent of breastfed infants, whose mothers were vaccinated against rubella after childbirth, contracted rubella [18].

A 2013 article describes a case of measles and rubella vaccination in a healthy 31-year-old male. Ten days later, he was hospitalized with a diagnosis of viral encephalitis, and another three days later, he died. The

RA27/3 rubella vaccine strain was isolated from both his brain tissue and cerebrospinal fluid [19].

In a Canadian study, 24% of infants had lymphadenopathy (swollen lymph nodes), 4.6% had a rash, and 3.3% had conjunctivitis after receiving the MMR vaccine [20]. In another study, the MMR vaccine was found to increase the risk of lymphadenopathy by 1.4–3.1 times, and the risk of parotitis by 2.5–5.7 times [21].

Problematic Components

One of the components used in MMR and MMRV, as well as in some other vaccines, is gelatin. Gelatin for vaccines is produced from porcine bones. This, of course, is a problem for Jews and Muslims.

Jews solve this issue very simply. Pork is prohibited for oral consumption, but the Torah does not say anything about the intramuscular administration of pork. The Sages of the Talmud did not write anything against the intramuscular or subcutaneous intake of pork either, and what is not prohibited is permitted.

Muslims took this issue more seriously and held a special seminar dedicated to this issue in Kuwait in 1995, in the presence of the WHO Regional Office for the Eastern Mediterranean. They concluded that processing transforms gelatin from an impure substance (haram) into a pure substance (halal) and bones, tendons, and skin of an impure animal become clean gelatin, which can even be used in food.

Despite the fact that MMR contains egg protein, this vaccine is not contraindicated to those allergic to eggs. It is believed that the component that causes anaphylactic shock from the MMR vaccine is gelatin [22].

Christians are not concerned about the pork in vaccines, but they are concerned about the aborted fetal cells. The Vatican condemns using aborted cell tissue and viruses from aborted fetuses and encourages Catholics to lobby for the development of alternative vaccines and to oppose in any way possible the use of vaccines with aborted cells. Given the lack of alternatives, the Vatican allows using these vaccines but insists that it is the duty of every Catholic to fight for a change in the current situation. The Vatican allows refusing vaccination if it does not lead to any significant risks [23].

Statistics

In 1966–1968, prior to the beginning of vaccination, 10–14 cases of congenital rubella syndrome were recorded in the US annually. In 1969–70, after vaccination began, the incidence increased to 62–67 cases annually and remained above the initial level until the 1980s [24]. That is, to prevent a dozen of cases of congenital rubella, eight million children are vaccinated each year.

One thousand one hundred fifty deaths or permanent disability cases after MMR or MMRV vaccine have been registered with VAERS between 2000 and 2018 (i.e., 60 cases per year on average). Considering that only 1–10% of all cases get registered with VAERS, there may be as many as 600–6,000 cases of death or disability per year.

Conclusions

Rubella is a harmless disease in childhood, but it is dangerous in the early stages of pregnancy. Vaccination causes a shift in the incidence towards adulthood when the risk of complications is significantly higher.

Rubella is far from being the only virus that can cause impaired fetal development, but it is one of the few that have a vaccine developed against it.

Vaccination is significantly more dangerous for infants and children than the disease itself. From the point of view of the population, it seems that vaccination causes more deaths and permanent disability cases than both rubella and congenital rubella.

Endnotes

1. Rubella. CDC Pink Book
2. Banatvala JE et al. Rubella. *Lancet.* 2004;363(9415):1127-37
3. Plotkin SA et al. Studies of immunization with living rubella virus. Trials in children with a strain cultured from an aborted fetus. *Am J Dis Child.* 1965;110(4):381-9
4. Hutton J. Does rubella cause autism: a 2015 reappraisal? *Front Hum Neurosci.* 2016;10:25
5. Best JM. Rubella vaccines: past, present and future. *Epidemiol Infect.* 1991;107(1):17-30
6. Silasi M et al. Viral infections during pregnancy. *Am J Reprod Immunol.* 2015;73(3):199-213
7. Galazka A. Rubella in Europe. *Epidemiol Infect.* 1991;107(1):43-54

8. Panagiotopoulos T et al. Increase in congenital rubella occurrence after immunisation in Greece: retrospective survey and systematic review. *BMJ.* 1999;319(7223):1462-7

9. Pandolfi E et al. Global seroprevalence of rubella among pregnant and childbearing age women: a meta-analysis. *Eur J Public Health.* 2017;27(3):530-7

10. Pebody RG et al. Immunogenicity of second dose measles-mumps-rubella (MMR) vaccine and implications for serosurveillance. *Vaccine.* 2002;20(7-8):1134-40

11. Gabutti G et al. Epidemiology of measles, mumps and rubella in Italy. *Epidemiol Infect.* 2002;129(3):543-50

12. Fefferman NH et al. Dangers of vaccine refusal near the herd immunity threshold: a modelling study. *Lancet Infect Dis.* 2015;15(8):922-6

13. Demicheli V et al. Vaccines for measles, mumps and rubella in children. *Cochrane Database Syst Rev.* 2012(2):CD004407

14. Erlewyn-Lajeunesse M et al. Anaphylaxis following single component measles and rubella immunisation. *Arch Dis Child.* 2008;93(11):974-5

15. Allen AD. Is RA27/3 rubella immunization a cause of chronic fatigue? *Med Hypotheses.* 1988;27(3):217-20

16. Howson CP et al. Chronic arthritis after rubella vaccination. *Clin Infect Dis.* 1992; 15(2):307-12

17. Geier DA et al. A one year followup of chronic arthritis following rubella and hepatitis B vaccination based upon analysis of the VAERS database. *Clin Exp Rheumatol.* 2002; 20(6):767-71

18. Losonsky GA et al. Effect of immunization against rubella on lactation products. *J Infect Dis.* 1982;145(5):654-66

19. Gualberto FA et al. Fulminant encephalitis associated with a vaccine strain of rubella virus. *J Clin Virol.* 2013;58(4):737-40

20. Freeman TR et al. Illness after measles-mumps-rubella vaccination. *CMAJ.* 1993; 149(11):1669-74

21. Dos Santos BA et al. An evaluation of the adverse reaction potential of three measles-mumps-rubella combination vaccines. *Rev Panam Salud Publica.* 2002;12(4):240-6

22. Pool V et al. Prevalence of anti-gelatin IgE antibodies in people with anaphylaxis after measles-mumps rubella vaccine in the United States. *Pediatrics.* 2002;110(6):e71

23. Pontifical Academy for Life. Moral Reflections on Vaccines Prepared from Cells Derived from Aborted Human Fetuses. *National Catholic Bioethics Quarterly.* 2006;6:541–8

24. Summary of Notifiable Diseases, United States, 1995. *CDC*

Chapter Fifteen

CHICKENPOX

The further a society drifts from the truth,
the more it will hate those that speak it.

— **George Orwell**

J ust recently, chickenpox was a harmless childhood disease, but it
becomes more dangerous year after year, and soon will come the time
when it will be even more dangerous than measles, which is already
more dangerous than Ebola.

Chickenpox (varicella) is caused by the varicella-zoster virus. The
same virus also causes herpes zoster (shingles). According to the CDC,
chickenpox is a mild disease in healthy children, however, in adults it is
more severe, and the risk of complications is higher. Children suffering
from lymphoma, leukemia, and HIV also face a higher risk of
complications. Prior to the introduction of vaccination, the fatality rate for
varicella among children was one in 100,000, and among adults 25 in
100,000. Adults accounted for 5% of the chickenpox cases, but 35% of the
deaths. Chickenpox is highly contagious: less than measles, but more than
mumps and rubella. Chickenpox during pregnancy can occasionally cause
birth defects. The risk of congenital varicella syndrome due to a mother's
infection is less than 2% [1]. Chickenpox during delivery is very dangerous
for the infant, and its fatality rate is 30%. Varicella vaccination started in the
US in 1995. In the early 2000s, varicella outbreaks were registered in

schools where almost all children have been vaccinated. As a result, the second dose of the vaccine was introduced in 2006. The vaccine produces fewer antibodies than natural infection [2].

The authors of the review published in 2013 state that "For many years, little serious medical attention was paid to varicella, which was considered to be little more than a rite of childhood... Varicella resembles poliomyelitis in that serious disease is at least a partial function of the advancement of civilization in the developed world. The medically forgettable nature of varicella changed radically when Sydney Farber introduced effective chemotherapy and began, for the first time in the history of humankind, to cure childhood cancers. The joy of that success, however, was unexpectedly turned to despair when a child who was surviving treatment for malignancy was killed by varicella, which can be deadly in an immunocompromised host. After the use of drugs that compromised immunity entered common usage, varicella could no longer be considered a benign rite of childhood. Instead, it was a disease to be feared and avoided... During the 20 to 30 years that followed the pioneering work of Farber, cancer chemotherapy became more common, complex, and intense. Organ and bone marrow transplantation came into use, while steroids and antimetabolites were employed to treat many autoimmune diseases. The resulting spread of immunodeficiency meant that not only varicella but also herpes zoster became a significant clinical problem. Medical successes in all age groups caused longevity in the United States to increase. Again, varicella zoster virus (VZV) tempered the benefits of advances of medical progress; the incidence of herpes zoster and its complications increased in tandem with age. It thus became necessary to control VZV, which had become an increasingly dangerous virus" [3].

Vaccine strain of the virus is produced by serial passages through human or animal cell cultures, which is meant to attenuate the wild virus. But how can one be sure that as a result of this procedure, the virus was truly attenuated? The hypothesis that chickenpox and shingles are caused by the same virus was proposed in 1909. In 1932, in order to test this hypothesis, researchers extracted vesicular fluid from shingles patients and injected it into children who have not been exposed to varicella. Fifty percent of children got chickenpox, but the rash was less severe than usual. That is, if an airborne virus is administered by injection, it causes an atypical disease. Therefore, it is impossible to conclude that the vaccine strain of the virus is attenuated only on the basis of it causing mild symptoms. It is also possible that the injected dose of the virus was not enough to cause the usual symptoms.

In a 1990 study, the researchers vaccinated children with leukemia against varicella and examined how often those who developed post-vaccination rash infected their healthy siblings. It turned out that only 17% of the siblings were infected. Since the wild strain of the virus infects 80%, the authors concluded that the vaccine strain is indeed attenuated [4].

Effectiveness

According to a Yale University study, the effectiveness of the vaccine in the first year after vaccination is 97%, but with time it decreases to 84% [5]. Vaccination at the age of under 14 months is three times less effective than vaccination after the age of 14 months [6]. Despite that, in most countries, the vaccine is given at 12 months old.

According to a 2014 study, vaccine effectiveness in South Korea was 54%, and despite the vaccination coverage of above 97%, it had almost no effect on varicella incidence, unlike in other countries. **Most varicella cases were reported among the vaccinated. The vaccine had no effect on the course of the disease [7].**

A 2002 article describes the varicella outbreak in a daycare, where 66% of children had been vaccinated. The effectiveness of the vaccine was 44%. After three years, the effectiveness decreased by 2.6 times. Vaccinated children had less rash than those unvaccinated. The primary case occurred in a healthy child who had been vaccinated three years previously and who infected more than 50 percent of his classmates with no history of varicella. The boy himself was infected by his sister, who had herpes zoster. Vaccine effectiveness was much lower than what was determined during clinical trials. The authors state that this is most probably due to the fact that during clinical trials, children who do not develop antibodies are revaccinated or excluded from the analysis of vaccine efficacy or are analyzed separately. This leads to an overestimated efficacy rate [8]. In a meta-analysis of 14 studies of chickenpox outbreaks, the effectiveness of one dose was 72% [9].

In an outbreak of chickenpox in the American school, where 97% of children had been vaccinated, the effectiveness of one dose and two doses was almost the same [10]. In a similar study in China, it turned out that among the unvaccinated children, 14% got infected. Among those vaccinated with one dose, 1.6% got infected, and among those vaccinated with two doses, 2% [11]. A Canadian study found that 62% of the unvaccinated ten-year-old children that have not had chickenpox (or did not know whether they have had it), had chickenpox antibodies, which suggests that most chickenpox cases are asymptomatic [12].

Herpes Zoster

After the infection, the varicella virus remains in the neurons of the spinal ganglia in the inactive form. Decades later, it may reactivate as a result of waning cell-mediated immunity and cause **herpes zoster**. One of the potential dangers of vaccination, which is often neglected, is that if exposure to varicella actually reduces the rate of reactivation of the virus, then mass vaccination could increase the incidence of herpes zoster. Robert Hope-Simpson, in 1965, was the first one to hypothesize that exposure to varicella reduces the risk of reactivation by boosting specific immunity to the virus (**exogenous boosting**). A study conducted in England in 1991 found that the incidence of herpes zoster is 25% lower among adults living with children. This figure is most likely underestimated, as many adults not currently living with children may have done so in the recent past. Exposure to varicella is estimated to boost immunity to herpes zoster for an average of 20 years. Based on this data, the authors built a mathematical model and concluded that mass vaccination would cause a shingles epidemic, which will last for 30–50 years. More than 50% of those aged 10– 44 years will get shingles, and only 46 years later, the incidence of shingles will decrease to the level of the pre-vaccine era. These figures are probably underestimated since the authors assume that herpes zoster does not occur in those vaccinated, which, as we know, is not the case [13].

According to a study in *the Lancet*, contact with varicella cases is associated with a decrease in the risk of herpes zoster by 71%. This figure is probably underestimated since varicella is contagious before the onset of the rash. Contact with shingles patients does not decrease the risk of shingles because shingles are less contagious than chickenpox. Pediatricians suffer from herpes zoster much less frequently than dermatologists and psychiatrists [14]. A Japanese study found that the incidence of herpes zoster was 50–85% lower among pediatricians and family practitioners than the general public [15].

Herpes zoster ophthalmicus (HZO) accounts for 15% of all herpes zoster cases. The number of HZO cases in Boston increased by 2.7 times between 2007 and 2013. The average age of patients decreased from 61 to 56 years [16]. The same was found in another study in Oklahoma, where the average age of HZO patients decreased from 65.5 to 59 years within eight years [17].

The incidence of varicella in Massachusetts declined by 79% between 1998 and 2003, but the incidence of herpes zoster increased by 90% [18]. The same happened in Taiwan, where the incidence of varicella decreased from 2001 to 2009, and the incidence of herpes zoster increased. It is interesting to note that the incidence of chickenpox is higher during the winter months, while the incidence of shingles is higher during the summer months [19].

After the introduction of vaccination in Australia, the incidence of herpes zoster increased by 2–6% annually among adults over 20 years of age [20]. By 2012, the incidence doubled among those under 50 years of age and tripled among those over 50 [21]. In the United States, the incidence of varicella decreased fourfold, and hospital costs associated with it decreased by $100 million annually. However, hospital costs associated with herpes zoster increased by more than $700 million annually by 2004 [22]. Medical costs associated with varicella zoster virus are four to five times higher for those with herpes zoster compared to those with varicella. Modest increases in the number of herpes zoster cases would be sufficient to outweigh any benefits caused by reductions in varicella incidence, morbidity, and mortality. A 2013 article states that for years the CDC opposed the publication of findings about increased herpes zoster incidence after the introduction of varicella vaccination and threatened to sue the researcher, who wanted to publish this data [23].

A 2002 article states that herpes zoster is much more painful than varicella. The number of years of quality life lost is ten times higher for shingles patients than for chickenpox patients. Thus, an increase in shingles incidence will bring serious consequences to public health and will eliminate the benefits of reduced varicella incidence [24].

Due to an increase in the herpes zoster incidence, a vaccine against it was licensed in 2006. It contains the same virus as the varicella vaccine but has 14 times more viral particles. The effectiveness is 70% for 50-year-olds, 64% for 60-year-olds, and 18% for 80-year-olds during the first three years. How long the protective effect lasts is unknown. The shingles vaccine is ineffective for people over 80 years of age, and more than doubles the risk of serious adverse effects [25].

A 2006 article explains why the UK does not vaccinate against varicella:

1. Chickenpox is more dangerous in adulthood than in childhood. Fatality, as well as the risk of pneumonia and encephalitis due to varicella, increase with age.

2. Vaccination will lead to an increase in neonatal and congenital varicella since mothers would not get exposure in childhood.

3. Vaccination can lead to an increase in the incidence of shingles.

Therefore, the UK is being cautious and waits to see what happens in the countries that do vaccinate [26]. Most other European countries also do not vaccinate against varicella.

Benefits Of Varicella

According to several studies which were cited in chapter 12, chickenpox in childhood is associated with a 33% decrease in the risk of heart attack, 47–50% decrease in the risk of lymphoma, 34% decrease in the risk of ovarian cancer, and 34% decrease in the risk of other types of cancer. Chickenpox also decreases the risk of Parkinson's disease. Here are a few more studies.

According to a 2012 study, having chickenpox before eight years of age is associated with a decrease in the odds of asthma by 88%, allergic rhinoconjunctivitis by 84%, atopic dermatitis by 43%, and allergic sensitization by 89%. In those who have had varicella, the level of IgE (antibodies responsible for allergic reactions) remains low for more than ten years after the disease [27]. According to another study, chickenpox in childhood is associated with a 45% decrease in the odds of atopic dermatitis and a 96% decrease in the odds of severe atopic dermatitis. Varicella vaccine, despite being a live one, does not provide protection from asthma or allergies. The authors conclude that the varicella vaccine might have contributed to a sharp increase in the incidence of atopic dermatitis. Studies proving the economic benefits of varicella vaccination did not take this into account [28].

In a German study, herpes type infection (including varicella) in the first three years of life is associated with a 50% decrease in the risk of asthma. Having five to seven viral infections in the first three years of life is associated with a 68% decrease in the risk of asthma, and eight or more viral infections are associated with an 84% decrease. Having rhinitis two or more times during the first year of life decreases the risk of asthma by 48% [29]. According to another German study, varicella in childhood is associated with a decrease in the risk of cancer by 34%. Having three common colds per year decreases the risk of cancer by 77–82%, and viral gastroenteritis by 57%. High frequency of infections decreases the risk of cancer by 53% [30].

Varicella is associated with a 47% decrease in the risk of glioma (brain tumor) among people under the age of 40, and a 21% decrease for people of all ages [31]. According to another study, varicella is associated with a 60% decrease in the risk of glioma, and herpes zoster with a 50% decrease [32]. This data has been confirmed in several other studies [31]. It is also known that the varicella virus kills cancer cells [33].

Safety

According to a 2000 study, the vaccine strain of the virus remains in the body and reactivates periodically upon a decrease of immunity. This could have negative long-term consequences. The virus reactivates with a probability of 19–41% in children with low titers. A wild strain of the virus reactivates with the same probability in immunocompromised people. Since immunity against the virus provided by the vaccination is weaker than that from the actual disease, the long-term effect of frequent virus reactivation on singles and other complications is unknown [34].

According to an American study, the MMRV vaccine increases the risk of febrile seizures twofold, as compared to separate vaccines (MMR and varicella). MMRV increases the risk of febrile seizures sevenfold, and MMR separately fourfold [35]. Similar results were obtained in studies in Canada and Germany [36–37].

Those recently vaccinated against chickenpox can be contagious to others. For example, in the case described in a 1997 article, a 12-month-old boy was vaccinated, developed a rash from the vaccine strain of varicella, and infected his pregnant mother, who had to have an abortion [38]. The inverse case is reported when a mother, who was vaccinated after childbirth, infected the infant, even though she did not get sick herself [39]. Another article reports a case of two brothers: after getting vaccinated, one of them got shingles from the vaccine and then infected his vaccinated brother, who got varicella [40].

A 2018 Harvard Medical School study reports that some children develop shingles at the vaccination site several years after vaccination [41]. In a study in New York, 69% of the 32 shingles cases were caused by the vaccine strain of varicella [42].

Statistics

It is usually argued that vaccines are completely safe and that serious adverse effects occur in one in a million vaccinated individuals. How are such statistics obtained? Here is an example for the varicella vaccine. Authors from the FDA and the CDC analyzed VAERS from 1995 to 1998. Fourteen deaths were recorded in this period. To calculate the probability of death after vaccination, they used the number of vaccines sold for this period (9.7 million) and concluded that the probability of death is one in a million (they round it up a little, as, in fact, it comes up to one in 700,000). But they did not take into account that only 1–10% of all adverse effects get registered with VAERS and that the number of vaccine doses sold does not equal the number of doses administered. Moreover, 9.7 million doses sold is not an exact figure, but a CDC estimate. A total of 6,574 adverse events have been registered with VAERS, 4% of which were serious. However, among children under four years of age, there were 6% of serious adverse events, among children under three years of age 9%, and among children under one year of age, who got vaccinated by mistake, 14%. A total of 271 serious adverse events have been registered, that is, one in every 36,000. These figures should be adjusted by a factor of 10–100 (i.e., the real number is between 1:3600 and 1:360), and considering that the number of administered doses was lower than the number of doses sold, which is quite possibly overestimated, they should be further adjusted by an additional factor [43].

According to VAERS, between 1998 and 2017, 140 people died after vaccination in the USA (almost all of them were children), and 580 people became permanently disabled. Considering that VAERS registers 1–10% of all adverse effects, it turns out that 70–700 children die each year after vaccination, and 290–2,900 become permanently disabled.

Given that four million children are born each year in the US, and the vaccination coverage is about 90% [44], the probability of death after vaccination is 1:5,200 to 1:52,000, and the probability of disability is 1:1,200 to 1:12,000. Before the introduction of vaccination, the probability of a child's death due to varicella was 1:100,000, and this required a medically damaged immune system.

Conclusions

Varicella is a harmless childhood disease, which can cause complications in very rare cases, such as those where the immune system has been suppressed by chemotherapy or other medications.

Vaccination causes a shift in the incidence towards adulthood, increasing the risk of complications, cancer, and allergic diseases. Vaccination has also caused an increase in the incidence of shingles.

In healthy children, vaccination risks are significantly higher than the risks of natural infection.

Endnotes

1. Ghosh S et al. Pregnancy and varicella infection: a resident's quest. *Indian J Dermatol Venereol Leprol*. 2013;79(2):264-7

2. Varicella. CDC Pinkbook

3. Gershon AA et al. Pathogenesis and current approaches to control of varicella-zoster virus infections. *Clin Microbiol Rev*. 2013;26(4):728-43

4. Tsolia M et al. Live attenuated varicella vaccine: evidence that the virus is attenuated and the importance of skin lesions in transmission of varicella-zoster virus. *J Pediatr*. 1990;116(2):184-9

5. Vázquez M et al. Effectiveness over time of varicella vaccine. *JAMA*. 2004;291(7):851-5

6. Galil K et al. Younger age at vaccination may increase risk of varicella vaccine failure. *J Infect Dis*. 2002;186(1):102-5

7. Oh SH et al. Varicella and varicella vaccination in South Korea. *Clin Vaccine Immunol*. 2014;21(5):762-8

8. Galil K et al. Outbreak of varicella at a day-care center despite vaccination. *N Engl J Med*. 2002;347(24):1909-15

9. Bayer O et al. Metaanalysis of vaccine effectiveness in varicella outbreaks. *Vaccine*. 2007;25(37-38):6655-60

10. Gould PL et al. An outbreak of varicella in elementary school children with two-dose varicella vaccine recipients—Arkansas, 2006. *Pediatr Infect Dis J*. 2009;28(8):678-81

11. Suo L et al. Varicella outbreak in a highly-vaccinated school population in Beijing, China during the voluntary two-dose era. *Vaccine*. 2017;35(34):4368-73

12. Boulianne N et al. Most ten-year-old children with negative or unknown histories of chickenpox are immune. *Pediatr Infect Dis J*. 2001;20(11):1087-8

13. Brisson M et al. Exposure to varicella boosts immunity to herpes-zoster: implications for mass vaccination against chickenpox. *Vaccine*. 2002;20(19-20):2500-7

14. Thomas SL et al. Contacts with varicella or with children and protection against herpes zoster in adults: a case-control study. *Lancet*. 2002;360(9334):678-82

15. Terada K et al. Incidence of herpes zoster in pediatricians and history of reexposure to varicella-zoster virus in patients with herpes zoster. *Kansenshogaku Zasshi.* 1995;69(8):908-12

16. Davies EC et al. Herpes zoster ophthalmicus: declining age at presentation. *Br J Ophthalmol.* 2016;100(3):312-4

17. Chan AY et al. Factors associated with age of onset of herpes zoster ophthalmicus. *Cornea.* 2015;34(5):535-40

18. Yih WK et al. The incidence of varicella and herpes zoster in Massachusetts as measured by the Behavioral Risk Factor Surveillance System (BRFSS) during a period of increasing varicella vaccine coverage, 1998-2003. *BMC Public Health.* 2005;5:68

19. Wu PY et al. Varicella vaccination alters the chronological trends of herpes zoster and varicella. *PloS One.* 2013;8(10):e77709

20. Jardine A et al. Herpes zoster in Australia: evidence of increase in incidence in adults attributable to varicella immunization? *Epidemiol Infect.* 2011;139(5):658-65

21. Kelly HA et al. Decreased varicella and increased herpes zoster incidence at a sentinel medical deputising service in a setting of increasing varicella vaccine coverage in Victoria, Australia, 1998 to 2012. *Euro Surveill.* 2014;19(41)

22. Patel MS et al. Herpes zoster-related hospitalizations and expenditures before and after introduction of the varicella vaccine in the United States. *Infect Control Hosp Epidemiol.* 2008;29(12):1157-63

23. Goldman GS et al. Review of the United States universal varicella vaccination program: herpes zoster incidence rates, cost-effectiveness, and vaccine efficacy based primarily on the Antelope Valley Varicella Active Surveillance Project data. *Vaccine.* 2013; 31(13):1680-94

24. Edmunds WJ et al. Varicella vaccination: a double-edged sword? *Commun Dis Public Health.* 2002;5(3):185-6

25. Fried RE. Herpes zoster. *N Engl J Med.* 2013;369(18):1766

26. Welsby PD. Chickenpox, chickenpox vaccination, and shingles. *Postgrad Med J.* 2006; 82(967):351-2

27. Silverberg JI et al. Chickenpox in childhood is associated with decreased atopic disorders, IgE, allergic sensitization, and leukocyte subsets. *Pediatr Allergy Immunol.* 2012;23(1):50-8

28. Silverberg JI et al. Association between varicella zoster virus infection and atopic dermatitis in early and late childhood: a case-control study. *J Allergy Clin Immunol.* 2010;126(2):300-5

29. Illi S et al. Early childhood infectious diseases and the development of asthma up to school age: a birth cohort study. *BMJ.* 2001;322(7283):390-5

30. Abel U et al. Common infections in the history of cancer patients and controls. *J Cancer Res Clin Oncol.* 1991;117(4):339-44

31. Amirian ES et al. History of chickenpox in glioma risk: a report from the glioma international case-control study (GICC). *Cancer Med.* 2016;5(6):1352-8

32. Wrensch M et al. Does prior infection with varicella-zoster virus influence risk of adult glioma? *Am J Epidemiol.* 1997;145(7):594-7

33. Leske H et al. Varicella zoster virus infection of malignant glioma cell cultures: a new candidate for oncolytic virotherapy? *Anticancer Res.* 2012;32(4):1137-44

34. Krause PR et al. Varicella vaccination: evidence for frequent reactivation of the vaccine strain in healthy children. *Nat Med.* 2000;6(4):451-4

35. Klein NP et al. Measles-mumps-rubella-varicella combination vaccine and the risk of febrile seizures. *Pediatrics*. 2010;126(1):e1-8

36. MacDonald SE at al. Risk of febrile seizures after first dose of measles–mumps–rubella–varicella vaccine: a population-based cohort study. *CMAJ*. 2014;186(11):824–9

37. Schink T et al. Risk of febrile convulsions after MMRV vaccination in comparison to MMR or MMR+V vaccination. *Vaccine*. 2014;32(6):645-50

38. Salzman MB et al. Transmission of varicella-vaccine virus from a healthy 12-month-old child to his pregnant mother. *J Pediatr*. 1997;131(1 Pt 1):151-4

39. Kluthe M et al. Neonatal vaccine-strain varicella-zoster virus infection 22 days after maternal postpartum vaccination. *Pediatr Infect Dis J*. 2012;31(9):977-9

40. Brunell PA et al. Chickenpox attributable to a vaccine virus contracted from a vaccinee with zoster. *Pediatrics*. 2000;106(2):E28

41. Song H et al. Herpes zoster at the vaccination site in immunized healthy children. *Pediatr Dermatol*. 2018;35(2):230-3

42. LaRussa P et al. Viral strain identification in varicella vaccinees with disseminated rashes. *Pediatr Infect Dis J*. 2000;19(11):1037-9

43. Wise RP et al. Postlicensure safety surveillance for varicella vaccine. *JAMA*. 2000;284(10):1271-9

44. Hill HA et al. Vaccination coverage among children aged 19-35 months - United States, 2015. *MMWR*. 2016;65(39):1065-71

Chapter Sixteen

POLIO

When you inoculate children with a polio vaccine,
you don't sleep well for two or three months.

— Jonas Salk

E ven though poliomyelitis has not been observed in developed
countries for decades, for some reason, it continues to incite terror.
Poliovirus is one of many intestinal viruses (enteroviruses) and, like
most of them, it spreads through the fecal-oral route. There are three
different serotypes of poliovirus. Polio vaccines are divided into two types:
IPV—inactivated (Salk vaccine), and **OPV**—live oral (Sabin vaccine).
According to the CDC, the vaccines contain fetal bovine serum, and the
virus for both of them is grown in green monkey kidney cells. OPV also
contains polysorbate 80, and IPV contains aluminum.

Ninety-six percent of cases of poliovirus infections are
asymptomatic or are accompanied by mild symptoms that disappear
within a few days. Only 1–5% of cases are accompanied by aseptic
meningitis, which disappears in two to ten days. Flaccid paralysis occurs
in less than 1% of infected children, and in the majority, it disappears
completely [1].

A Bit Of History

Albert Sabin, who subsequently developed the live vaccine, writes in his 1947 article that although sporadic cases of paralysis were also observed in ancient times, polio epidemics suddenly appeared only at the beginning of the 20th century. Some scientists believed that poliomyelitis simply began to be diagnosed better, but Sabin does not agree with that and believes that such epidemics of paralysis could not have been missed in the past. Moreover, he writes that polio is yet unknown in large parts of the world. Epidemics are mainly rampant in large cities, in countries with good sanitary and hygienic conditions, but are not observed in other countries with similar climatic conditions. For example, in China only rare, sporadic cases have been recorded, even though excellent Western-trained physicians work in many Chinese cities, and they could not have missed such outbreaks in the native population if they had occurred. Paralytic poliomyelitis remains practically dormant most of the year, and then seems to explode during the late summer and early autumn, and it always begins in large cities.

Even though American, British, and Australian soldiers in the Philippines, Japan, China, and the Middle East suffered from polio, cases of paralysis were virtually non-existent among the local population. Poliomyelitis was the leading cause of death among US soldiers in the Philippines, while there were no epidemics among the local population, 90% of which had antibodies to poliovirus. Soldiers in the US suffered from poliomyelitis ten times more than soldiers based abroad. Sabin personally observed an outbreak of poliomyelitis among American marines in China, while there was no outbreak among the native population. A British physician, who worked in China for 25 years, often saw paralytic poliomyelitis among foreigners, but rarely among the Chinese. Other researchers have confirmed this observation [2].

Xavante is a Native American tribe in Brazil, which was virtually untouched by civilization. A 1964 study found that they were all infected with poliovirus, and almost all of them had antibodies to all three serotypes, but they had neither paralytic polio nor any symptoms of the disease. They also had antibodies to other diseases—measles, pertussis, influenza, salmonella, but most of the infections were subclinical [3].

A 1995 article published by the Mayo Clinic reports that polio diagnosis during the 1950s epidemics was based on the paralytic symptoms or cerebrospinal fluid testing. If the patient had flaccid paralysis, he was diagnosed with "paralytic poliomyelitis." And if the lymphocyte count in the cerebrospinal fluid was elevated, then it was "non-paralytic poliomyelitis." **It is known today that these kinds of laboratory findings are typical for viral meningitis, but are in no way diagnostic of poliomyelitis.** This caused an over-diagnosis of poliomyelitis during the epidemics. Only when the epidemics were winding down, the specific viral studies became readily available.

Any type of paralysis such as peripheral neuropathy, stroke, brain or spinal cord tumor, multiple sclerosis, hysterical paralysis, and many other diseases could have been diagnosed as polio. It was difficult to reject a polio diagnosis because of the generous financial assistance available to polio patients, which was not available to patients with other types of paralysis. Many kinds of medicines were advocated for the treatment of poliomyelitis, including strychnine, curare, cobra venom, and various antibiotics. Reports of their efficacy were based on anecdotal information but were propounded with certitude. A commonly advocated therapy was the irradiation of the muscles or spinal cord. In the 20th century, it became commonplace to splint and cast patients who had acute poliomyelitis. Paralyzed patients lay in plaster body casts for months at a time. Prolonged casting led to the atrophy of muscles, which were already not paralyzed. The stringent isolation of hospitalized patients, depriving them of contact with family and friends, was often remembered as the most stressful event of the illness. This isolation was interpreted as abandonment by many patients. The fear of polio led to the avoidance of polio patients, even by medical personnel.

Contemporary newspapers documented the anxiety and mass hysteria that is remembered by the patients who survived polio. Polio was the sword of Damocles that hung over every child and young adult. In the late summer and early fall, newspapers displayed headlines that reported on each new outbreak of poliomyelitis. One typical small-town newspaper reported in September and October 1948 that because of the polio epidemic, "the whole town must be closed as far as children are concerned, they must be kept strictly in their own yards." The town was sprayed with DDT, and it was suggested that each family should carry out an intensive spraying program [4].

Effectiveness

The word "poliomyelitis" means "inflammation of the gray bone marrow" in Greek. This term appeared in the 19th century when nothing was yet known of the poliovirus [5]. What is called "poliomyelitis" today is not what the term was used for before the late 1950s. **The word "poliomyelitis" meant a symptom back then. Today it means a symptom caused by a specific virus.**

During the polio epidemics in Michigan in 1958, only 25% of paralyzed patients had poliovirus in their blood. **In most of them, paralysis was not caused by poliovirus.** Coxsackie virus and echoviruses were the reason for more cases of nonparalytic poliomyelitis and aseptic meningitis, than poliovirus. Eleven patients paralyzed due to poliovirus have been vaccinated with at least three doses [6].

During the clinical trials of IPV, Jonas Salk published an article in which he claimed that all the virus in the vaccine was inactivated, but he did not provide data on all vaccine batches. Paul Meier, a well-known scientist, believed that there was something wrong with the data, so the National Fund for Childhood Paralysis (NFIP) formed an advisory committee to deal with it. "And they reformed it five or six times. Each time somebody didn't agree, they dropped them and got somebody who might agree. By the time they were done forming the committee, everybody on it was distinguished, but very agreeable," recalls Meier. After the clinical trials, NFIP gave the committee two hours to review the materials. "The NFIP was quite powerful. They had anybody engaged in public health, pediatric groups, all supporting the vaccine. Almost everybody said it was an excellent vaccine and it should be immediately released for vaccine injections." Six companies were then licensed to produce the Salk vaccine [7].

Two weeks after the license was issued, some of the children vaccinated with Cutter Laboratories vaccine got paralyzed. The vaccine was recalled, but 380,000 children had already been vaccinated with it. Subsequently, it turned out that 40,000 of them developed polio, 200 got paralyzed, and ten died because the vaccine was not completely inactivated and contained live poliovirus. Wyeth Laboratories also produced one batch of the vaccine that paralyzed and killed several children. Other companies had difficulties with virus inactivation as well. A very small amount of formaldehyde did not kill the virus, while too much made the vaccine useless. Residues of various substances in the vaccine protected the viral particles from the formaldehyde [8].

Because the other manufacturers went around to various newspapers and threatened to cut their advertising, all the blame was dumped on Cutter Laboratories. Even though Cutter's negligence was not proved, the court ruled that Cutter was liable to pay compensation. Over time, this led to an abundance of lawsuits against vaccine manufacturers, which resulted in a law being passed in 1986, according to which it became impossible to sue vaccine manufacturers in the United States. Since then, the compensation can only be received by filing a lawsuit with a special federal court, which is financed by a tax on every vaccine dose.

However, one loophole remained. If the special court dismisses the claim, then it is possible to file a lawsuit against the company with a regular court. Paul Offit, who is already familiar to us, proposes to close this loophole since these lawsuits cost the companies millions of dollars and deter them from the introduction of new vaccines [9].

In 1960, polio experts in the US held a panel reporting the following facts, which allow one to come to a conclusion whether the vaccine had any effect on the decrease in polio incidence in the mid-1950s:

1. In 1955, when the Salk vaccine was licensed, the definition of polio was changed. While a 24-hour paralysis was previously enough for a diagnosis of poliomyelitis, from 1955, the paralysis had to last for at least 60 days. "Coxsackie viruses' infections and aseptic meningitis, which were previously considered as polio, were distinguished from paralytic poliomyelitis. Prior to 1954 large numbers of these cases were mislabeled as paralytic poliomyelitis. Thus, simply by changes in diagnostic criteria, the number of paralytic cases was predetermined to decrease in 1955-1957, whether or not any vaccine was used... This change in definition meant that in 1955 we started reporting a new disease, namely, paralytic poliomyelitis with a longer lasting paralysis."

The definition of epidemic also changed. "Prior to the introduction of the Salk vaccine the NFIP defined an epidemic as 20 or more cases of polio per year per 100,000 population. On this basis there were many epidemics through the United States yearly. Presently a community is considered to have an epidemic when it has 35 cases of polio. The present higher rate has resulted in not a real but a semantic elimination of epidemics."

2. "For every case of known paralytic polio we have about a thousand cases of subclinical polio infections."

3. "One of the most obvious pieces of misinformation being delivered to the American public is that 50% rise in paralytic poliomyelitis in 1958 and the real accelerated increase in 1959 have been caused by persons failing to be vaccinated. This represents a certain amount of 'double talk' and an unwillingness to face facts and to evaluate the true effectiveness of the Salk vaccine. It is double talk from the standpoint of logical reasoning: If the Salk vaccine is to take credit for the decline from 1955-1957, how can those individuals who were vaccinated several years ago contribute to the increase in 1958 and 1959? Are not these persons still vaccinated? The number of persons over two years of age in 1960 who have not been vaccinated cannot be more, and must be considerably less, than the number who had no vaccination in 1957. Yet, a recent Associated Press release to warn about the impending threat referring to the idea that the 'main reason is that millions of children and adults have never been vaccinated'. If they were not vaccinated, undoubtedly many more than were reported were unvaccinated during 1955, 1956, and 1957 when the same officials were claiming that reduction in rates was due to the vaccine."

4. "The Salk vaccine was used in 400,000 persons in a single field trial in a study which *assumed* safety and was primarily designed to determine effectiveness... The field trials in 1954 showed that the vaccine used was 72% effective in preventing paralytic poliomyelitis within one year, but completely ineffective in preventing nonparalytic poliomyelitis. However, for the 1955 vaccine, certain changes in the manufacture and testing for safety were introduced. To insure 'absolute safety' an extra filtration step was introduced. The result of that change as well as preceding ones, upon the effectiveness of the present vaccine is unknown... The second filtration step was picked out of thin air with no experimentation to back it up. Because it was thought that residual live virus particles encased in a mass of killed particles were getting through, the filtration step was introduced in the hope that it would remove this aggregate. We've known for years, however, that any time you introduce an additional filtration step you lose antigen. Actually, the Israelis found they lose from 10 to 30-fold in virus content by a second filtration step. If you have a small amount of antigen to start with, additional filtration will only reduce it further."

5. "In 1954, 10 of the 48 lots of vaccine produced for field trial use were positive for live virus... The real cause for alarm was the knowledge that there was no correlation of positive test results among 3 different laboratories. Notwithstanding, on the basis of Dr. Salk's report of no

adverse effects following the vaccination of 7,507 children with commercially prepared vaccines, the 1954 field trials were allowed to proceed... In 1953, experienced investigators failed to produce a safe vaccine by the Salk formula. Their findings were dismissed by the backers of Salk vaccine.

"The general theory that Salk was working on was a very simple and old one: that the inactivation of poliovirus by formalin would proceed in a straight-line, first-order reaction. This means that in x hours in contact with formalin, half of the virus particles would be inactivated, that an equal number of additional hours would inactivate another half of the *remaining* live virus particles and so on... Although this theory applies to many cases, whether it applies to the Salk vaccine remains an empirical question. What troubled me greatly was that it appeared from actual data which Salk presented that the theory did not apply. Assuming there was some error in my understanding or in Salk's, I inquired of the people who knew about this. The answer I consistently received was 'I see what you mean. I haven't thought about it very carefully myself, but there are many important and competent people who are taking care of this. Don't worry. After all, this is merely a paper for the public and not the real technical goods.' The answer as it emerged later, of course, was no one was taking care of it.

"The triple safety checking of the vaccine was used in the field trials by the manufacturer, Dr. Salk's laboratory, and the Public Health Service was dropped in the licensing procedure. Most of the lots distributed in 1955 were tested only by the manufacturer. It was no surprise, then, that we had a spring outbreak of vaccine-induced cases. The only surprise was that there weren't more."

6. "From experience we know that it is wise to have a highly virulent strain for good antibody response... The virulent strain, however, was responsible for the vaccine-induced outbreaks in the spring of 1955. In Idaho, where the people were polio virgins, the vaccine caused numerous cases of polio. In New Mexico, Arizona, and elsewhere, were natural immunity was present, there were few or no cases."

7. "Laboratory findings are another reason why I am getting nervous. If polio antibodies mean anything in respect to protection, then I am forced to conclude that much of the Salk vaccine we have been using is useless. For two years now we have done antibody titrations on children who have received three or more doses of Salk vaccine. These titrations show that over 50% do not have antibodies to types I and III and that 20% lack

antibodies to type II poliovirus. This is very disturbing fact. When a phenomenon like this occurs two years in a row, one has reason to believe that the material we are injecting is not an antigenic preparation."

8. "In 1956, New York State Health Department reported that there was a 600-fold variation in the potency of commercial Salk vaccine on the market... In 1957, the largest producer of Salk vaccine in the United States had several million dollars worth of vaccine on hand which did not pass the minimum potency requirements of the USPHS (Public Health Service). Subsequently, the Division of Biological Standards reinterpreted the minimum requirements to make possible the commercial utilization of this vaccine."

9. In comparing the incidence among vaccinated and unvaccinated people, they forgot to count 101,000 unvaccinated children, which led to an overestimated effectiveness.

> "If the vaccine was not as effective, one might wonder why the tremendous reduction occurred in the 1955, 1956, and 1957 reported rates. Here, again, much of this reduction was a statistical artifact."

10. It is very difficult to convince doctors to diagnose non-paralytic poliomyelitis in those vaccinated. In 1956–57, it turned out that most cases of non-paralytic poliomyelitis were actually Coxsackie virus and echovirus.

11. During the 1958 epidemic in Israel, there was no difference in the incidence among vaccinated and unvaccinated. During the epidemic in Massachusetts, there were more paralytic cases in the triple vaccinated than in the unvaccinated.

12. Studies of inactivated vaccines against Rocky Mountain spotted fever, epidemic typhus fever, and Japanese encephalitis have shown that when the number of viral particles in a vaccine was less than 100 million, vaccinated guinea pigs and mice died before the unvaccinated controls. The low antigen vaccine caused sensitization, only increasing the susceptibility to the disease. This is an immunologic fact confirmed by the Public Health Service. That is, **insufficient potency of the vaccine does more harm than good**. This is probably what happened in Massachusetts, where 47% of paralysis cases were observed among those vaccinated with three doses and only in 37% of the unvaccinated group.

13. "Not all lots were checked by laboratories other than the manufacturers'. They were random sampled. The director of the Laboratory of Biological Controls was aware of safety testing problems but was unsuccessful in obtaining a clarification from Dr. Salk... He did not want to grant the license, but his decision was overruled."

14. "It is hard to convince the public that something is good. Consequently, the best way to push forward a new program is to decide on what you think the best decision is and not question it thereafter, and further, not to raise questions before the public or expose the public to open discussion of the issues" [10].

> In 1952, 3,145 people died of poliomyelitis during the largest epidemic in the US. In that same year, 200,000 people died of cancer, and 20,000 died of tuberculosis. And since any kind of paralysis was counted as polio back then, the actual number of deaths due to poliomyelitis caused by poliovirus was much lower.

It is believed that the "iron lungs" disappeared thanks to the polio vaccine. Respiratory muscle paralysis, which is why these iron lungs were used, is not caused just by the poliovirus, so the iron lungs did not actually go anywhere. They simply do not look so terrible nowadays, thanks to modern technology. The ventilator, for example, is one of the substitutes of the iron lungs.

Poliomyelitis, of course, did not go anywhere either. After all, only a small number of poliomyelitis cases were caused by poliovirus. Poliomyelitis simply has different names today, such as transverse myelitis, Guillain-Barré syndrome, acute flaccid paralysis, and so on. One thousand four hundred cases of transverse myelitis are diagnosed each year in the US, and the cause of it remains unknown.

Acute Flaccid Myelitis

An outbreak of a new, strange disease among children began in the US in 2014, a disease very similar to polio. It was named Acute Flaccid Myelitis (AFM) and was supposedly caused by enteroviruses. In 2014 there were 1,153 cases of serious infection, 14 deaths, and 120 cases of paralysis. The CDC has no idea what this disease is. Moreover, they refuse to discuss it and to report the number of cases registered and in which states they occurred. AFM deaths get attributed to other diseases. In an internal correspondence, which the CDC reluctantly provided a year and a half after the request, this disease is being called the poliomyelitis of the 21st century. The situation is similar to what was happening in the early 20th century. Millions of people were infected with poliovirus, but only in a small fraction of them did it cause paralysis.

AFM causes more serious complications than measles, Ebola and Zika combined, but nonetheless, no statistics on this disease are being collected, and the physicians are not required to report it to the CDC [11]. AFM outbreaks are reported not only in the US but also in other countries. AFM is actively discussed in medical literature, but only a small number of people have heard of it. Since there is no vaccine for this disease, there is no point in creating a panic about it in the population.

Provocation Poliomyelitis

Between 1970 and 1984, Romania participated in a safety study of the live attenuated oral poliovirus vaccine coordinated by the WHO. It turned out that, for unexplained reasons, the risk of vaccine-associated paralytic poliomyelitis (VAPP) was five to 17 times higher in Romania than in any other country in the study. It was first believed that the OPV vaccine in Romania was too virulent, but when it was replaced with another vaccine, the VAPP incidence did not change. It turned out that 86% of paralyzed children received intramuscular injections 30 days before the onset of paralysis (17 injections on average), as compared to 51% of non-paralyzed children (three injections on average). Each additional injection increased the risk of paralysis by 13%. Paralysis was observed eight times more often in those who received one injection, and 182 times more often in those who received over ten injections compared to those who did not receive any injections. The authors conclude that 86% of VAPP cases might have been prevented by the elimination of intramuscular injections within 30 days after exposure to oral poliovirus vaccine [12].

The fact that injections and vaccines provoke paralysis was known back in 1950. During the polio epidemic in Melbourne in 1949, some children developed paralytic poliomyelitis shortly after they had been given an injection of diphtheria and pertussis vaccine. Doctors denied any link. It turned out, however, that such a link existed, since in most cases, paralysis developed precisely in the inoculated limb. The authorities thought for a long time whether the public and doctors should be informed of these facts and decided to inform about the pertussis vaccine, but not about the diphtheria vaccine. The announcements did not receive any unfavorable comments from the press, and the future of vaccination was not called into question [13].

In 1950, poliomyelitis following prophylactic injections was recognized in Australia, the UK, and later in the US. Epidemiological analysis showed a causal relationship which was later confirmed by animal experiments. By giving the injections to children in the winter months, provocation poliomyelitis was reduced to a minimum. The authors of a 1985 article reviewed the literature and concluded that the risk of paralysis due to injections might increase by 25 times and that multiple injections, especially of arsenic and penicillin, significantly increase the risk of paralysis [14].

> An experiment on mice was conducted in 1998. It was found that skeletal muscle injury from injections can indeed lead to a rapid progression of poliovirus-induced paralysis. Also, the mechanism of how it enters the nervous system has been described.

Other human enteroviruses also have the propensity to cause poliomyelitis, although the mechanism by which these viruses reach and enter motor neurons is currently unknown [15].

Nothing changed since the 1950s, however. There was a large poliomyelitis outbreak in Oman in 1988–1989, despite the 87% vaccination coverage. No correlation between the number of vaccine doses and odds of paralysis was found. However, a significantly higher proportion of paralyzed children received their last DTP injection within the 30-day period preceding the onset of paralysis. In 25–35% of children, the paralysis was attributable to the DTP injection [16]. In 1993, 89% of 152 children with paralytic poliomyelitis in Pakistan received an unnecessary injection 48 hours or less before paralysis, and there was an almost complete correlation between the area of paralysis and the site of injection. Other studies in Pakistan showed a similar pattern [17]. The same was observed in India [14].

Tonsillectomy (removal of tonsils) is associated with an increase in the risk of poliomyelitis by 2.6 times in the following 30 days. The risk of bulbar and bulbospinal forms of poliomyelitis (the most dangerous ones) increased by 16 times [18].

Pesticides

The author of the article published in 1949, reports that "During a period of more than two years, numerous cases of a curious syndrome complex, apparently never before reported, have been observed throughout the United States... It has been widely attributed to infection with a thus far illusory "virus X."

The syndrome is accompanied by acute gastroenteritis, nausea, vomiting, abdominal pain, diarrhea, runny nose, cough, persistent sore throat, joint pain, muscle weakness, fatigue, and paralysis. It turned out later that all these symptoms were caused by DDT. Paralysis from DDT is similar to poliomyelitis.

"Despite the fact that DDT is a highly lethal poison for all species of animals, the myth has become prevalent among the general population that it is safe for man in virtually any quantity. Not only is it used in households with reckless abandon, so that sprays and aerosols are inhaled, the solutions are permitted to contaminate the skin, bedding and other textiles are saturated, and food and food utensils are contaminated, but DDT is also widely used in restaurants and food processing establishments and as an insecticide on crops. Cattle, sheep and other food animals are extensively dusted with it and large areas are indiscriminately sprayed from airplanes for mosquito control. DDT is difficult and usually completely impossible to remove from contaminated foods, and it accumulates in the fat and appears in the milk of animals who feed on sprayed pasture or on contaminated fodder or who lick the DDT from their hides. As DDT is a cumulative poison (in animals repeated small doses are as lethal as single large ones) it is inevitable that large scale intoxication of the American population would occur" [19].

The high toxicity of DDT, and even its ability to cause paralysis, was already known in 1945, but that did not prevent it from being widely used in the 50s and 60s. DDT was only banned in the USA in 1972, after causing an almost complete extinction of eagles, pelicans, and other birds [20]. Poliovirus multiplies much faster in human cells treated with DDT. Other insecticides have a similar effect [21].

Another insecticide, which was widely used before DDT, was arsenic, the poisoning by which also causes paralysis [22].

Other causes of polio-like paralytic syndromes include snake, spider, scorpion and tick bites, organophosphorus insecticides, as well as enteroviruses and other infections.

There was an outbreak of a polio-like disease in Bulgaria in 1975, which turned out to be enterovirus 71. Similar outbreaks have also been reported in California and Hungary [23]. In the 1930s, epidemics of "polio" caused by bacteria in milk were observed [24].

A 1952 article analyzes dozens of cases and outbreaks of poliomyelitis, in which paralysis was caused by poisoning with lead, arsenic, mercury, cyanide, pesticides, carbon monoxide, etc. It is also reported that ascorbic acid, which effectively treats poliomyelitis, has been used to treat poisoning. The author writes that earlier epidemics of pellagra and beriberi were observed, and so it was believed that these were infectious diseases. Since poliomyelitis was legally categorized as a contagious and infectious disease in 1911, only specialists in virology dealt with it, while general practitioners and clinicians could not participate in the research. It is also the reason why studies determining whether poisoning could cause poliomyelitis are not being funded [25].

India

An article published in the *Science* journal in 2006 reports that in the Indian states of Bihar and Uttar Pradesh, children under five years of age were receiving, on average, 15 doses of the polio vaccine, compared to ten doses in the rest of India. Only 4% of children were reported to have received fewer than three doses, of whom 90% were under six months old. This level of vaccine coverage should have already eliminated the infection. The authors investigated the efficacy of the vaccine and concluded that the estimated protective efficacy was just 9% per dose in those states [26]. A 1997 study reported that 54% of children with paralytic poliomyelitis had received at least three doses of the vaccine [27].

The authors of a 2012 article write that "It was hoped that following polio eradication, immunization could be stopped. However, the synthesis of polio virus in 2002, made eradication impossible." Therefore, the global eradication campaign for polioviruses would have to be continued indefinitely. Getting poor countries to spend their scarce resources on an impossible dream over the last ten years was unethical. Moreover, despite the fact that there has not been a single case of poliomyelitis in India for a year now, there has been a huge increase in cases of non-polio acute flaccid paralysis (NPAFP). Forty-seven thousand five hundred new cases have been registered in 2011, which is 12 times higher than expected. In the states of Uttar Pradesh and Bihar, which have pulse polio rounds nearly every month, the NPAFP rate is 25- and 35-fold higher than the international norms. Clinically, NPAFP is no different from poliomyelitis, but it is twice as deadly. The number of NPAFP cases is directly proportional to the number of vaccine doses received. Although this data was collected officially, it was never examined. From India's point of view, $2.5 billion spent on eradication might have been better spent on water, sanitation, and routine vaccination. It would then have been possible to control or eliminate poliovirus, as it happened in developed countries. The authors suggest that the huge bill of $8 billion spent on the program is a small sum to pay if the world learns to be wary of such vertical programs in the future [28].

A 2018 article reports that the incidence of non-polio acute flaccid paralysis in India is significantly higher than expected (13.3 instead of 1–2 per 100,000). In 2004, it was 3.11 per 100,000, but in 2005 it has more than doubled. This was exactly the year when a new, live vaccine, which contained five times more virus, was introduced. After 2011, when the number of vaccination campaigns began to decrease, the NPAFP incidence began to decrease as well. The authors analyzed the data from the years 2000 to 2017 and concluded that out of 640,000 cases of paralysis in children, 491,000 were associated with polio vaccination [29].

Treatment

It was discovered back in the 1930s that vitamin C could help prevent paralysis from poliovirus [30]. Rhesus monkeys infected with poliovirus that avoided paralysis had higher levels of vitamin C than the ones that were paralyzed [31]. A 1955 article describes several cases of successful treatment of acute poliomyelitis with large doses of vitamin C (10g every three hours). The symptoms were resolved in several days [32].

A 1949 article reports on 60 patients with poliomyelitis. All of them received 1–2g of vitamin C intravenously every two to four hours. They were all clinically well in 72 hours. Three patients had a relapse, and their treatment was continued for two more days. The level of vitamin C in the urine of patients with poliomyelitis was lower than in healthy controls [33].

Safety

In 1960, it turned out that kidney cells of rhesus macaques, which were used to grow the vaccine viruses, were infected with Simian Virus 40 (SV40), which caused cancer tumors in hamsters. Later, dozens of studies have been published, which found this virus in human tumors. SV40 is found in mesotheliomas, brain tumors, breast carcinomas, colon cancer, lymphomas, and osteosarcomas, etc. Malignant mesothelioma (MM) is an aggressive cancer, resistant to conventional therapies; about 90% of those diagnosed with this disease die within two years. The incidence of MM is increasing in the Western world; in the US, approximately 3,000 cases are diagnosed annually, compared with almost none before 1950. Exposure to asbestos is considered to be its main cause, but SV40 plays the role of co-carcinogen, acting synergistically with asbestos and causing malignant transformation. The virus is usually found in tumors, but not in the healthy tissue surrounding them.

> Since 1963, the manufacturers have switched from the macaque kidneys to kidneys of other monkeys and began to test vaccines for SV40. However, they tested poorly, and in some countries, including USSR and Eastern European countries, vaccines were contaminated until 1978, and possibly later. In Italy, contaminated vaccines were used until 1999, and in China and some other countries, they might still be in use.

In the US, about 90% of children and 60% of adults were immunized with polio vaccines between 1955 and 1961, and, therefore, are potentially infected. SV40-positive tumors were found in people in the US, Canada, China, Japan, Europe, and New Zealand, but not in Finland, Turkey, Yugoslavia, and Austria—countries that did not use SV40-contaminated vaccines. However, despite the abundance of studies proving the carcinogenicity of SV40, no one is in a hurry to recognize the link. The topic is considered controversial; it is not funded or supported by reviewers, which is why researchers switch to other fields, and the entire SV40 research area has been paralyzed for many years. However, even studies that allegedly do not confirm the link between SV40 and tumors, in fact, detect small amounts of SV40, or find DNA of the virus instead of a virus protein. It is then argued whether the presence of DNA is a sufficient carcinogenic factor. After SV40 was removed from the vaccines, it did not go anywhere, as it multiplies in human cells, is present in semen and is transmitted sexually, as well as from mother to child [34].

In 1963, vaccine manufacturers switched from rhesus macaque kidney cells to Cercopithecus monkey kidney cells. This change eliminated SV40 as a potential contaminant of this vaccine's cell substrate but has intermittently raised concerns about other potential simian adventitious agents. In a 2002 study, the FDA found DNA of simian cytomegalovirus in several lots of the oral polio vaccine manufactured prior to 1992 [35]. In addition to the Cercopithecus monkey kidney cells, African green monkey kidney cells were also used in vaccine production. Nearly half of the vaccines based on these cells were contaminated with simian cytomegalovirus [36]. In 1996, Japanese researchers tested 43 lots of live virus vaccines (MMR and OPV) produced by different manufacturers and found pestivirus RNA in 28% of the lots [37].

The committee of the Institute of Medicine spent 18 months reviewing all available scientific and medical data, and in 1993 has concluded that OPV increases the risk of Guillain-Barré syndrome in adults by 3.5 times [38].

An article published in the *New England Journal of Medicine* in 1988 reported that children born to mothers who received an inactivated polio vaccine between 1959 and 1965 had a 13 times higher risk of neural tumors. This was not due to SV40, but probably due to some other, still undetected infection in vaccines [39].

In a 2018 Mexican study, some children in three villages were given a live polio vaccine. The authors investigated how the vaccine virus spreads. On the first day after vaccination, vaccinated children already started to infect the unvaccinated. Some vaccinated children continued to shed the virus 70 days after vaccination. No correlation between the distance to the home of the vaccinated child and infection was found. That is, the risk of infection for the unvaccinated child was the same regardless of the distance to the house of the vaccinated child. The authors conclude that the only way to avoid infection is to avoid using a live vaccine or to ensure strict control measures for the **vaccinated** children, such as quarantine or strict hygiene protocols, and that this finding supports the global cessation of OPV use [40].

Safety studies of IPOL inactivated vaccine lasted for just 48 hours. Additionally, the vaccine was administered together with the DTP vaccine

[41]. According to VAERS, about 1,000 people died, and more than 500 people became permanently disabled after the OPV vaccine in the US since 1980; that is, since the time when the last case of poliomyelitis from the wild-type virus has been recorded. During the same time, more than 750 people died, and more than 600 became permanently disabled after the IPV vaccine. These figures do not include the combination of vaccines and represent only about 1–10% of all cases.

In 2019, 176 cases of wild poliomyelitis were registered worldwide (in Afghanistan and in Pakistan), and another 367 cases of circulating vaccine virus. **The probability of contracting poliovirus is virtually zero nowadays. It is only possible to get infected from a live vaccine.**

Conclusions

Poliovirus is one of the hundreds of intestinal viruses, which has been completely harmless for centuries, but suddenly, in the late 19th – early 20th century, it began to penetrate the nervous system and cause paralysis. Official science still does not answer the questions of why it happened, why most places with increased hygiene suffered at first, and why places with poor hygiene became more affected later on—even though the answer lies on the surface and is described in hundreds of scientific articles. There is no evidence that the virus suddenly mutated, much less that all three of its serotypes mutated at the same time, from which it follows that the reason for the sudden virulence of the virus lies in the changing ecological conditions. Vaccines, injections of arsenic and antibiotics, removal of tonsils, insecticides, and pesticides—all of these are factors that led to the spread of the intestinal virus into the nervous system, and to its sudden virulence.

A study of 568 thousand children in Taiwan found that children infected with enteroviruses had a 56% lower risk of developing leukemia [42]. There are currently trials being conducted on the use of poliovirus for the treatment of glioblastoma (brain tumor) [43].

Vaccination destroyed an almost harmless virus, and in return, it seems to have caused epidemics of much more serious diseases.

Endnotes

1. Polio. CDC Pink Book

2. Sabin AB. The epidemiology of poliomyelitis; problems at home and among the Armed Forces abroad. *JAMA*. 1947;134(9):749-56

3. Neel JV et al. Studies on the Xavante Indians of the Brazilian Mato Grosso. *Am J Hum Genet*. 1964;16(1):52-140

4. Mulder DW. Clinical observations on acute poliomyelitis. *Ann N Y Acad Sci*. 1995;753:1-10

5. Sturge WA. Three cases of acute anterior poliomyelitis (acute spinal paralysis) in adults. *BMJ*. 1879;1(962):849-51

6. Brown GC et al. Laboratory data on the Detroit poliomyelitis epidemic-1958. *JAMA*. 1960;172:807-12

7. Meier P. A conversation with Paul Meier. Interview by Harry M Marks. *Clin Trials*. 2004; 1(1):131-8

8. Juskewitch JE et al. Lessons from the Salk polio vaccine: methods for and risks of rapid translation. *Clin Transl Sci*. 2010;3(4):182-5

9. Offit PA. The Cutter incident, 50 years later. *N Engl J Med*. 2005;352(14):1411-2

10. The present status of polio vaccine. *Ill Med J*. 1960;118:84-93

11. Mystery Virus. Full Measure with Sharyl Attkisson. 2017 Jun 4

12. Strebel PM et al. Intramuscular injections within 30 days of immunization with oral poliovirus vaccine—a risk factor for vaccine-associated paralytic poliomyelitis. *N Engl J Med*. 1995;332(8):500-6

13. McCloskey BP. The relation of prophylactic inoculations to the onset of poliomyelitis. 1950. *Rev Med Virol*. 1999;9(4):219-226

14. Wyatt HV et al. Unnecessary injections and paralytic poliomyelitis in India. *Trans R Soc Trop Med Hyg*. 1992;86(5):546-9

15. Gromeier M et al. Mechanism of injury-provoked poliomyelitis. *J Virol*. 1998;72(6):5056-60

16. Sutter RW et al. Attributable risk of DTP (diphtheria and tetanus toxoids and pertussis vaccine) injection in provoking paralytic poliomyelitis during a large outbreak in Oman. *J Infect Dis*. 1992;165(3):444-9

17. Wyatt HV. Unnecessary injections and poliomyelitis in Pakistan. *Trop Doct*. 1996; 26(4):179-80

18. Anderson J. Poliomyelitis and recent tonsillectomy. *J Pediatr*. 1945;27(1):68–70

19. Biskind MS. DDT poisoning and elusive virus X; a new cause for gastro-enteritis. *Am J Dig Dis*. 1949;16(3):79-84

20. Gabliks J et al. Effects of insecticides on mammalian cells and virus infections. *Ann N Y Acad Sci*. 1969;160(1):254-71

21. Gabliks J. Responses of cell cultures to insecticides. 3. Altered susceptibility to poliovirus and diphtheria toxin. *Proc Soc Exp Biol Med*. 1965;120(1):172-5

22. Bencko V et al. The history of arsenical pesticides and health risks related to the use of Agent Blue. *Ann Agric Environ Med*. 2017;24(2):312-6

23. Gear JH. Nonpolio causes of polio-like paralytic syndromes. *Rev Infect Dis*. 1984;6 Suppl 2:S379-84

24. Rosenow E. An institutional outbreak of poliomyelitis apparently due to a streptococcus in milk. *J Infect Dis.* 1932;50(5/6):377-425

25. Scobey RR. The poison cause of poliomyelitis and obstructions to its investigation. *Arch Pediatr.* 1952;69(4):172-93

26. Grassly NC et al. New strategies for the elimination of polio from India. *Science.* 2006; 314(5802):1150-3

27. Srinivasa DK et al. Poliomyelitis trends in Pondicherry, south India, 1989-91. *J Epidemiol Community Health.* 1997;51(4):443-8

28. Vashisht N et al. Polio programme: let us declare victory and move on. *Indian J Med Ethics.* 2012;9(2):114-7

29. Dhiman R et al. Correlation between non-polio acute flaccid paralysis rates with pulse polio frequency in India. *Int J Environ Res Public Health.* 2018;15(8)

30. Jungeblut CW. Inactivation of poliomyelitis virus in vitro by crystalline vitamin C (ascorbic acid). *J Exp Med.* 1935;62(4):517-21

31. Jungeblut CW et al. Vitamin C content of monkey tissues in experimental poliomyelitis. *J Exp Med.* 1937;66(4):479-91

32. Greer E. Vitamin C in acute poliomyelitis. *Med Times.* 1955;83(11):1160-1

33. Klenner FR. The treatment of poliomyelitis and other virus diseases with vitamin C. *South Med Surg.* 1949;111(7):209-14

34. Qi F et al. Simian virus 40 transformation, malignant mesothelioma and brain tumors. *Expert Rev Respir Med.* 2011;5(5):683-97

35. Sierra-Honigmann AM et al. Live oral poliovirus vaccines and simian cytomegalovirus. *Biologicals.* 2002;30(3):167-74

36. Baylis SA et al. Simian cytomegalovirus and contamination of oral poliovirus vaccines. *Biologicals.* 2003;31(1):63-73

37. Sasaki T et al. Application of PCR for detection of mycoplasma DNA and pestivirus RNA in human live viral vaccines. *Biologicals.* 1996;24(4):371-5

38. Stratton KR et al. Adverse events associated with childhood vaccines other than pertussis and rubella. Summary of a report from the Institute of Medicine. *JAMA.* 1994;271(20):1602-5

39. Rosa FW et al. Absence of antibody response to simian virus 40 after inoculation with killed-poliovirus vaccine of mothers of offspring with neurologic tumors. *N Engl J Med.* 1988;318(22):1469

40. Jarvis CI et al. Spatial analyses of oral polio vaccine transmission in an community vaccinated with inactivated polio vaccine. *Clin Infect Dis.* 2018;67(suppl_1):S18-25

41. IPOL vaccine package insert

42. Lin JN et al. Risk of leukaemia in children infected with enterovirus: a nationwide, retrospective, population-based, Taiwanese-registry, cohort study. *Lancet Oncol.* 2015; 16(13):1335-43

43. Brown MC et al. Oncolytic polio virotherapy of cancer. *Cancer.* 2014;120(21):3277-86

Chapter Seventeen

INFLUENZA

No amount of evidence will ever persuade an idiot.
— Mark Twain

I t is believed that influenza kills more people than all other vaccine-preventable diseases combined. Therefore, if there is any point in getting vaccinated at all, then it should be against influenza.

Vaccine virus is grown either in fertilized chicken eggs or in dog kidney cells. Thimerosal (mercury preservative) is no longer used in children's vaccines, but it is still added to the multidose vials. In addition, the vaccine usually contains polysorbate 80. Twice a year, the WHO decides which strains should be included in the new vaccines. Preference is given to the strains that multiply well in eggs. Since the viruses mutate in the process of growing, the strain chosen by WHO does not always correspond to the strain in the vaccine [1]. Each egg yields one dose of the vaccine, and vaccine manufacturers use a million fertilized eggs per day [2].

There are three types of flu viruses: A, B, and C. Type A influenza subtypes are determined by the surface antigens hemagglutinin (H) and neuraminidase (N). There are 18 hemagglutinin antigens, and nine neuraminidase antigens in total. Three types of hemagglutinin are of particular importance to humans: H1, H2, and H3, as they play a role in virus attachment to cells, as well as two types of neuraminidase (N1 and N2) that play a role in the virus's ability to enter cells. The vaccine usually contains one strain of each of the virus types: A(H1N1), A(H3N2), and B. Quadrivalent flu vaccines, containing an additional strain of type B virus, became available in 2013 [3]. Type C is rarely reported in humans. As the virus strains change every year, so do the flu vaccines; therefore, the vaccine's effectiveness is impossible to access before the flu season begins.

Effectiveness

How is vaccine effectiveness calculated? There is a variety of ways. The majority of them are based on observational studies when all hospitalized patients presenting symptoms of acute respiratory infection are tested for influenza. However, these tests take into consideration only the strains contained in the vaccine. In other words, vaccine effectiveness is usually measured only among hospitalized patients, or among the already sick, and it is measured only for vaccine strains, and not for all influenza (or influenza-like) morbidity. This clearly does not result in an adequate evaluation of effectiveness.

In addition, most studies do not take vaccination in previous seasons into the account. For instance, vaccine effectiveness for the 2016/17 season among hospitalized elderly people was 17%. Among those who also received vaccination in the previous season, vaccine effectiveness was -2% (negative). The median age of hospitalized patients was 80 years old, and 94% of them were suffering from other diseases, which predisposed them to respiratory infections [4]. During the 2014/15 season, the effectiveness of vaccine against A(H3N2) strain in Canada was estimated at 53% for those who were vaccinated only in that season. Among those who had also been vaccinated in the previous season, the effectiveness was negative: -32%. Among those who were vaccinated for the third year in a row, the vaccine effectiveness was -54%. The average vaccine effectiveness was -17% [5]. Vaccine effectiveness during 2004–2013 was 65% for those who were vaccinated only in that season. For those who were vaccinated frequently, the effectiveness was 24%. The effectiveness of the vaccine against type B influenza was 75% for those vaccinated only in that season, and 48% for those who were vaccinated frequently [6]. During the 2010/11 season, the vaccine effectiveness was negative (-45%) among those who were vaccinated two years in a row. Among those who got vaccinated in that season only, the effectiveness was 62%. Among those who were infected at home, the effectiveness was -51%. Among adults who were infected at home, the effectiveness was -283% (i.e., the vaccine increased the risk of influenza almost fourfold) [7]. A 2019 study found that repeated vaccinations produce less effective antibodies than the first vaccination [8].

Analysis of influenza vaccine effectiveness for pregnant women in 1997–2002 showed that vaccination did not have any impact on influenza morbidity [9]. According to another study, flu vaccination during pregnancy does not reduce the risk of respiratory infections in infants [10].

A 2005 review reported that according to observational studies, influenza vaccination in the elderly reduces winter mortality risk from any cause by 50%.

> Influenza vaccination coverage among the elderly increased from 20% in the 1970s to 65% in 2001. Paradoxically, influenza-related mortality in this age group also increased during this period.

The authors conclude that "Because fewer than 10% of all winter deaths are attributable to influenza in any season, observational studies substantially overestimate vaccination benefit" [11]. An article published in the journal *Vaccine* in 2009 reported that more than 90% of influenza mortality falls on seniors above 70 years old. However, there are no randomized studies that document influenza vaccine benefits in seniors. Some research shows that vaccination apparently prevented mortality more effectively before the influenza season than during the influenza season, which demonstrates selection bias. Nevertheless, studies with such flaws still get published in influential medical journals. Despite the claims made by observational studies that vaccination reduces all-cause winter mortality by approximately 50%, increased vaccine coverage did not result in the reduction of either influenza-related mortality or all-cause winter mortality [12].

The largest study on the effectiveness of the influenza vaccine for the elderly was published in 2020. The authors analyzed 170 million hospital admissions and more than seven million deaths in England and found that the vaccine is ineffective and reduces neither morbidity nor mortality [13].

The author of the analysis of literature on the effect of vaccination of health care workers (HCW) on patients writes that the studies aiming to prove the widespread belief that HCW vaccination decreases patient morbidity and mortality are heavily flawed, and vaccination recommendations are biased. **No reliable published evidence shows that** vaccination of healthcare workers brings substantial benefit to their patients—neither in reducing patient morbidity or mortality and nor even in increasing patient vaccination rates. The author concludes that "The arguments for uniform healthcare worker influenza vaccination are not supported by existing literature. The decision whether to get vaccinated should, except possibly in extreme situations, be that of the individual healthcare worker, without legal, institutional, or peer coercion" [14].

A 2017 article analyzes four randomized studies of the impact of HCW vaccination. According to these studies, the vaccination of eight health care workers saves one patient from death, which means that vaccination of health care workers saves 687,000 lives a year in the US, which is more people than died during the epidemic of 1918. The article goes on to explain how the authors of the research are playing with statistics in order to get these completely insane results, and conclude that even according to the most optimistic estimates, at least 6,000–32,000 hospital workers would need to be vaccinated before a single patient death could potentially be prevented. In addition, according to these studies, it turns out that 90% of the people die from the flu without the presence of respiratory symptoms, and that the number of people saved by flu vaccination is greater than the total number of people who contract influenza. Authors conclude that current scientific data is inadequate to support the ethical implementation of enforced HCW influenza vaccination to reduce patients' risk, and that the resources may be better used on something that is more evidence-based [15].

The Unvaccinated

A study that lasted for eight seasons found that the risk of hospitalization due to influenza in vaccinated children was 3.7 times higher than in the unvaccinated [16]. In a 2012 randomized placebo-controlled trial, the risk of virologically confirmed non-influenza infections in vaccinated children was 4.4 times higher than in the unvaccinated. There was also no statistically significant difference in the risk of confirmed seasonal influenza infection between the vaccinated and the unvaccinated. The authors conclude: "Being protected against influenza, vaccine recipients may lack temporary non-specific immunity that protects against other respiratory viruses" [17]. According to a 2014 Australian study, influenza-vaccinated children were 1.6 times more likely than the unvaccinated children to have a non-influenza illness within 13 weeks of vaccination, while the risk of influenza was the same in both groups [18]. A 2018 study reports that those vaccinated against influenza for two consecutive seasons exhale six times more influenza viral particles than the unvaccinated. The authors speculate that certain types of prior immunity promote lung inflammation, airway closure, and aerosol generation [19].

An article in *JAMA*, published in 2000, reports on the results of a randomized, double-blind, placebo-controlled trial of the economic benefits of influenza vaccination. In the first year of the study, the strain was not predicted correctly, and the vaccine was ineffective. Vaccinated people missed 45% more working days due to illness than the unvaccinated, and visited physicians 378% more often. In the second year, the strain was predicted correctly, and the unvaccinated missed 32% more working days than the vaccinated and attended physicians 47% more often. In both seasons, vaccination led to losses. The authors conclude that vaccination may not provide overall economic benefits in most years [20].

The authors of a 2006 study wanted to test how influenza vaccination affects herd immunity. Children were immunized at school with a live vaccine. Families of the vaccinated children had significantly fewer influenza-like symptoms than families of the unvaccinated children, but, paradoxically, families of the vaccinated had higher rates of hospitalization. There was no difference in the number of missed school days between the vaccinated and the unvaccinated [21].

According to a 2014 study, influenza vaccination did not reduce the risk of subsequent hospital admission among patients who had influenza. The authors conclude that these findings do not support the hypothesis that vaccination reduces influenza illness severity [22].

Many people believe that influenza vaccination can cause influenza. Authors of a 2018 study set out to disprove this belief. However, they found that the incidence of influenza among the vaccinated and the unvaccinated was similar, and the incidence of non-influenza respiratory infections among vaccinated children was 71% higher compared to the unvaccinated [23].

Systematic Reviews

The Cochrane systematic review of the effectiveness of influenza vaccines **for children** included 75 studies. For children over the age of two, the efficacy of the live vaccine was 33%, and of the inactivated vaccine, it was 36%. For children under the age of two, the efficacy of the vaccine was practically zero. There is no evidence that the vaccine reduces mortality, hospitalization, serious complications, or disease transmission. The authors were surprised to find only one safety study for the inactivated vaccine. It was conducted in 1976 and included 35 children. They believe that it is rather strange that the vaccine is recommended to all children, despite the almost complete absence of safety studies. They found ten safety studies of the attenuated live vaccine, but they could not analyze the data, because manufacturers refused to provide all the information about the adverse effects. The authors note that all vaccine studies were of poor quality [24].

The Cochrane systematic review of the effectiveness of influenza vaccines **for adults** included 90 studies. Less than 10% of the studies were of good quality. The authors concluded that vaccination has a very modest effect. It is necessary to vaccinate 40 people to prevent one case of acute respiratory illness, and 71 people to prevent one case of influenza. Vaccination did not affect the number of hospitalizations with influenza or the number of missed workdays. There is no evidence that vaccination reduces the risk of serious complications [25].

The Cochrane systematic review of the effectiveness of influenza vaccines **for the elderly** included 75 studies. All of the studies were of such low quality that the authors could not conclude anything [26].

The authors of a Cochrane systematic review of the effectiveness of influenza vaccination **of medical personnel** working with the elderly concluded that there is no evidence that the vaccination reduces the number of influenza cases, the number of complications, or the mortality among the elderly [27].

The Cochrane systematic review of 259 influenza vaccine trials concluded that 70% of studies were of low quality and overly optimistic in their findings. In only 18% of the studies, the data presented support the authors' conclusions.

> In 82% of the studies, the conclusions were not supported by data. Let that sink in.

In high-quality studies, the results and conclusions were in agreement 16 times more often. High-quality studies concluded that vaccines are effective 25 times less often. Studies funded by the government were two times less likely to conclude that vaccines are effective. Industry-funded studies are more often published in prestigious medical journals, regardless of the quality of the study or the number of participants. The authors conclude that studies with conclusions in favor of vaccines are of significantly lower methodological quality [28].

In a 2006 article published in *the BMJ*, Tom Jefferson, the head of the Cochrane Vaccines Field, states that "Evidence from systematic reviews shows that inactivated vaccines have little or no effect. Most studies are of poor methodological quality. Little comparative evidence exists on the safety of these vaccines. Reasons for the current gap between policy and evidence are unclear, but given the huge resources involved, a re-evaluation should be urgently undertaken." Again, these are the thoughts expressed by the head of the Cochrane Vaccines Field. The very same one who believes that despite the lack of good-quality evidence, any further research on the topic of aluminum adjuvants is not recommended [29]. Because of his views, he was ostracized by his colleagues and had to have lunch by himself during a pandemic preparation conference [30].

Heterosubtypic Immunity

Infection with influenza type A virus increases the immune response to other, potentially more dangerous virus strains. This is called heterosubtypic immunity. Vaccination has the opposite effect. In a 2009 study, mice were vaccinated against seasonal influenza and then infected with pandemic avian influenza. The vaccinated mice died, but the unvaccinated mice survived. The authors conclude that during the next pandemic, children that received the annual flu shot would be at higher risk of developing severe illness and a fatal outcome [31].

In another study, some of the mice were infected with seasonal influenza, and a month later, all the mice were infected with lethal avian flu. Almost all mice that were previously infected with seasonal influenza survived. All the mice that were not previously infected died [32]. According to a study published in the journal *Science* in 2016, influenza in childhood provides profound, lifelong protection against severe infection and death from the more dangerous virus subtypes [33].

Original Antigenic Sin

Due to the influenza virus's constant mutation, the immune system response to it is subject to the "original antigenic sin" (this effect is described in detail in chapter 9). Upon encounter of a new virus strain, the immune system produces more antibodies against older viral strains at the expense of the response with novel, protective antibodies. This exacerbates the severity of the infection [34].

According to a 2011 study, vaccine effectiveness does not monotonically decrease with the antigenic distance between the vaccine strain and the circulating strain. The minimal vaccine effectiveness falls at some intermediate antigenic distance between the vaccine strain and the circulating strain. Since the vaccine effectiveness at this intermediate antigenic distance is lower than the effectiveness at a larger antigenic distance, the original antigenic sin may cause an increased susceptibility to the virus among the vaccinated [35]. This phenomenon may possibly explain why, during the years when the vaccine strain is predicted incorrectly, the vaccine is not only of little benefit but, in fact, exacerbates the severity of the disease [20]. Vaccine strain is correctly predicted in less than 50% of cases.

According to a 2008 study, if vaccination provides partial or imperfect immunity, it can significantly affect the mutation of the virus and accelerate its evolution. This has been demonstrated in chickens. Chickens vaccinated against influenza had two times more virus mutations compared to the unvaccinated chickens. The authors conclude that in seasons with high vaccination coverage, mutant strains of the virus should be expected [36].

Swine Flu

Seasonal influenza vaccination in 2009 increased the risk of pandemic swine flu infection by 2.5 times among children in Canada. These results were confirmed in five other studies [37]. This was also tested on ferrets. Some ferrets were vaccinated with a seasonal flu vaccine and then infected with the swine flu. It turned out that for the vaccinated ferrets, the flu was indeed more severe than for the unvaccinated ones [38].

Soldiers that received influenza vaccination in the previous season had a significantly higher risk of contracting the pandemic swine flu [39].

Young piglets that received influenza vaccination had significantly more complications when they were infected with the swine flu. The antibodies produced by the vaccine helped the new influenza strain penetrate the lungs [40].

The risk of narcolepsy among those vaccinated with the swine flu vaccine was 17 times higher compared to the unvaccinated [41]. These results were confirmed in two studies in England [42–43]. A similar Swedish study found increased psychiatric comorbidity in children and adolescents with narcolepsy caused by this vaccine [44].

Safety

A 2011 Dutch study found that annual vaccination against influenza hampers the development of the virus-specific CD8$^+$ T cell responses. The authors conclude that "This may render young children who have not previously been infected with an influenza virus more susceptible to infection with a pandemic influenza virus of a novel subtype" [45].

According to a 2017 study, vaccination against influenza during pregnancy increased the risk of miscarriage twofold in the next 28 days. Among those who were also vaccinated against swine flu in the last season, the risk of miscarriage was 7.7 times higher [46]. According to VAERS analysis, in the 2009–10 season, when two influenza vaccines had been used (seasonal and pandemic), the risk of miscarriage was 11 times higher compared to the 2008–9 season and six times higher compared to the 2010–11 season.

As proof of the safety of influenza vaccination during pregnancy, three studies are frequently cited. The first one involved 56 women, and the second one 180. In these studies, a thimerosal-free vaccine was used. The third study involved 2,291 women, but miscarriages were not included in the analysis. Medical literature reports that the mean rate of miscarriages after the flu vaccine is 1.9 per million pregnant women vaccinated. However, this data does not take into account that a negligible number of all side effects is registered in VAERS [47].

According to a 2017 study, the influenza vaccine during the first trimester of pregnancy was associated with an increase in the risk of autism by 20%. However, after correction for multiple testing, the statistical significance disappears, and the authors conclude that this association could be due to chance [48].

An Italian study found that influenza vaccine induced platelet activation and may transiently increase the risk of cardiovascular events [49].

Statistics

The CDC claims that around 36,000 Americans die from influenza every year. However, they also include pneumonia-related deaths into this statistic, even though pneumonia is not always caused by influenza. For example, antacids also increase the risk of pneumonia, but they are not included in the same statistics. According to the National Center for Health Statistics (which is part of the CDC), on average, influenza causes 1,348 deaths yearly.

Prior to 2003, the CDC stated that the annual death toll due to influenza was 20,000. Then the article was published in *JAMA*, which increased this number by 80% based on a statistical model, even though flu-related mortality in the '90s was 30% lower than in the '80s.

"In 2003, the demand for flu vaccines was low, 'the manufacturers were telling us that they weren't receiving a lot of orders for vaccine for use in November or even December' said Dr. Nowak, associate director for communications of the CDC's National Immunization Program, on NPR. 'It really did look like we needed to do something to encourage people to get a flu shot'" [50]. In his presentation, Dr. Nowak explains precisely how the media and medical experts should scare the population to increase vaccine coverage: "Fostering demand, particularly among people who don't routinely receive an annual influenza vaccination, requires creating concern, anxiety, and worry."

A 2005 US National Institutes of Health study of over 30 influenza seasons "could not correlate increasing vaccination coverage after 1980 with declining mortality rates in any age group" [51]. A 2013 article claims that influenza vaccines have a zero chance of benefitting most recipients since the majority of Americans do not annually contract influenza. **Only 7% of influenza-like illnesses are caused by influenza.** The retrospective studies quoted by the CDC may be heavily confounded by "healthy user bias" (the higher tendency for healthier people to get vaccinated compared to people who are less healthy). Given the current poor vaccine performance, influenza does not deserve to be called a "vaccine-preventable disease" [52].

In his 2013 article in *the BMJ*, the editor of the journal, Peter Doshi, writes: "Promotion of influenza vaccines is one of the most visible and aggressive public health policies today. Twenty years ago, in 1990, 32 million doses of influenza vaccine were available in the United States. Today around 135 million doses of influenza vaccine annually enter the US market, with vaccinations administered in drug stores, supermarkets — even some drive-throughs. This enormous growth has not been fueled by popular demand but instead by a public health campaign that delivers a straightforward, who-in-their-right-mind-could-possibly-disagree message: influenza is a serious disease, we are all at risk of complications from influenza, the flu shot is virtually risk free, and vaccination saves lives. Through this lens, the lack of influenza vaccine availability for all 315 million US citizens seems to border on the unethical. Yet across the country, mandatory influenza vaccination policies have cropped up, particularly in healthcare facilities, precisely because not everyone wants the vaccination, and compulsion appears the only way to achieve high vaccination rates. Closer examination of influenza vaccine policies shows that although proponents employ the rhetoric of science, the studies underlying the policy are often of low quality, and do not substantiate officials' claims. The vaccine might be less beneficial and less safe than has been claimed, and the threat of influenza appears overstated."

> In 1960, the CDC recommended vaccination only for the elderly. In 1984, they began to recommend the vaccination for healthcare workers, and in 1987 those who lived in the same house as the elderly got included in the campaign. In 1997, vaccination of pregnant women in the second and third trimesters started. In 2000, vaccination of people over 50 years of age. In 2004, vaccination was introduced for pregnant women in the first trimester, children at the age of six months to two years, as well as anyone who comes into contact with them. In 2006, the recommendation expanded to include children under five years of age and anyone in contact with them. In 2008, the vaccination was introduced for all children under 18 years of age, and for the rest of the population in 2010, except for infants under six months old.

Based on the observational study that was funded by the National Vaccine Program Office and the CDC, the CDC claims that influenza vaccine reduces all-cause mortality in the elderly by 48%. "If true, these statistics indicate that influenza vaccines can save more lives than any other single licensed medicine on the planet. Perhaps there is a reason CDC does not shout this from the rooftop: it's too good to be true. Since at least 2005, non-CDC researchers have pointed out the seeming impossibility that influenza vaccines could be preventing 50% of all deaths from all causes when influenza is estimated to only cause around 5% of all wintertime deaths.

"If the observational studies cannot be trusted, what evidence is there that influenza vaccines reduce deaths of older people — the reason the policy was originally created? Virtually none. There has only been one randomized trial of influenza vaccines in older people — conducted two decades ago — and it showed no mortality benefit. This means that influenza vaccines are approved for use in older people despite any clinical trials demonstrating a reduction in serious outcomes. Approval is instead tied to a demonstrated ability of the vaccine to induce antibody production, without any evidence that those antibodies translate into reductions in illness." And since today, the influenza vaccine is a standard of care thanks to the CDC's guidelines, it would be unethical to conduct placebo-controlled trials at this point [53].

In 2002 the CDC started encouraging vaccination of children between six months and two years old; in 2004, this encouragement turned into a recommendation. From that point on, a child receives two doses of the vaccine during the first year of his life. In 2009 children received an additional vaccine against swine flu. Below is a graph of influenza-related mortality in children under five years old in 1996–2014.

From the graph of influenza-related deaths in children under five years old, it could be argued that influenza vaccination has led to an increase in mortality from influenza.

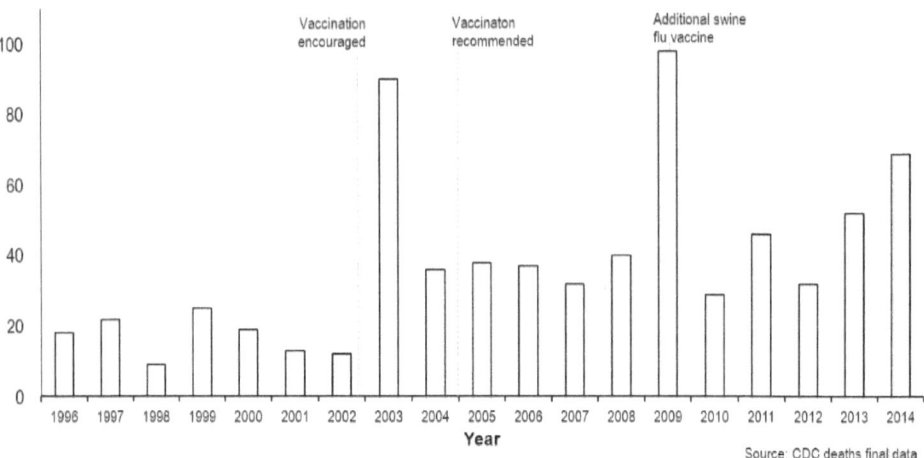

Influenza death cases among children in the US (1996-2014)

Source: CDC deaths final data

In 2010, the recommendation was extended to all people over six months old. From the graph of influenza-related deaths in all age groups, it can be concluded that influenza vaccination has led to an increase in mortality from influenza.

Influenza death cases in the US (1996-2014)

Source: CDC deaths final data

To put things into perspective, more than 3,000 people in the United States die every year from malnutrition, 40,000 from poisoning, 30,000 from alcohol, 50,000 from drugs, 40,000 from suicide, 80,000 from diabetes, 90,000 from Alzheimer's, and 200,000–400,000 from medical errors [54].

According to VAERS, more than 900 people have died after the flu shot since 2000, and more than 2,700 have become permanently disabled. Given that only 1–10% of serious side effects are reported in VAERS, it is plausible that the flu vaccine took the lives of more people than the flu.

Influenza Benefits, Treatment, And Prevention

In a study conducted in six countries, those who reported a history of infectious diseases (e.g., colds, flu) showed a 30% reduction in the risk of glioma (brain tumor) development [55].

The authors of a 2015 review concluded that "Biased, poor-quality, mostly unpublished evidence suggests that Tamiflu and Relenza shorten the duration of influenza symptoms by 0.6 to 0.7 of a day. Pneumonia and hospitalizations rates are not decreased. These products are not recommended if symptoms have lasted longer than 48 hours" [56]. Mortality risk 12 hours after taking Tamiflu was 1.9 times higher than after taking Relenza, and the risk of complications was six times higher [57]. According to a systematic review of eight animal studies, antipyretics (aspirin, paracetamol, diclofenac) taken during influenza increase mortality by 34% [58].

In a small, randomized, double-blind, placebo-controlled trial of treatment of influenza with elderberry extract, it was shown that elderberry extract shortened the duration of influenza by four days compared to the placebo [59]. For comparison, Tamiflu shortens influenza by 17 hours, at the same time increasing the risk of psychiatric complications and renal insufficiency. However, governments spend millions of dollars to stock up on Tamiflu, and nobody is stocking up on the elderberry.

Megadoses of vitamin C (1g every hour for six hours, then thrice a day) administered before or after the appearance of cold and flu symptoms reduced the symptoms by 85% [60]. There is strong evidence that large doses of zinc contribute to the reduction of common cold duration [61]. Some probiotics also contribute to a reduction in the incidence of influenza [62].

Vitamin D

There are many hypotheses as to why respiratory infections are so widespread only during a certain season: low temperatures, dry air, crowding together indoors in winter, traveling patterns, seasonality of ultraviolet (UV) radiation from the sun that might kill pathogens, circannual rhythms of hormones like the "dark hormone" melatonin, etc. Authors of a 2009 study analyzed the annual death numbers of influenza and pneumonia in Norway for the time period of 1980–2000 and compared them with UVB radiation level and vitamin D levels produced by it.

> Influenza-related mortality starts to increase two months after the vitamin D levels have reached their minimum. This, however, may be caused by the fact that disease usually starts weeks prior to death.

Generally, there is no distinct seasonal pattern of influenza in the tropics, but starting from latitudes between 20 and 30 degrees north, distinct seasons of influenza are present. This seems surprising at first sight. However, at 25 degrees north, the rate of vitamin D synthesis in human skin in late June is about five times larger than in late December. Authors conclude that high numbers of winter influenza and pneumonia deaths are related to low vitamin D levels in this season [63]. In a British study winter, mortality was inversely related to hours of sunlight. Every additional hour of sunlight reduced mortality by 2.9%. Mortality from the respiratory diseases showed the greatest decrease due to sunshine [64]. According to a systematic review and meta-analysis of 11 studies, vitamin D reduces the risk of respiratory tract infections by 36% [65].

Conclusions

Numerous studies have established that influenza vaccine effectiveness is very low and that due to the effects of the heterosubtypic immunity and the original antigenic sin, its effectiveness can even become negative, especially for those who are vaccinated year after year.

Influenza mortality statistics are artificially overestimated and distorted.

The vast majority of acute respiratory infections are caused not by influenza, but by other viruses.

Endnotes

1. Harding AT et al. Rationally designed influenza virus vaccines that are antigenically stable during growth in eggs. *mBio*. 2017;8(3)

2. Buckland BC. The development and manufacture of influenza vaccines. *Hum Vaccin Immunother*. 2015;11(6):1357-60

3. Influenza. CDC Pink Book

4. Rondy M et al. Low 2016/17 season vaccine effectiveness against hospitalised influenza A(H3N2) among elderly: awareness warranted for 2017/18 season. *Euro Surveill*. 2017;22(41)

5. Skowronski DM et al. A perfect storm: impact of genomic variation and serial vaccination on low influenza vaccine effectiveness during the 2014-2015 season. *Clin Infect Dis*. 2016;63(1):21-32

6. McLean HQ et al. Impact of repeated vaccination on vaccine effectiveness against influenza A(H3N2) and B during 8 seasons. *Clin Infect Dis*. 2014;59(10):1375-85

7. Ohmit SE et al. Influenza vaccine effectiveness in the community and the household. *Clin Infect Dis*. 2013;56(10):1363-9

8. Khurana S et al. Repeat vaccination reduces antibody affinity maturation across different influenza vaccine platforms in humans. *Nat Commun*. 2019;10(1):3338

9. Black SB et al. Effectiveness of influenza vaccine during pregnancy in preventing hospitalizations and outpatient visits for respiratory illness in pregnant women and their infants. *Am J Perinatol*. 2004;21(6):333-9

10. France E et al. Impact of maternal influenza vaccination during pregnancy on the incidence of acute respiratory illness visits among infants. *Arch Pediatr Adolesc Med*. 2006;160(12):1277-83

11. Simonsen L et al. Impact of influenza vaccination on seasonal mortality in the US elderly population. *Arch Intern Med*. 2005;165(3):265-72

12. Simonsen L et al. Influenza vaccination and mortality benefits: new insights, new opportunities. *Vaccine*. 2009;27(45):6300-4

13. Anderson ML et al. The effect of influenza vaccination for the elderly on hospitalization and mortality: an observational study with a regression discontinuity design. *Ann Intern Med*. 2020;172(7):445-52

14. Abramson ZH. What, in fact, is the evidence that vaccinating healthcare workers against seasonal influenza protects their patients? A critical review. *Int J Family Med*. 2012;2012:205464

15. De Serres G et al. Influenza vaccination of healthcare workers: critical analysis of the evidence for patient benefit underpinning policies of enforcement. *PloS One*. 2017;12(1):e0163586

16. Joshi AY et al. Effectiveness of trivalent inactivated influenza vaccine in influenza-related hospitalization in children: a case-control study. *Allergy Asthma Proc*. 2012; 33(2):e23-7

17. Cowling BJ et al. Increased risk of noninfluenza respiratory virus infections associated with receipt of inactivated influenza vaccine. *Clin Infect Dis*. 2012;54(12):1778-83

18. Dierig A et al. Epidemiology of respiratory viral infections in children enrolled in a study of influenza vaccine effectiveness. *Influenza Other Respir Viruses.* 2014;8(3):293-301

19. Yan J et al. Infectious virus in exhaled breath of symptomatic seasonal influenza cases from a college community. *PNAS.* 2018;115(5):1081-6

20. Bridges CB et al. Effectiveness and cost-benefit of influenza vaccination of healthy working adults: a randomized controlled trial. *JAMA.* 2000;284(13):1655-63

21. King JC et al. Effectiveness of school-based influenza vaccination. *N Engl J Med.* 2006; 355(24):2523-32

22. McLean HQ et al. Influenza vaccination and risk of hospitalization among adults with laboratory confirmed influenza illness. *Vaccine.* 2014;32(4):453-7

23. Rikin S et al. Assessment of temporally-related acute respiratory illness following influenza vaccination. *Vaccine.* 2018;36(15):1958-64

24. Jefferson T et al. Vaccines for preventing influenza in healthy children. *Cochrane Database Syst Rev.* 2012(8):CD004879

25. Demicheli V et al. Vaccines for preventing influenza in healthy adults. *Cochrane Database Syst Rev.* 2014(3):CD001269

26. Jefferson T et al. Vaccines for preventing influenza in the elderly. *Cochrane Database Syst Rev.* 2010(2):CD004876

27. Thomas RE et al. Influenza vaccination for healthcare workers who care for people aged 60 or older living in long-term care institutions. *Cochrane Database Syst Rev.* 2016(6):CD005187

28. Jefferson T et al. Relation of study quality, concordance, take home message, funding, and impact in studies of influenza vaccines: systematic review. *BMJ.* 2009;338:b354

29. Jefferson T. Influenza vaccination: policy versus evidence. *BMJ* 2006;333(7574):912-5

30. Brownlee S et al. Does the Vaccine Matter? *The Atlantic.* 2009 Nov

31. Bodewes R et al. Vaccination against human influenza A/H3N2 virus prevents the induction of heterosubtypic immunity against lethal infection with avian influenza A/H5N1 virus. *PloS One.* 2009;4(5):e5538

32. Kreijtz JH et al. Infection of mice with a human influenza A/H3N2 virus induces protective immunity against lethal infection with influenza A/H5N1 virus. *Vaccine.* 2009;27(36):4983-9

33. Gostic KM et al. Potent protection against H5N1 and H7N9 influenza via childhood hemagglutinin imprinting. *Science.* 2016;354(6313):722-6

34. Kim JH et al. Original antigenic sin responses to influenza viruses. *J Immunol.* 2009;183(5):3294-301

35. Pan K. Understanding original antigenic sin in influenza with a dynamical system. *PloS One.* 2011;6(8):e23910

36. Boni MF. Vaccination and antigenic drift in influenza. *Vaccine.* 2008;26 Suppl 3:C8-14

37. Janjua NZ et al. Seasonal influenza vaccine and increased risk of pandemic A/H1N1-related illness: first detection of the association in British Columbia, Canada. *Clin Infect Dis.* 2010;51(9):1017-27

38. Skowronski DM et al. Randomized controlled ferret study to assess the direct impact of 2008-09 trivalent inactivated influenza vaccine on A(H1N1)pdm09 disease risk. *PloS One.* 2014;9(1):e86555

39. Crum-Cianflone NF et al. Clinical and epidemiologic characteristics of an outbreak of novel H1N1 (swine origin) influenza A virus among United States military beneficiaries. *CLin Infect Dis.* 2009;49(12):1801-10

40. Khurana S et al. Vaccine-induced anti-HA2 antibodies promote virus fusion and enhance influenza virus respiratory disease. *Sci Transl Med.* 2013;5(200):200ra114

41. Trogstad L et al. Narcolepsy and hypersomnia in Norwegian children and young adults following the influenza A(H1N1) 2009 pandemic. *Vaccine.* 2017;35(15):1879-85

42. Stowe J et al. Risk of narcolepsy after AS03 adjuvanted pandemic A/H1N1 2009 influenza vaccine in adults: a case-coverage study in England. *Sleep.* 2016;39(5):1051-7

43. Miller E et al. Risk of narcolepsy in children and young people receiving AS03 adjuvanted pandemic A/H1N1 2009 influenza iaccine: retrospective analysis. *BMJ.* 2013;346:f794

44. Szakács A et al. Psychiatric comorbidity and cognitive profile in children with narcolepsy with or without association to the H1N1 influenza vaccination. *Sleep.* 2015; 38(4):615-21

45. Bodewes R et al. Annual vaccination against influenza virus hampers development of virus-specific CD8+ T cell immunity in children. *J Virol.* 2011;85(22):11995-2000

46. Donahue JG et al. Association of spontaneous abortion with receipt of inactivated influenza vaccine containing H1N1pdm09 in 2010-11 and 2011-12. *Vaccine.* 2017; 35(40):5314-22

47. Goldman GS. Comparison of VAERS fetal-loss reports during three consecutive influenza seasons: was there a synergistic fetal toxicity associated with the two-vaccine 2009/2010 season? *Hum Exp Toxicol.* 2013;32(5):464-75

48. Zerbo O et al. Association Between Influenza Infection and Vaccination During Pregnancy and Risk of Autism Spectrum Disorder. *JAMA Pediatr.* 2017;171(1):e163609

49. Lanza GA et al. Inflammation-related effects of adjuvant influenza A vaccination on platelet activation and cardiac autonomic function. *J Intern Med.* 2011;269(1):118-25

50. Doshi P. Are US flu death figures more PR than science? *BMJ.* 2005;331:1412

51. Doshi P. Trends in recorded influenza mortality: United States, 1900-2004. *Am J Public Health.* 2008;98(5):939-45

52. Doshi P. Influenza vaccines: time for a rethink. *JAMA Intern Med.* 2013;173(11):1014-6

53. Doshi P. Influenza: marketing vaccine by marketing disease. *BMJ.* 2013;346:f3037

54. Makary MA et al. Medical error-the third leading cause of death in the US. *BMJ.* 2016; 353:i2139

55. Schlehofer B et al. Role of medical history in brain tumour development. Results from the international adult brain tumour study. *Int J Cancer.* 1999;82(2):155-60

56. Korownyk C et al. Antiviral medications for influenza. *Can Fam Physician.* 2015;61(4):351

57. Hama R et al. Oseltamivir and early deterioration leading to death: a proportional mortality study for 2009A/H1N1 influenza. *Int J Risk Saf Med.* 2011;23(4):201-15

58. Eyers S et al. The effect on mortality of antipyretics in the treatment of influenza infection: systematic review and meta-analysis. *J R Soc Med.* 2010;103(10):403-11

59. Zakay-Rones Z et al. Randomized study of the efficacy and safety of oral elderberry extract in the treatment of influenza A and B virus infections. *J Int Med Res.* 2004; 32(2):132-40

60. Gorton HC et al. The effectiveness of vitamin C in preventing and relieving the symptoms of virus-induced respiratory infections. *J Manipulative Physiol Ther.* 1999; 22(8):530-3

61. Hemilä H. Zinc lozenges may shorten the duration of colds: a systematic review. *Open Respir Med J.* 2011;5:51-8

62. Waki N et al. Oral administration of Lactobacillus brevis KB290 to mice alleviates clinical symptoms following influenza virus infection. *Lett Appl Microbiol.* 2014;58(1):87-93

63. Moan J et al. Influenza, solar radiation and vitamin D. *Dermatoendocrinol.* 2009;1(6):307-9

64. Cannell JJ et al. Epidemic influenza and vitamin D. *Epidemiol Infect.* 2006;134(6):1129-40

65. Bergman P et al. Vitamin D and respiratory tract infections: a systematic review and meta-analysis of randomized controlled trials. *PloS One.* 2013;8(6):e65835

Chapter Eighteen

HAEMOPHILUS INFLUENZAE (HIB)

In a time of universal deceit,
telling the truth is a revolutionary act.
— George Orwell

H aemophilus influenzae, pneumococcus, and meningococcus are the three main types of bacteria that can cause meningitis and other invasive diseases. Bacterial meningitis, unlike viral meningitis, can be very dangerous.

Haemophilus influenzae is a bacterium, which was initially believed to be the cause of influenza (hence the name). The bacterium forms a polysaccharide capsule around itself. There are six serotypes of H. influenzae (*a-f*) that differ by capsule type. The vaccine exists only for serotype *b* (Hib), which caused 95% of H. influenzae infections in the pre-vaccine era. There are also noncapsulated strains. According to the CDC, one in 200 children developed invasive Hib disease in the pre-vaccine era. Hib was isolated from the nasopharynx of 0.5–3% of healthy infants and children but was not common in adults. Almost all cases of H. influenzae occurred in children under five years of age, and two-thirds occurred in children under 18 months of age. Invasive infection can cause meningitis, epiglottitis, pneumonia, arthritis, and cellulitis. The fatality rate of meningitis is 3–6%, while neurologic consequences are observed in 15–30% of survivors. The exact mechanism of bacterial invasion of the bloodstream is unknown. In the pre-vaccine era, most children acquired natural immunity by five to six years of age through asymptomatic infection by Hib bacteria.

The first Hib vaccine (polysaccharide) was used from 1985 to 1988, but was ineffective. A *conjugate* vaccine has been used since 1988 [1]. Conjugate vaccines are a special category of vaccines. The H. influenzae bacterium capsule is a carbohydrate (polysaccharide). Creating an effective polysaccharide vaccine turned out to be impossible since the immune system does not develop antibodies to carbohydrates very well. To solve this problem, a protein was attached to the polysaccharide (diphtheria or tetanus toxoids are usually used for that), and in that way, the immune system develops carbohydrate antibodies together with the protein antibodies. Other conjugate vaccines are pneumococcal and meningococcal vaccines. All of them contain aluminum.

Risk Factors

Breastfeeding has a protective effect from Hib meningitis, which lasts for five to ten years. A short breastfeeding period (less than 13 weeks) increases the risk of Hib almost fourfold. It has been shown that breast milk has an inhibiting effect on the attachment of bacteria to the nasopharyngeal mucosa. In Sweden, following a decrease in the number of breast-fed infants, the incidence of Hib increased, and when their percentage increased again, the incidence of Hib decreased [2]. Among children over one year of age, a short breastfeeding period is associated with an eightfold increase in the risk of Hib. Each additional week of breastfeeding decreased the risk of Hib by 5%. The protective effect of breastfeeding begins from 13 weeks of exclusive breastfeeding and lasts for months and years [3]. The protective effect of breastfeeding against Hib infection has been identified in other studies. Among children under the age of six months, exclusive breastfeeding is associated with a 90% decrease in the risk of Hib. Attending daycare, previous hospitalizations, and passive smoking are associated with an increased Hib risk. Other risk factors include crowding, low socioeconomic status, low parental education levels, several chronic diseases, and chemotherapy [1].

Effectiveness And Strain Replacement

Polysaccharide Hib vaccine was licensed in the US in 1985. A clinical trial in Finland found that the vaccine is not efficacious in children under the age of two years and has 80% efficacy for two- to three-year-olds. Prior to licensing, the only efficacy study on 16,000 children in the US did not prove the vaccine to be effective. The vaccine was thus licensed based on the Finnish efficacy data, only for children over two years of age, even though most cases occurred in children under one year of age. Once the vaccine was licensed, conducting a randomized study turned out to be impossible. However, since Hib is a rare disease, conducting this kind of study is difficult anyway, as it requires many participants. An observational study in Minnesota found that the effectiveness of this vaccine is negative, and it increases the risk of H. influenzae by 58%. Other studies have found that the vaccine increases the risk of H. influenzae in the first week after vaccination [4].

The conjugate vaccine is quite effective against serotype *b*, but as in the case of HPV, vaccine strains simply get replaced by other strains and other bacteria. The next chapter will show that the decrease in the incidence of Hib caused an increase in the incidence of pneumococcus. Following that, vaccination against pneumococcus was introduced in 2000, which, in turn, increased the incidence of H. influenzae and streptococcus.

Hib incidence in Manitoba (Canada) decreased due to vaccination, but then it began to increase again, and in 2006 already reached the pre-vaccine level. If previously only 10% of cases were in those over ten years old, now 56% of invasive disease cases occur in individuals aged ten and over. Similar changes in epidemiology are also observed in the US. The authors compared their research data to the official incidence data and found that only three in 17 Hib cases between 2000–2004 were officially registered. They conclude that Hib incidence rate is significantly underestimated and that the incidence of infection with other H. influenzae serotypes is, most likely, also underestimated [5].

In Ontario, another Canadian province, vaccination led to a 57% decrease in the Hib incidence by 2007, but the incidence of infections with serotype *f* (Hif) increased by three times, and with noncapsulated strains by 2.4 times. Hib incidence decreased by 7% annually in children under the age of five, and the incidence of noncapsulated strains increased by 7% annually in children of five to 19 years of age. Overall, the incidence of H. influenzae virtually did not change [6]. By 2015, serotype *a* (Hia) incidence in Ontario was already 76% higher than the incidence of Hib in the pre-vaccine era [7]. In 1989, before Hib conjugate vaccines were introduced in Canada, 24 cases of invasive Hib were reported in the province of British Columbia. In 2008–2009, 45–53 cases a year were reported. Serotype *b* incidence decreased, and serotype *a* incidence increased. Previously, mostly children got infected, but now adults are getting the disease as well [8].

After the introduction of vaccination, Hib incidence among adults in England decreased, but the overall incidence of H. influenzae infections increased due to a sharp increase in the incidence of noncapsulated strains, especially among the elderly [9]. After Hib incidence among adults reached its low point in 1998, it started to increase again and reached pre-vaccine levels by 2003. The level of Hib antibodies in adults decreased after the introduction of the vaccine. The same happened among children. At first, Hib incidence decreased sharply but then began to increase sharply, despite the high vaccination coverage. The number of cases among children has been doubling every year since 1998, and most of the cases occur among those fully vaccinated [10].

One year after the introduction of vaccination in Brazil, Hib meningitis incidence decreased by 69%. However, the incidence of H. influenzae type *a* (Hia) meningitis increased eightfold. Clinically, the virulence of Hia strains was indistinguishable from that of Hib [11]. Before the introduction of the vaccine, Hib incidence in Alaska was the highest in the world. It decreased sharply due to vaccination, but H. influenzae incidence of other serotypes increased, mostly of serotype *a* and of noncapsulated strains [12].

The incidence of Hib cases in Illinois between 1996 and 2004 increased by 2.5 times overall, and by 3.5 times among the elderly. The number of cases of infection with noncapsulated strains increased by 657%. In 1996, noncapsulated strains were responsible for 17% of cases, whereas in 2004, they were already responsible for 71% of the cases [13]. However, after the introduction of vaccination in Israel, H. influenzae incidence decreased by 90% by 1996 and remained low in the subsequent years [14].

Hib incidence in the Netherlands decreased substantially after the introduction of the vaccine and reached a minimum in 1999, but then started to increase again. This is probably because "natural boosting" became less common due to the disappearance of bacteria, which leads to a decrease in immunity and an increase in susceptibility to the invasive infection [15]. According to another theory, it could also be because vaccination destroyed strains with a thin capsule and left strains with a thicker capsule [16].

The graph of the H. influenzae incidence in the US is also indicative. The incidence has been decreasing until the mid-90s, after which it has been steadily increasing.

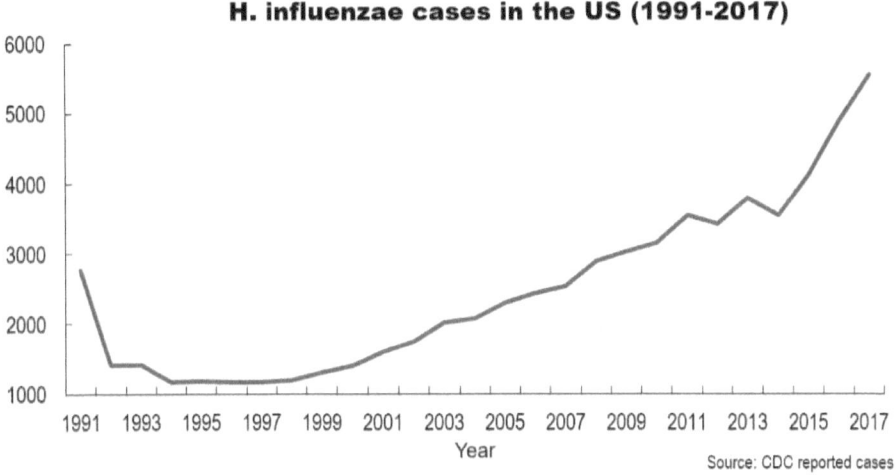

H. influenzae cases in the US (1991-2017)

Source: CDC reported cases

Safety

In a clinical trial in Finland (116,000 children), Hib vaccine was associated with a 26% increase in the risk of type 1 diabetes. Diabetes developed 38 months after vaccination. The vaccine was also tested on mice prone to diabetes. Vaccinated mice developed diabetes at a higher rate compared to the control group. Other studies found a similar increased risk of diabetes, but since these studies were small, the results were not statistically significant [17]. In an article published in *BMJ*, it is claimed that just this adverse effect alone (increased risk of type 1 diabetes) exceeds the benefit of the vaccine, which should prevent seven deaths and seven to 26 disability cases per 100,000 vaccinated. Instead, the vaccine adds 31 children with diabetes for every 100,000 vaccinated.

After the introduction of Hib vaccination in the US and England, diabetes incidence increased dramatically, especially among children under four. The authors conclude that the potential risk of the vaccine exceeds the potential benefit [18]. Hib vaccine increases the risk of development of GAD autoantibodies sixfold, and the risk of IA-2 autoantibodies development threefold. These autoantibodies are considered to be autoimmune markers of the development of type-1 diabetes [19].

According to VAERS, more than 1,900 people died after receiving the vaccine between 1991 to 2010, and about 1,200 people became permanently disabled (this is just 1–10% of all cases). One hundred sixty people died from all serotypes of H. influenzae during the same period [20].

According to a British study, the DPT-Hib vaccine often leads to cardiorespiratory events in preterm infants, especially if the vaccine is given before the age of 70 days. Adverse events were reported in 38% of infants [21]. In another study, DPT and Hib vaccines increased the risk of apnea (respiratory arrest) and bradycardia (decreased heart rate) in preterm infants [22]. A Swiss study claims that the Hib vaccine sometimes causes Guillain-Barré syndrome [23].

A 1990 study found that the risk of Hib infection during the first week after vaccination increases by six times. According to the CDC study, the risk of Hib in the first week after vaccination increases by 1.8 times [24]. This happens because the antibody titers decrease two to three days after the vaccination, and then increase again on day seven post-vaccination [25]. That is, in case of an asymptomatic Hib infection, vaccination can cause an invasive infection. The term "negative phase" was introduced in 1901 to describe the decrease in bactericidal activity, which was observed for 21 days after typhoid vaccination. This phenomenon was also observed in clinical trials of conjugate and non-conjugate Hib vaccines: for those who already had Hib antibodies, the concentration of antibodies decreased after vaccination. This phenomenon is believed to occur with all four of the existing vaccines. It is believed that the decrease in the number of antibodies happens because the existing antibodies get attached to vaccine antigens. If this happens during asymptomatic colonization, the risk of invasive disease increases [26].

Conclusions

An invasive H. influenzae infection is a dangerous, but very rare and opportunistic infection. That is, the bacterium itself is harmless, but becomes dangerous if there is an immune deficiency.

A longer breastfeeding period significantly decreases the risk of infection.

Vaccination is effective against serotype *b*, but this has led to the replacement of vaccine strain with other serotypes, and as a result, the overall incidence of invasive infections has not decreased and may have even increased.

Endnotes

1. Haemophilus influenzae type b. *CDC Pink Book*

2. Silfverdal SA et al. Protective effect of breastfeeding: an ecologic study of Haemophilus influenzae meningitis and breastfeeding in a Swedish population. *Int J Epidemiol*. 1999;28(1):152-6

3. Silfverdal SA et al. Protective effect of breastfeeding on invasive Haemophilus influenzae infection: a case-control study in Swedish preschool children. *Int J Epidemiol*. 1997;26(2):443-50

4. Osterholm MT et al. Lack of efficacy of Haemophilus b polysaccharide vaccine in Minnesota. *JAMA*. 1988;260(10):1423-8

5. Tsang RS et al. Characterization of invasive Haemophilus influenzae disease in Manitoba, Canada, 2000-2006: invasive disease due to non-type b strains. *Clin Infect Dis*. 2007;44(12):1611-4

6. Adam HJ et al. Changing epidemiology of invasive Haemophilus influenzae in Ontario, Canada: evidence for herd effects and strain replacement due to Hib vaccination. *Vaccine*. 2010;28(24):4073-8

7. Eton V et al. Epidemiology of invasive pneumococcal and Haemophilus influenzae diseases in Northwestern Ontario, Canada, 2010-2015. *Int J Infect Dis*. 2017;65:27-33

8. Shuel M et al. Invasive Haemophilus influenzae in British Columbia: non-Hib and non-typeable strains causing disease in children and adults. *Int J Infect Dis*. 2011;15(3):e167-73

9. Sarangi J et al. Invasive Haemophilus influenzae disease in adults. *Epidemiol Infect*. 2000;124(3):441-7

10. McVernon J et al. Trends in Haemophilus influenzae type b infections in adults in England and Wales: surveillance study. *BMJ*. 2004;329(7467):655-8

11. Ribeiro GS et al. Prevention of Haemophilus influenzae type b (Hib) meningitis and emergence of serotype replacement with type a strains after introduction of Hib immunization in Brazil. *J Infect Dis*. 2003;187(1):109-16

12. Bruce MG et al. Haemophilus influenzae serotype a invasive disease, Alaska, USA, 1983-2011. *Emerg Infect Dis*. 2013;19(6):932-7

13. Dworkin MS et al. The changing epidemiology of invasive Haemophilus influenzae disease, especially in persons > or = 65 years old. *Clin Infect Dis*. 2007;44(6):810-6

14. Bamberger EE et al. Pediatric invasive Haemophilus influenzae infections in Israel in the era of Haemophilus influenzae type b vaccine: a nationwide prospective study. *Pediatr Infect Dis J*. 2014;33(5):477-81

15. Spanjaard L et al. Increase in the number of invasive Haemophilus influenzae type b infections. *Ned Tijdschr Geneeskd*. 2005;149(49):2738-42

16. Schouls L et al. Two variants among Haemophilus influenzae serotype b strains with distinct bcs4, hcsA and hcsB genes display differences in expression of the polysaccharide capsule. *BMC Microbiol*. 2008;8:35

17. Classen JB et al. Clustering of cases of insulin dependent diabetes (IDDM) occurring three years after hemophilus influenza B (HiB) immunization support causal relationship between immunization and IDDM. *Autoimmunity*. 2002;35(4):247-53

18. Classen JB et al. Association between type 1 diabetes and hib vaccine. Causal relation is likely. *BMJ*. 1999;319(7217):1133

19. Wahlberg J et al. Vaccinations may induce diabetes-related autoantibodies in one-year-old children. *Ann N Y Acad Sci*. 2003;1005:404-8

20. Reported Cases and Deaths from Vaccine Preventable Diseases, United States.

21. Sen S et al. Adverse events following vaccination in premature infants. *Acta Paediatr*. 2001;90(8):916-20

22. Sánchez PJ et al. Apnea after immunization of preterm infants. *J Pediatr*. 1997; 130(5):746-51

23. Gervaix A et al. Guillain-Barré syndrome following immunisation with Haemophilus influenzae type b conjugate vaccine. *Eur J Pediatr*. 1993;152(7):613-4

24. Sood SK et al. Disease caused by Haemophilus influenzae type b in the immediate period after homologous immunization: immunologic investigation. *Pediatrics*. 1990;85(4 Pt 2):698-704

25. Daum RS et al. Serum anticapsular antibody response in the first week after immunization of adults and infants with the Haemophilus influenzae type b-Neisseria meningitidis outer membrane protein complex conjugate vaccine. *J Infect Dis*. 1991; 164(6):1154-9

26. Greenberg-Kushnir N et al. Haemophilus influenzae type b meningitis in the short period after vaccination: a reminder of the phenomenon of apparent vaccine failure. *Case Rep Infect Dis*. 2012;2012:950107

Chapter Nineteen

PNEUMOCOCCUS

If I were to remain silent, I'd be guilty of complicity.
— **Albert Einstein**

P neumococcus is a common bacterium that, like H. influenzae, can lead to meningitis and other invasive diseases. After the introduction of the vaccine against Hib, the incidence of H. influenzae temporarily decreased, and the incidence of pneumococcal infection increased. However, if the fatality rate of H. influenzae meningitis is 3%, the fatality rate of pneumococcal meningitis is 19% [1].

According to the CDC, pneumococcus (Streptococcus pneumoniae) lives in the nasopharynx of 5–90% of healthy people. Among school-aged children, 20–60% may be colonized, among military personnel 50–60%, and among adults without children, 5–10% may be colonized. S. pneumoniae can lead to pneumonia, bacteremia, and meningitis. Accurate statistics on pneumococcus are not collected, but it is estimated that every year 400,000 people are hospitalized with pneumococcal pneumonia (fatality rate 5–7%), 12,000 with bacteremia (fatality rate 20%, and 60% among the elderly), and 3,000–6,000 with meningitis (fatality rate 8% among children and 22% among adults). There are 92 serotypes of pneumococcus. The ten most common serotypes are estimated to account for 62% of invasive disease worldwide. The first pneumococcal conjugate vaccine was licensed in 2000 and included seven serotypes. In 2010, a vaccine against 13 serotypes was licensed. There is also a 23-valent polysaccharide pneumococcal vaccine (licensed in 1983) that is used today for the elderly. The vaccine contains aluminum and polysorbate 80 [2].

Risk Factors

Breastfeeding is associated with a 73% reduction in the risk of invasive pneumococcal disease [3]. Infants who were not breastfed were 17 times more likely to be admitted to hospital with pneumonia (not only of pneumococcal type) than those being exclusively breastfed. Among non-breastfed infants under three months old, the risk was 61 times higher [4].

Smoking is associated with a fourfold increase in the risk of invasive pneumococcal disease in adults and passive smoking with a 2.5-fold increase [5]. Diabetes increases the risk by 3.4 times, chronic heart disease by six times, cancer by 23 times, AIDS by 48 times, and alcohol abuse by 11 times. The risk of death from pneumococcal infection in patients with a chronic condition is two to eight times higher [6]. The use of antibiotics is associated with an increased subsequent risk of pneumococcal infection, as well as H. influenzae infection, meningitis, Staphylococcus aureus skin infections, Salmonella and Campylobacter, typhoid fever, recurrent boils, mastitis, respiratory infections, and urinary tract infections [7].

In a study in Texas, people with low income suffered from invasive infections two times more often than people with medium income, and three times more often than people with high income [8]. Similar results were obtained in a study in Maryland. African Americans get pneumococcal infection three times more often than white Americans. Among patients aged 18 years and older, the median age of African Americans with invasive pneumococcal infections was 27 years less than that of whites. AIDS increases the risk of pneumococcal infection by 100–300 times. The authors conclude that it is necessary to provide pneumococcal vaccine to young adults in poor urban areas with a high HIV prevalence. However, it is difficult to vaccinate only risk groups. This approach has failed with hepatitis B vaccination, which necessitated a shift in policy towards universal immunization [9].

In the US, the incidence of invasive pneumococcal infection among children under six years of age is three to eight times higher than in Europe. This difference arises because US practice guidelines recommend blood culture (and antibiotics) for all children aged three to 36 months with a fever of 39°C (102.2°F) or greater and elevated white blood cell counts, while in Europe a similar test is usually done only for hospitalized children. Since most cases of invasive pneumococcal infection are in the form of temporary bacteremia that does not require hospitalization, they are, for the most part, not diagnosed in European countries [10].

Pneumococcus And Haemophilus Influenzae

Between 1992 and 1994, the incidence of pneumococcal infection in Finland increased by two times among children under two years of age and three times among children under 16 years of age. The authors attribute this to the disappearance of Hib [11]. In 1994, 22% of pneumococcal pneumonia cases in the United States were accompanied by complications. In 1999, the number of pneumonia cases with complications increased to 53% [12].

During five years after the introduction of Hib vaccination, the incidence of pneumococcal bacteremia in Philadelphia doubled (from 38 to 73 cases per year), the incidence of H. influenzae bacteremia has decreased from 34 to nine cases per year, and the incidence of meningococcal bacteremia has not changed (three cases per year). The incidence of pneumococcal meningitis increased by 50%, the incidence of H. influenzae meningitis has decreased by 70%, and the incidence of meningococcal meningitis has not changed [13].

In vitro, pneumococcus has a bactericidal effect on the H. influenzae bacteria. Pneumococcus produces hydrogen peroxide, which kills the H. influenzae. Pneumococcus also has an inhibitory effect on the meningococcus, which also dies when exposed to hydrogen peroxide. Other bacteria that produce hydrogen peroxide are lactobacilli and oral streptococci. Staphylococcus aureus, N. gonorrhoeae (a bacterium that causes gonorrhea), and diphtheria are also among the bacteria that hydrogen peroxide kills or inhibits [14].

Although in vitro pneumococcus kills H. influenzae, in vivo in mice, it turned out to be the opposite. Even though pneumococcus and H. influenzae live separately in the nasopharynx, in the case of joint colonization, pneumococcus quickly disappears, and only the H. influenzae remains. It turns out that H. influenzae somehow affects neutrophils (a type of phagocyte), which kill pneumococcal bacteria. Neutrophils alone do not kill pneumococci as effectively as in the presence

223

of an H. influenzae. How exactly H. influenzae affects neutrophils is still unknown. The authors conclude that manipulations such as antibiotics or vaccines, which are meant to diminish the presence of a single pathogen, may inadvertently alter the competitive interactions of complex microbial communities [15].

Pneumococcus And Staphylococcus Aureus

A clinical study of pneumococcal vaccine in the Netherlands found that colonization with vaccine serotypes of pneumococcus negatively correlates with Staphylococcus aureus colonization. No correlation was found between non-vaccine serotypes and Staphylococcus aureus. The incidence of acute otitis media caused by Staphylococcus aureus increased after vaccination [16]. Another study in Israel also found that colonization with pneumococcus, specifically vaccine-type strains, is negatively associated with Staphylococcus aureus carriage in children [17]. Hydrogen peroxide produced by pneumococcus also kills Staphylococcus aureus [18]. Pneumococcal vaccination temporarily increases Staphylococcus aureus colonization in children [19].

A Yale University study found that pneumococcus colonization negatively correlates with H. influenzae and Staphylococcus aureus colonization. The authors conclude that elimination of pneumococcus and H. influenzae due to vaccination may increase the risk of otitis media due to colonization with Staphylococcus aureus, and that "The public health impact of a given intervention strategy may be hard to predict, and caution should be used when designing control strategies that target nasopharyngeal colonization" [20].

MRSA—methicillin-resistant staphylococcus aureus, also called a superbug—is an intractable infection that is resistant to most antibiotics. Before the 1980s, it was rarely registered. In the 1980s, it was only possible to get infected in hospitals, and in the 1990s, it became possible to get infected outside of hospitals [21]. Each year, about 11,000 Americans die from Staphylococcus aureus, and 5,500 die from MRSA [22]. Three times fewer people die from pneumococcal infections.

Effectiveness

The pneumococcal polysaccharide vaccine was licensed in the US in 1977. It is usually given to the elderly, various chronic patients, and other risk groups. In a 1994 review, the authors analyze all published studies and conclude that there is no evidence that this vaccine is effective for any population group. The FDA licensed the vaccine based on the studies from the 1930s and 1940s, studies from South African gold mines, and among residents of New Guinea highland communities. Randomized trials sponsored by the NIH failed to show any benefit of the vaccine. The vaccine is least effective for those risk groups for which it is intended—the elderly and the immunocompromised patients [23]. According to the Cochrane systematic review, a polysaccharide vaccine is effective against invasive infections but does not reduce mortality, which suggests that even if the vaccine decreases the risk of death from pneumococcus, it increases mortality from other causes [24].

In a study published in 2006, the authors report that after the introduction of the conjugate vaccine, the incidence of pneumococcal bacteremia significantly decreased among the elderly, and only slightly among children. The incidence of pneumococcal meningitis fell threefold. This is what the authors report in the abstract. What they are not focusing on is that **the total incidence of bacterial meningitis has not changed, and the incidence of bacteremia has only increased [25].**

Pleural empyema is a complication of pneumonia (accumulation of pus in the cavities surrounding the lungs), which occurs in 3% of cases of pneumonia, and in a third of cases of pneumococcal pneumonia. The incidence of pleural empyema in the United States increased by 70% between 1997 and 2006, despite a decrease in the incidence of bacterial pneumonia and pneumococcal infections. Among children under five years of age, hospitalization due to pleural empyema increased by 100%. Although the rate of bacterial pneumonia decreased by 13%, and the rate of invasive pneumococcal disease has decreased by 50%, the rate of complicated pneumonia increased by 44% [26].

In a randomized trial in the Philippines, conjugate vaccine efficacy against pneumonia was 23%, and the efficacy against very severe pneumonia was negative: -27% (no statistical significance). The vaccinated showed 2.4 times more serious adverse events from all causes, and 3.6 times more serious adverse events from pneumonia, compared with the placebo group [27].

Strain Replacement

In response to antibiotics and vaccination, pneumococcus rapidly mutates. Pneumococcal bacteria can change their serotype [28]. After the introduction of vaccination in the United States, a new serotype appeared (35B), which had been rarely seen before, but which is now responsible for an increasing number of pneumococcal infections. This serotype is five times more deadly than other serotypes and is often non-responsive to antibiotics [29].

After vaccination was introduced in Barcelona, the incidence of invasive pneumococcal disease among children aged two years and younger increased by 58%, and among children aged two to four years by 135%. The incidence of vaccine serotypes decreased by 40%, but of non-vaccine serotypes increased by 531%. The incidence of pneumonia and empyema among children under five years of age increased by 320% [30]. After vaccination began in Salt Lake City, the incidence of pneumococcal infection decreased by 27% between 1997 and 2003. The incidence of vaccine serotypes decreased from 73% to 50%. The number of cases from non-vaccine serotypes increased threefold. Children with non-vaccine serotypes had longer hospital stays. The proportion of cases of empyema complications increased from 16% to 30%, and the proportion of severe cases increased from 57% to 71% [31].

In the first three years after the introduction of routine vaccination, the incidence of pneumococcal infection in Native Alaskan children younger than two years decreased by 67%. However, over the next two years, it increased by 82%. The disease rate from vaccine serotypes decreased by 96%, but from non-vaccine serotypes, it increased by 140%. The proportion of cases complicated by pleural empyema increased sixfold. The proportion of cases with pneumonia and bacteremia increased from 40% to 57% [32].

In British Columbia, the incidence of invasive pneumococcal infection among children under five years old declined by 78% between 2002 and 2010 but increased among children over five years old, adults, and the elderly. Vaccine strains were replaced by non-vaccine strains. The overall incidence has not changed [33]. In West Virginia, the incidence of invasive pneumococcal infection among children decreased by 50% between 1996 and 2010, but among adults, it increased by a third. The overall incidence slightly increased [34].

In Northern France, the incidence of pneumococcal meningitis among children under 18 years of age increased twofold between 2005 and 2008. The incidence among children under two years of age increased sixfold. Vaccination coverage during this time increased from 56% to 90%. In 2008, the incidence of pneumococcal meningitis reached the same level as in the pre-vaccine era [35]. In Philadelphia, the annual rate of disease due to vaccine serotypes declined by 29% per year, but the rate of disease due to non-vaccine serotypes increased by 13% per year, yielding an overall 7% increase in the annual rate of disease among adults [36].

There are dozens of more studies published in the scientific literature that testify to the replacement of the vaccine pneumococcus serotypes by non-vaccine ones and to the replacement of pneumococcus by H. influenzae and other bacteria. All studies show a decrease in the incidence of vaccine serotypes and an increase in the incidence of non-vaccine serotypes, but there are also studies according to which, despite the replacement of strains, the overall incidence of pneumococcal infections (or the incidence in some populations) has decreased.

Safety

Between 2000 and 2018, more than 1,700 deaths from pneumococcal vaccine were reported to VAERS. Fifteen thousand people were hospitalized, and more than 1,600 became permanently disabled.

In a confidential report that Pfizer provided to the European Medicines Agency, the following is reported among other things:

1. In the first half of 2011, 22 deaths were recorded after the Prevenar-13 vaccine. In most cases, death occurred shortly after vaccination.

2. During the two-year period, 1691 cases of adverse events were recorded, of which 18% were neurological. Among children who received only Prevenar-13, 9% of the adverse events were neurological. Among those who received Prevenar-13 along with another vaccine, 21% of the adverse events were neurological. Among those who received Prevenar-13 with Infanrix Hexa, 34% of the adverse events were neurological [37].

Another confidential report that analyzes the clinical trials of the 13-valent vaccine which Wyeth (subsequently Pfizer) provided to the European Medicines Agency states:

1. Prevenar-13 clinical safety studies included 1,365 children. Of these, 493 infants and 287 children received the tested vaccine. Prevnar vaccine was used as a placebo.

2. Among those who received the vaccine subcutaneously, fewer than 8% used antipyretics after vaccination. Among those who received the vaccine intramuscularly, antipyretics were used by 80%. Loss of appetite was observed in fewer than 19% in the subcutaneous group, and in more than 54% in the intramuscular group. Irritability: less than 37% in the subcutaneous group, and more than 88% in the intramuscular group. Drowsiness: fewer than 41% in the subcutaneous group, and more than 70% in the intramuscular group. Sleep disturbance: fewer than 24% in the subcutaneous group, and more than 45% in the intramuscular group. However, the manufacturer recommends this vaccine to be administered intramuscularly.

3. Adverse reactions were reported in 83–92%. In one study, serious adverse events were observed in 11% of children. Most of them were infections requiring hospitalization. All of them were deemed unrelated to the vaccine. The vast majority of serious adverse reactions were among infants. In total, 35 serious complications were recorded in 25 children from the group of 780 children receiving the 13-valent vaccine. That is, the total percentage of serious complications in the two studies was 3.2%. The percentage of complications from pneumococcus itself is much lower [38].

Conclusions

Like H. influenzae, pneumococcus is an opportunistic bacterium, which lives in the nasopharynx in most people.

Longer breastfeeding period significantly decreases the risk of infection.

The incidence of pneumococcal infection increased after the introduction of H. influenzae vaccination.

Vaccination has caused the replacement of vaccine strains with other strains, as well as the increase in the incidence of H. influenzae and other infections.

Endnotes

1. Wenger JD et al. Bacterial meningitis in the United States, 1986: report of a multistate surveillance study. *J Infect Dis*. 1990;162(6):1316-23

2. Pneumococcal. *CDC Pink Book*

3. Levine OS et al. Risk factors for invasive pneumococcal disease in children: a population-based case-control study in North America. *Pediatrics*. 1999;103(3):E28

4. César JA et al. Impact of breast feeding on admission for pneumonia during postneonatal period in Brazil: nested case-control study. *BMJ*. 1999;318(7194):1316-20

5. Nuorti JP et al. Cigarette smoking and invasive pneumococcal disease. *N Engl J Med*. 2000;342(10):681-9

6. Kyaw MH et al. The influence of chronic illnesses on the incidence of invasive pneumococcal disease in adults. *J Infect Dis*. 2005;192(3):377-86

7. Malik U et al. Association between prior antibiotic therapy and subsequent risk of community-acquired infections: a systematic review. *J Antimicrob Chemother*. 2018; 73(2):287-96

8. Pastor P et al. Invasive pneumococcal disease in Dallas County, Texas: results from population-based surveillance in 1995. *Clin Infect Dis*. 1998;26(3):590-5

9. Harrison LH et al. Invasive pneumococcal infection in Baltimore, Md: implications for immunization policy. *Arch Intern Med*. 2000;160(1):89-94

10. Hausdorff WP et al. Geographical differences in invasive pneumococcal disease rates and serotype frequency in young children. *Lancet*. 2001;357(9260):950-2

11. Baer M et al. Increase in bacteraemic pneumococcal infections in children. *Lancet*. 1995;345(8950):661

12. Tan TQ et al. Clinical characteristics of children with complicated pneumonia caused by Streptococcus pneumoniae. *Pediatrics*. 2002;110(1 Pt 1):1-6

13. Foster JA et al. Rising rate of pneumococcal bacteremia at the Children's Hospital of Philadelphia. *Pediatr Infect Dis J*. 1994;13(12):1143-4

14. Pericone CD et al. Inhibitory and bactericidal effects of hydrogen peroxide production by Streptococcus pneumoniae on other inhabitants of the upper respiratory tract. *Infect Immun*. 2000;68(7):3990-7

15. Lysenko ES et al. The role of innate immune responses in the outcome of interspecies competition for colonization of mucosal surfaces. *PLoS Pathog*. 2005;1(1):e1

16. Bogaert D et al. Colonisation by Streptococcus pneumoniae and Staphylococcus aureus in healthy children. *Lancet*. 2004;363(9424):1871-2

17. Regev-Yochay G et al. Association between carriage of Streptococcus pneumoniae and Staphylococcus aureus in Children. *JAMA*. 2004;292(6):716-20

18. Regev-Yochay G et al. Interference between Streptococcus pneumoniae and Staphylococcus aureus: in vitro hydrogen peroxide-mediated killing by Streptococcus pneumoniae. *J Bacteriol*. 2006;188(13):4996-5001

19. van Gils EJ et al. Effect of seven-valent pneumococcal conjugate vaccine on Staphylococcus aureus colonisation in a randomised controlled trial. *PLoS One*. 2011; 6(6):e20229

20. Pettigrew MM et al. Microbial interactions during upper respiratory tract infections. *Emerg Infect Dis*. 2008;14(10):1584-91

21. Calfee DP. The epidemiology, treatment, and prevention of transmission of methicillin-resistant Staphylococcus aureus. *J Infus Nurs.* 2011;34(6):359-64

22. Klein E et al. Hospitalizations and deaths caused by methicillin-resistant Staphylococcus aureus, United States, 1999-2005. *Emerg Infect Dis.* 2007;13(12):1840-6

23. Hirschmann JV et al. The pneumococcal vaccine after 15 years of use. *Arch Intern Med.* 1994;154(4):373-7

24. Moberley S et al. Vaccines for preventing pneumococcal infection in adults. *Cochrane Database Syst Rev.* 2013:CD000422

25. Shah SS et al. Trends in invasive pneumococcal disease-associated hospitalizations. *Cin Infect Dis.* 2006;42(1):e1-5

26. Li ST et al. Empyema hospitalizations increased in US children despite pneumococcal conjugate vaccine. *Pediatrics.* 2010;125(1):26-33

27. Lucero MG et al. Efficacy of an 11-valent pneumococcal conjugate vaccine against radiologically confirmed pneumonia among children less than 2 years of age in the Philippines: a randomized, double-blind, placebo-controlled trial. *Pediatr Infect Dis J.* 2009;28(6):455-62

28. Croucher NJ et al. Rapid pneumococcal evolution in response to clinical interventions. *Science.* 2011;331(6016):430-4

29. Olarte L et al. Emergence of Multidrug-Resistant Pneumococcal Serotype 35B among Children in the United States. *J Clin Microbiol.* 2017;55(3):724-34

30. Muñoz-Almagro C et al. Emergence of invasive pneumococcal disease caused by nonvaccine serotypes in the era of 7-valent conjugate vaccine. *Clin Infect Dis.* 2008; 46(2):174-82

31. Byington CL et al. Temporal trends of invasive disease due to Streptococcus pneumoniae among children in the intermountain west: emergence of nonvaccine serogroups. *Clin Infect Dis.* 2005;41(1):21-9

32. Singleton RJ et al. Invasive pneumococcal disease caused by nonvaccine serotypes among alaska native children with high levels of 7-valent pneumococcal conjugate vaccine coverage. *JAMA.* 2007;297(16):1784-92

33. Sahni V et al. The epidemiology of invasive pneumococcal disease in British Columbia following implementation of an infant immunization program. *Can J Public Health.* 2012;103(1):29-33

34. Norton NB et al. Routine pneumococcal vaccination of children provokes new patterns of serotypes causing invasive pneumococcal disease in adults and children. *Am J Med Sci.* 2013;345(2):112-20

35. Alexandre C et al. Rebound in the incidence of pneumococcal meningitis in northern France: effect of serotype replacement. *Acta Paediatr.* 2010;99(11):1686-90

36. Metlay JP et al. Exposure to children as a risk factor for bacteremic pneumococcal disease: changes in the post-conjugate vaccine era. *Arch Intern Med.* 2010;170(8):725-31

37. Prevenar 13 PSUR 04 - Response to RSI Neurological Events. 2012

38. Prevenar 13 (EMEA/H/C/001104) Article 46 of Pediatric Regulation 1901/2006

Chapter Twenty

MENINGOCOCCUS

The remedy is worse than the disease.
— **Francis Bacon**

Meningococcus is the third type of bacteria that can cause meningitis and bacteremia. The incidence of meningococcal infection is significantly lower than the incidence of pneumococcal and H. influenzae infections, but since the meningococcal vaccine is the newest licensed vaccine, meningococcus has recently become the biggest horror story.

According to the CDC, there are 13 serogroups of meningococcus, but invasive infections are caused mainly by the following five: A, B, C, W, Y. Sixty percent of invasive infections in children are caused by serogroup B. The fatality rate of invasive infections is 10–15% and the fatality rate of meningococcemia (meningococcal sepsis) is up to 40%. Ninety-eight percent of cases are sporadic, and only 2% happen as a result of outbreaks.

The first meningococcal vaccine (polysaccharide) was introduced in 1974. Like other polysaccharide vaccines, it is ineffective for infants. The first meningococcal conjugate vaccines (Menactra and Menveo) were licensed in 2005 and 2010 for adolescents over 11 years of age. Both vaccines protect from ACWY serogroups. The vaccines were expected to be effective for ten years, but it turned out that the antibody titers decrease after three to five years already, and those vaccinated at 11 years old will no longer be protected at the age of 16–21 years when the risk of meningococcal infection is higher. As a result, a booster dose was added for the 16 years olds in 2010. In 2014–15, two vaccines against serogroup B were licensed: Bexsero (GSK) and Trumenba (Pfizer) [1].

It was believed previously that the highest incidence of invasive infection is among children of six to 24 months old, but recent data indicates that the highest incidence is among infants under the age of six months, who lack maternal antibodies. Most cases of the infection happen due to serogroup B, but since the capsule of this serogroup contains a molecule, which is very similar to the glycoproteins in the brain, polysaccharide vaccines for this group poorly induce antibody production and can cause an autoimmune response due to the molecular mimicry mechanism. To go around that, vaccines based on the *outer membrane proteins* were developed. However, meningococcal outer membrane proteins are able to change antigens, which can lead to vaccine ineffectiveness. Since meningococcal infection is a rare disease, all meningococcal vaccines were licensed based on immunogenicity only (i.e., the level of antibodies), and not based on the clinical efficacy [2].

An article published by the CDC in 2010 reported that between 1998 and 2007, the incidence of meningococcal infection decreased by 64% in the US. On average, the incidence was one in 200,000 in the population during these years, and by 2007 it decreased to one in 300,000. The highest incidence was among infants under one year of age (one in 20,000). Fifty percent of the cases in them were caused by serogroup B. The fatality rate of meningococcal infection is 11%, and it increases with age. The fatality rate among the elderly is 24% and among infants 3–6%. Most cases are observed in January and February, and the least in August. The authors conclude that before the introduction of the vaccine, the incidence of meningococcal disease in the US decreased to a historic low, and there was no significant decrease in the incidence among adolescents after the introduction of vaccination, because the vaccine uptake among adolescents was only 32% [3].

(The idea that runs through almost all studies: If there was no significant decrease in the incidence after the introduction of a vaccine, it was because the coverage was insufficient, but if there was a decrease, it was, obviously, due to the vaccination, even if only 2% had been vaccinated.)

As a result of asymptomatic colonization of meningococcus, meningococcal antibodies are produced within several weeks. Infants under six months of age are protected by their mothers' antibodies, and the concentration of antibodies in the blood of infants is higher than in the blood of their mothers. Natural immunity to meningococcus is usually acquired in childhood [4].

A 2004 review reported that 10% of the population are carriers of meningococcal bacteria. Among children, less than 3% are infected, but 24–37% are infected among ages 15–24. A high level of colonization is also observed in the military. For example, more than 70% were meningococcus carriers among Norwegian soldiers.

A recent study showed that the number of meningococcus carriers, determined by conventional methods (bacterial cultures), might be underestimated. Results from a different method (immuno-histochemistry) showed that 45% of people were carriers of meningococcus, while conventional methods found meningococcus only in 10% of them. About 50% of the strains found in carriers were noncapsulated. It was believed previously that noncapsulated strains were not pathogenic, but it turned out that meningococci are able to turn the production of capsules on and off with high frequency. There is evidence that the loss of a capsule enhances the ability of meningococci to colonize the nasopharynx and avoid the body's defense system. Chronic benign meningococcemia may develop in less than 1%. How these patients tolerate potentially lethal bacteria in the bloodstream for several weeks is unknown [5].

Meningococcal disease is most common in the "African meningitis belt," which includes sub-Saharan countries. However, there has not been a single case published about a traveler who has been affected. The CDC investigates an incidence of possible transmission of meningococcal disease on an aircraft approximately every six weeks. However, only two such cases are known so far [6].

Risk Factors

The risk of meningococcal infection for a child under 18 years of age increases by almost four times if his mother smokes. Active and passive smoking increases the risk of meningococcal infection in adults by 2.5 times, and chronic disease by 11 times [7]. When both parents smoke, the risk of meningococcal infection increases by eight times [8]. In Ghana, where meningococcal meningitis is much more common than in developed countries, cooking in wood-burning ovens is associated with a ninefold increase in the risk of infection [9].

The risk of meningococcal infection in homosexuals is four times higher than in heterosexuals. Forty-five percent of meningococcus patients reported having multiple partners and engagement in anonymous sex [10]. In New York and Southern California, the risk of meningococcal infection among homosexuals was 50 times higher than on average [11, 12]. Homosexuals are also significantly more likely to be carriers of meningococcal bacteria [13]. A new strain of meningococcus that can be transmitted sexually was discovered in 2016 [14]. According to the CDC, in 2016, 57% of men over 16 years of age infected with meningococcus reported having homosexual relationships [15]. HIV infection increases the risk of meningococcal infection by 11 times. A meningococcal infection outbreak among homosexuals began in New York in 2010. It was linked to mobile dating apps and attending gay bars [16].

In a British study, intimate kissing with multiple partners was associated with a 3.7-fold increase in the risk of meningococcal infection among adolescents. Preterm birth and a history of preceding illness was associated with a threefold increase in the risk of infection. Attending religious ceremonies was associated with 11 times lower risk of infection, and vaccination with eight times lower risk [17]. Marijuana use is associated with a fourfold increase in the risk of meningococcal infection and attending nightclubs with a threefold increase. Attending picnics or school dance decreased the risk by three to four times [18]. In the US, attending bars was associated with an eight times increase in the risk of infection, and kissing with more than one partner – with a 13 times increase [19].

In Chile, risk factors for meningococcal infection were crowding, low level of mother's education, low income, alcohol abuse, and chronic illness [20].

Effectiveness

According to the CDC, the clinical effectiveness of Menactra one year after vaccination is 91%, but it decreases to 58% in two to five years, and this effect has no statistical significance [21]. In England, the vaccine was added to the national immunization schedule for infants in 1999. Vaccine effectiveness was 93% during the first year after vaccination but became negative (-81%) after a year [22].

The highest incidence of meningococcal infection in Europe is observed in Norway, and 80% is due to serogroup B. A double-blind, randomized study (170,000 people) was conducted on an outer membrane vaccine (OMV). Aluminum hydroxide was used as a placebo. Vaccine effectiveness was only 57%, and the effect was insufficient to justify a public vaccination program [23].

In the clinical trial of the serogroup B vaccine in Chile (40,000 people), another meningococcal vaccine was used as a placebo. Vaccine efficacy was 51% (no statistical significance), and among children under five years old, the efficacy was negative: -23% [24].

The meningococcal serogroup B epidemic began in New Zealand in 1991. By 2001, it reached its peak and began to decline. By 2004, a special vaccine for the New Zealand strain was developed. Since conducting randomized trials during the epidemic was considered unethical, vaccination campaign for all children from the age of six weeks to 19 years was launched in 2004. By 2006, 80% of children had been vaccinated, and the campaign was discontinued. Eventually, it turned out that seven months after the third dose of the vaccine, the antibody titers in infants dropped to almost baseline [25].

Like pneumococcus, meningococcal bacteria are able to change their serogroup [26].

In 2004, there was an outbreak of meningococcal disease due to serogroup B in Québec. The authors conclude that "The emergence of this clone of serogroup B meningococci occurred after a mass vaccination against serogroup C meningococcal bacteria, suggesting possible capsule replacement" [27]. Thirty cases of meningococcal infection in vaccinated individuals were registered by the CDC in 2006–10. The fatality rate among them was the same as among the unvaccinated [1].

Colonization

Serogroup B meningococcal infection outbreak (two cases) occurred in a college in Rhode Island in early 2015. Both patients recovered. As a result of the outbreak, five three-dose vaccination campaigns were conducted for students and teachers on campus, as well as for their intimate partners. A total of about 4,000 people had been vaccinated with the newly licensed Trumenba vaccine. Since it was unknown how this vaccine affected colonization, the authors used this vaccination campaign to study this fact. They concluded that vaccination does not affect the colonization of meningococcus and herd immunity, and therefore, high vaccination coverage is necessary [28]. In a study of the colonization of meningococcus at other universities in Rhode Island and in Oregon, the vaccination had no effect on colonization either. In England, the colonization of meningococcus was examined before and after vaccination against serogroups ACWY, and it turned out that despite the 71% vaccination coverage, the colonization increased from 14% to 46%, and serogroup W colonization increased 11-fold, from 0.7% to 8% [29].

Safety

Menactra was licensed in January of 2005 and was recommended for 11- to 12-year-olds, as well as for college freshmen. Five cases of the Guillain-Barré syndrome were registered with VAERS among vaccinated freshmen between June 10th and July 25th of 2005. In one case, the vaccinated girl already had a history of Guillain-Barré syndrome twice before, at the ages of two and five years, both times within two weeks after vaccination. The CDC concluded that it might be a coincidence and recommended to continue vaccination [30]. According to a study published in 2017, the risk of Bell's palsy (facial paralysis) within 12 weeks of vaccination was five times higher for those who received a meningococcal vaccine with concomitant vaccines, as compared to the control group. However, the control group consisted of the same vaccinated subjects, just after the "risk window period of 12 weeks." This study design is called a "self-controlled case series" and is frequently used in order to justify vaccine safety. The risk of Hashimoto's disease was 5.5 times higher within the risk window, and the risk of epileptic seizures was three times higher. All these cases were later reviewed, some of them were excluded, and the authors concluded that there was no statistically significant correlation between the vaccine and these diseases [31].

During clinical trials of the Menveo vaccine, 5,700 patients received Menveo and five other vaccines, and 2,000 patients received other vaccines only. Sixteen percent of infants vaccinated with Menveo and other vaccines, and 13% of infants vaccinated only with the other vaccines, experienced severe systemic reactions. The authors played around with statistics and concluded that there was no difference between the two groups, and that the vaccine is completely safe. Also, the group vaccinated against meningococcus had twice as many deaths, but according to the authors, these deaths had no link to the vaccine whatsoever [32].

According to the analysis of the randomized trials, the incidence of serious adverse effects potentially associated with Bexsero is one in 185 cases. It is 4.5 times higher than the incidence of serious adverse effects from other vaccines [33]. Aluminum hydroxide, another meningococcal vaccine, or Japanese encephalitis vaccine were used as a placebo in Bexsero clinical trials. Serious adverse events were registered in 2.1% of those vaccinated. The vaccine does not protect against all serogroup B strains. Bexsero contains the largest amount of aluminum among all vaccines at 1,500 mcg. Hepatitis B vaccine, for example, contains 250 mcg [34].

In clinical trials of Menactra for infants, the control group received pneumococcal, hepatitis A, and MMRV vaccines. In clinical trials of the vaccine for children and adults, a meningococcal polysaccharide vaccine was used as a placebo. Serious adverse events were registered in 2–2.5% of the recipients. Irritability was observed in 60% of infants, and loss of appetite in 30%. It is reported that the vaccine might be linked with facial palsy, transverse myelitis, and acute disseminated encephalomyelitis [35].

Meningitec (conjugate vaccine against serogroup C) is used in France. At least 680 children were injured by this vaccine. They sued the company, and their lawyer ordered a laboratory test of the vaccine. It turned out that it contained nanoparticles of heavy metals, such as titanium, lead, and zirconium [36, 37].

Miscellaneous

Dr. Rodewald, the head of the vaccination department at the CDC, stated in 2004 that the CDC was not doing well with vaccination of adolescents, and therefore, intimidating parents with the consequences of not vaccinating their children will become part of the advertising campaign, and that meningococcal vaccine is perfect for this purpose. After the meningococcal vaccine, vaccines against tetanus, diphtheria, and pertussis, as well as the HPV and herpes vaccines, will need to be added to the immunization schedule. The article also states that vaccination is usually much cheaper than the cost of treatment, but not in the case of meningococcus. Vaccination will cost $3.5 billion per year, and each saved life will cost over a million dollars [38].

Statistics

When the meningococcal vaccine was added to the national immunization schedule in 2006, meningococcal infection incidence was one in 250,000 [39]. The mortality rate was one in 2.5 million [40].

In 2015, the incidence rate was one in a million. In 2014, only 43 people died of meningococcus in the US; five of them were children under five years of age. That is, the meningococcal mortality rate was one in seven million [41].

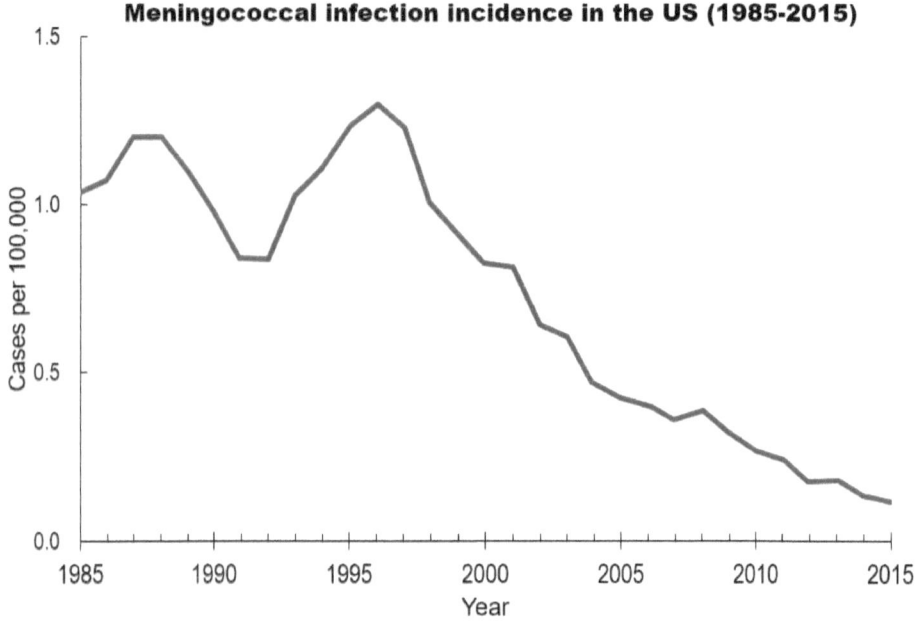

For comparison, 1,015 people died from H. influenzae infection in 2015, and 3,350 people died from pneumococcal infection.

The meningococcus mortality rate among children under five years of age in the US decreased by more than 90% since the mid-90s, despite the fact that vaccination for children had not been introduced yet.

As of 2019, VAERS has registered about 200 deaths and 500 permanent disability cases after the meningococcal vaccine. In 2016, seven children under three years of age died after vaccination, and 15 became permanently disabled. In the same year, nine children under five died from the meningococcal infection. Given that only 1–10% of all cases are registered in VAERS and that only children in high-risk groups are vaccinated, the meningococcal vaccine probably kills more people than meningococcal infection.

Conclusions

Like the previous two types of bacteria, meningococcal infection is a dangerous, but very rare disease, despite the fact that 10% of the population are carriers of meningococcal bacteria.

The meningococcal infection affects mainly the risk groups, such as homosexuals, those who are HIV positive, and patients with chronic diseases. Exposure to smoke as well as active and passive smoking increase the risk of carriage and infection.

An 85–90% decrease in the incidence happened prior to the introduction of vaccination.

The meningococcal vaccine contains huge amounts of aluminum and causes many more adverse effects than other vaccines.

Endnotes

1. Meningococcal. *CDC Pink Book*

2. Tan LK et al. Advances in the development of vaccines against Neisseria meningitidis. *N Engl J Med*. 2010;362(16):1511-20

3. Cohn AC et al. Changes in Neisseria meningitidis disease epidemiology in the United States, 1998-2007: implications for prevention of meningococcal disease. *Clin Infect Dis*. 2010;50(2):184-91

4. Goldschneider I et al. Human immunity to the meningococcus. II. Development of natural immunity. *J Exp Med*. 1969;129(6):1327-48

5. Manchanda V et al. Meningococcal disease: history, epidemiology, pathogenesis, clinical manifestations, diagnosis, antimicrobial susceptibility and prevention. *Indian J Med Microbiol*. 2006;24(1):7-19

6. Steffen R. The risk of meningococcal disease in travelers and current recommendations for prevention. *J Travel Med*. 2010;17 Suppl:9-17

7. Fischer M et al. Tobacco smoke as a risk factor for meningococcal disease. *Pediatr Infect Dis J*. 1997;16(10):979-83

8. Murray RL et al. Second hand smoke exposure and the risk of invasive meningococcal disease in children: systematic review and meta-analysis. *BMC Public Health*. 2012; 12:1062

9. Hodgson A et al. Risk factors for meningococcal meningitis in northern Ghana. *Trans R Soc Trop Med Hyg*. 2001;95(5):477-80

10. Folaranmi TA et al. Increased risk for meningococcal disease among men who have sex with men in the United States, 2012-2015. *Clin Infect Dis*. 2017;65(5):756-63

11. Simon MS et al. Invasive meningococcal disease in men who have sex with men. *Ann Intern Med*. 2013;159(4):300-1

12. Nanduri S et al. Outbreak of serogroup C meningococcal disease primarily affecting men who have sex with men - Southern California, 2016. *MMWR*. 2016;65(35):939-40

13. Russell JM et al. Pharyngeal flora in a sexually active population. *Int J STD AIDS*. 1995; 6(3):211-5

14. Taha MK et al. Evolutionary events associated with an outbreak of meningococcal disease in men who have sex with men. *PloS One*. 2016;11(5):e0154047

15. Enhanced meningococcal disease surveillance report. 2016. *CDC*

16. Invasive meningococcal disease among men who have sex with men. 2013. *ECDC*

17. Tully J et al. Risk and protective factors for meningococcal disease in adolescents: matched cohort study. *BMJ*. 2006;332(7539):445-50

18. Harrison LH et al. Risk factors for meningococcal disease in students in grades 9-12. *Pediatr Infect Dis J*. 2008;27(3):193-9

19. Mandal S et al. Prolonged university outbreak of meningococcal disease associated with a serogroup B strain rarely seen in the United States. *Clin Infect Dis*. 2013;57(3):344-8

20. Olea A et al. Case-control study of risk factors for meningococcal disease in Chile. *Emerg Infect Dis*. 2017;23(7):1070-8

21. Updated recommendations for use of meningococcal conjugate vaccines (ACIP), 2010. *MMWR*. 2011;60(3):72-6

22. Trotter CL et al. Effectiveness of meningococcal serogroup C conjugate vaccine 4 years after introduction. *Lancet*. 2004;364(9431):365-7

23. Bjune G et al. Effect of outer membrane vesicle vaccine against group B meningococcal disease in Norway. *Lancet*. 1991;338(8775):1093-6

24. Boslego J et al. Efficacy, safety, and immunogenicity of a meningococcal group B (15:P1.3) outer membrane protein vaccine in Iquique, Chile. *Vaccine*. 1995;13(9):821-9

25. Jackson C et al. Antibody persistence following MeNZB vaccination of adults and children and response to a fourth dose in toddlers. *Arch Dis Child*. 2011;96(8):744-51

26. Swartley JS et al. Capsule switching of Neisseria meningitidis. *PNAS*. 1997;94(1):271-6

27. Law DK et al. Invasive meningococcal disease in Quebec, Canada, due to an emerging clone of ST-269 serogroup B meningococci with serotype antigen 17 and serosubtype antigen P1.19 (B:17:P1.19). *J Clin Microbiol*. 2006;44(8):2743-9

28. Soeters HM et al. Meningococcal Carriage Evaluation in Response to a Serogroup B Meningococcal Disease Outbreak and Mass Vaccination Campaign at a College-Rhode Island, 2015-2016. *Clin Infect Dis*. 2017;64(8):1115-22

29. Oldfield NJ et al. Rise in group W meningococcal carriage in university students, United Kingdom. *Emerg Infect Dis*. 2017;23(6):1009-11

30. Guillain-Barré syndrome among recipients of Menactra meningococcal conjugate vaccine—United States, June-July 2005. *MMWR*. 2005;54(40):1023-5

31. Tseng HF et al. Safety of quadrivalent meningococcal conjugate vaccine in 11- to 21-year-olds. *Pediatrics*. 2017;139(1):e20162084

32. Abdelnour A et al. Safety of a quadrivalent meningococcal serogroups A, C, W and Y conjugate vaccine (MenACWY-CRM) administered with routine infant vaccinations: results of an open-label, randomized, phase 3b controlled study in healthy infants. *Vaccine*. 2014;32(8):965-72

33. Flacco ME et al. Immunogenicity and safety of the multicomponent meningococcal B vaccine (4CMenB) in children and adolescents: a systematic review and meta-analysis. *Lancet Infect Dis*. 2018;18(4):461-72

34. Bexsero vaccine package insert

35. Menactra vaccine package insert

36. Burgerminister J. Vaccin Meningitec: un lot jugé dangereux pour la santé. 2016

37. Condomines A. Vaccin Meningitec: des composants dangereux repérés par une analyse accablante. *LCI*. 2016 Apr 5

38. Harris G. Panel reviews new vaccine that could be controversial. *NY Times*. 2004 Oct 27

39. Adams DA et al. Summary of notifiable infectious diseases and conditions - United States, 2015. *MMWR*. 2017;64(53):1-143

40. Heron M et al. Deaths: final data for 2006. *Natl Vital Stat Rep*. 2009;57(14):1-134

41. Kochanek KD et al. Deaths: final data for 2014. *Natl Vital Stat Rep*. 2016;65(4):1-122

Chapter Twenty-One

ROTAVIRUS

Vaccination is a barbarous practice, and it is one of the most fatal of all the delusions of the world. Conscientious objectors to vaccination should stand alone, if need be, against the whole world, in defense of their conviction.

— **Mahatma Gandhi**

B efore the introduction of the vaccine, few people have heard of rotavirus infection, even though almost all children caught it at some point.

Rotavirus was discovered in 1973. When viewed under a microscope, it resembles a wheel, and this is how it got its name. The virus is the most common cause of gastroenteritis in infants and children. It is transmitted by the fecal-oral route. According to the CDC, the first infection after three months of age is usually the most severe. It can be asymptomatic, cause mild diarrhea, or it can cause severe diarrhea with fever and vomiting. The symptoms usually resolve within three to seven days. Similar symptoms can also be caused by other pathogens, so laboratory testing is required for confirmation. In temperate climates, the disease is more common during fall and winter periods.

There are currently two oral rotavirus vaccines: RotaTeq and Rotarix. Vaccines are 74–90% effective against the serotypes they contain. The duration of immunity is unknown. In clinical studies, among those who received RotaTeq vaccines, there were more cases of diarrhea and vomiting during the first week after vaccination, compared to those who got a placebo. During 42 days after vaccination, diarrhea, vomiting, otitis media, nasopharyngitis, and bronchospasm occurred more often in those vaccinated. In those vaccinated with Rotarix as opposed to a placebo group, cough and runny nose were observed more often during seven days after vaccination, and irritability and flatulence occurred more often during the month following vaccination [1]. In clinical trials of both vaccines, the respective vaccine without the antigen was used as a placebo [2, 3].

According to a 1996 review, the probability of diarrhea upon the first rotavirus infection is 47%. With subsequent infections, the probability of diarrhea decreases. Rotavirus diarrhea decreases the risk of diarrhea upon repeated infection by 77%, and the risk or severe diarrhea by 87%. Asymptomatic infection decreases the risk of subsequent infection by 38%. Two infections (symptomatic or asymptomatic) result in complete protection against moderate to severe diarrhea [4]. Re-infections after childhood are common, but symptoms are usually mild, if at all present.

Infected neonates often have no symptoms, and subsequent rotavirus infections among them are less frequent and less severe than in children not infected with rotavirus during the neonatal period. Asymptomatic infection in infants after the neonatal period is as protective as symptomatic infection, with protection lasting for at least two years. After early childhood, significant symptomatic infection is uncommon [5]. A short breastfeeding period increases the risk of rotavirus infection. Exclusive breastfeeding reduces the risk of rotavirus infection by 38% [6]. The level of zinc in the blood correlates with protection against rotavirus [7].

How Lethal Is Rotavirus?

The development of the rotavirus vaccine began in the '90s, which made the CDC wonder how many children actually die from it. They conducted a few studies to answer this question. A 1988 study reported that deaths from diarrhea (from any reason) account for 2% of all post-neonatal mortality. Between 1973 and 1983 in the US, 500 children annually died from diarrhea; on average, 50% of them died in hospitals. Diarrheal death rate decreases drastically with age, it is higher in winter than in summer, and it is believed that the rotavirus is responsible for excess winter deaths. It was estimated that 70–80 children die each year from rotavirus [8].

A 1995 study in the US reported that diarrheal deaths nationwide have declined by 75% from 1968 to 1985, but stabilized since then at about 300 deaths per year. The fatality rate among children was 1:17,000. From 1985 and on, half of them died at the age of under 1.5 months (that is, before the vaccination age). The authors conclude that a vaccine against rotavirus will have a measurable but small impact on mortality from diarrhea [9].

According to a 1996 article, it was estimated that 873,000 people die from rotavirus annually worldwide. However, similar information about diarrheal disease was not available for developed countries. Thus, the Institute of Medicine concluded that a rotavirus vaccine was not a priority for the United States after reviewing new vaccine priorities for developed countries. Since no child in the United States has ever been reported to have died with a diagnosis of rotavirus diarrhea, many pediatricians believed that it could never be severe or fatal. However, a review of national mortality data (in the previous studies) has provided cogent but indirect evidence that rotavirus has been a cause of death in American children. Based on the two previous studies, the authors estimate that 55,000 children are hospitalized due to rotavirus annually, and 20 children die (i.e., one in every 200,000). They believe that these children also have underlying illnesses or conditions. The authors conclude that less than 40 children each year die of rotavirus, although they never explain how they came up with 40 since they only counted 20 in the body of the article [10]. The CDC claims that 20–60 children die of rotavirus each year, but they do not explain where they got 60 from since their own studies estimated only 20 deaths [1].

The first rotavirus vaccine (Rotashield) was licensed in 1998 and contained four serotypes. It was withdrawn in 1999 because it was associated with intussusception. Intussusception is when part of the intestine folds onto itself, like a telescope. In 1998, the Rotarix vaccine was licensed. It contains one serotype. The isolated wild strain from an infected child was attenuated by 33 serial passages in African green monkey kidney cells. The vaccine strain multiplies well in the human intestines. In 1996, the RotaTeq vaccine was licensed. It contains five serotypes. Unlike the other live vaccines, RotaTeq is not an attenuated, but a *reassortant* vaccine. The rotavirus genome consists of 11 RNA segments. Some human rotavirus segments in the RotaTeq vaccine strains were replaced with bovine rotavirus segments. Vaccines, in which some human virus RNA segments were replaced by segments of animal virus strains, are called reassortant vaccines. This type of virus does not multiply well in the intestines, which is why RotaTeq has 100 times more virus particles than Rotarix. The Rotashield vaccine was also reassortant, but it used segments of the rhesus monkey virus [11].

Shedding

During the clinical trials of Rotashield, vaccine strains were detected in the stool of those who received a placebo a year after the beginning of the trial and were no longer detected 100 days after the end of the trial, which suggests the establishment of a community reservoir. Rotarix clinical trials found that about 50–80% of infants shed the virus after the first dose. A Singapore study found that approximately 80% of infants shed the virus on the seventh day after vaccination, and 20% continue to shed it one month after the vaccination. A study in the Dominican Republic revealed that 19% of unvaccinated twins were infected with a vaccine strain from their vaccinated siblings [12]. In RotaTeq vaccine studies, up to 87% of infants were shedding the virus after vaccination [13].

Vaccine virus shedding and transmission to the unvaccinated contacts have been primarily viewed as potential adverse events after vaccination with live-virus vaccines, but there is also a potential benefit. Infecting the unvaccinated will make them develop immunity, the same way as it happens with the polio vaccine. This will lead to significant benefits in poor countries, where the vaccination coverage is low, the mortality rate is high, and the number of immunocompromised people is low. In developed countries, where the rotavirus mortality rate is low, the number of immunocompromised people is high, and most regulatory bodies, physicians, and families wish to avoid the risk (particularly after the previous experience with Rotashield), shedding rotavirus vaccine strains that could be viewed as a potential liability. One gram of stool of an infected child contains 100 billion virus particles, and only ten particles may result in an infection. Therefore, adults who change infants' diapers are at risk of infection [11].

Effectiveness

According to a Cochrane systematic review, vaccination in developed countries reduces the risk of severe diarrhea by 40%, and the risk of severe rotavirus diarrhea by 86%. There was no evidence of the vaccine effect on mortality. Serious adverse events were reported in 4.6% of those vaccinated with Rotarix and 2.4% of those vaccinated with RotaTeq [14].

Within 15 months after the introduction of the vaccine in Brazil, G2P[4] rotavirus strain has replaced all other strains, even though it was only seen in 19–30% of cases prior to the vaccine introduction. Vaccine effectiveness against this strain was 77% among children of six to 11 months of age, and -24% (negative) among children over 12 months of age [15]. Another study reports that after the introduction of the vaccine in Brazil, usual rotavirus strains were replaced with the new GP12[8] strain [16]. Strain replacement also took place in Paraguay and Argentina. Effectiveness of the vaccine (Rotarix) among six- to 11-month-old children in Columbia was 79%, against severe cases of diarrhea 63%, and against very severe cases 67%. The effectiveness among children over 12 months of age was -40%, against severe cases -6%, and against very severe cases -156% (negative effectiveness). The overall effectiveness of the vaccine for all ages was -2%, -54% against severe cases, and -114% against very severe cases (negative effectiveness) [17].

In Central Australia, the effectiveness of two doses of Rotarix was 19% (no statistical significance), and the effectiveness of one dose was zero [18]. A 1995 study did not find a correlation between the antibody level developed and the clinical effectiveness of the vaccine [19]. Rotarix's effectiveness against rotavirus diarrhea in a Bangladeshi study was 41%, but its overall effectiveness against all types of diarrhea turned out to be negative (-2.2%) [20]. In Korea, the authors tested stool samples of 1,106 infants suffering from gastroenteritis and found group A rotavirus in 26% of them. Thirteen percent of the detected strains were vaccine strains [21].

Reassortment

Since the rotavirus genome consists of separate segments, when two different strains of the virus infect the same cell, they can exchange segments and create a new strain. This is the same as the reassortment process done in a laboratory, but it can also happen on its own.

A case of gastroenteritis in a seven-year-old girl was reported in Finland. A rotavirus strain was isolated from her stool sample. The strain was a reassortant of two other human-bovine strains from the RotaTeq vaccine. However, the girl has not been vaccinated against rotavirus.

Moreover, she has not been in contact with anyone who has been vaccinated. Her two brothers also had similar gastroenteritis symptoms, and they have also not been vaccinated or in contact with anyone who has been. The isolated reassortant strain of the virus turned out to be stable and very contagious. The authors believe that this new virus is most likely circulating in the community [22].

In Nicaragua, the researchers analyzed the genome of rotavirus taken from vaccinated children suffering from gastroenteritis and found new strains of the virus, which formed due to reassortment between the wild strain and the RotaTeq vaccine strains [23]. Reassortant viruses have previously been isolated, but only in those recently vaccinated with RotaTeq. Cases of new virus strains from reassortment of the wild virus with the Rotarix vaccine strain have also been reported [24].

A study in Finland found that 17% of children were shedding the virus after vaccination, and 37% of them were shedding a double reassortant virus. Some children were shedding the virus for a long time after the vaccination, from nine to 84 days after the last dose [25]. Among children in Australia who had diarrhea within two weeks of vaccination, 21% had been infected with the vaccine strain. Thirty-seven percent of the isolated vaccine strains were reassortant from two RotaTeq strains [26].

Safety

Type 1 diabetes incidence among children under 18 years of age in Israel has been increasing by 6% annually between 2000 and 2008. Among children under five years of age, it increased by 104% in six years. The authors suggested that viral infections could be one of the factors in the disease, which means that rotavirus vaccination might reduce the risk of diabetes. It turned out, however, that vaccination was associated with a sevenfold increase in the risk of type 1 diabetes [27, 28].

After the introduction of rotavirus vaccination in France, 508 adverse effects were registered (201 of them serious), and 47 cases of intussusception. Two of the infants with intussusception died, and one other died from necrotizing enterocolitis. In the five years preceding the vaccination, only one fatal case of intussusception has been reported. **Following these events, health authorities refused to recommend and reimburse rotavirus vaccines.** It is noteworthy that clinical trials have never demonstrated a reduction in all-cause mortality with these vaccines, neither in high nor in low-income countries [29].

In clinical trials of RotaTeq, the risk of epileptic seizures in those who were vaccinated was twice as high as compared to the "placebo" group. Kawasaki syndrome was registered in five patients vaccinated with RotaTeq and one patient from the "placebo" group. Among the preterm infants, adverse events were registered in 5.5% of the vaccinated and 5.8% of the "placebo" group [30]. In the clinical trial of Rotarix, the mortality rate was 0.19% among the vaccinated patients and 0.15% in the "placebo" group. The risk of Kawasaki syndrome among the vaccinated was 71% higher (no statistical significance) [31]. In the largest clinical trial of Rotarix (63,000 children), 2.7 times more deaths from pneumonia were registered in the vaccinated group, as compared to the "placebo" group [32]. The FDA believes that this is most likely a coincidence [33].

In 2010, a group of independent researchers accidentally found a porcine circovirus (PCV1) in the Rotarix vaccine, and the FDA decided to temporarily suspend vaccination [34]. At first, the FDA stated that RotaTeq did not contain a porcine virus, but two months later, it turned out that RotaTeq contained DNA of two porcine viruses (PCV1 and PCV2). The FDA assembled a committee, which concluded that these viruses were most likely harmless to humans and that the benefits of vaccination outweigh the hypothetical harm. The committee also recommended that manufacturers develop vaccines without porcine viruses. One week after detecting the viruses in RotaTeq, the FDA recommended pediatricians to resume vaccination with both vaccines. The manufacturers, however, are in no hurry to develop vaccines without the porcine viruses.

In a study published in 2014, the authors wanted to determine whether porcine viruses multiply in the human intestine. They did not find porcine viruses, but they did detect a baboon endogenous M7 virus in the RotaTeq vaccine, which probably got there from African green monkey kidney cells, in which the vaccine virus is grown [35]. The PCV2 porcine virus, which has been known for 40 years and was harmless, has suddenly mutated and spread throughout the world, causing disease in piglets and becoming deadly to pigs [36, 37].

Intussusception

RotaTeq vaccine is associated with a ninefold risk of intussusception (one in every 65,000) [38]. Rotarix increases the risk of intussusception by eight times [39]. Similar results were obtained in other studies. In Australia, Rotarix increased the risk of intussusception by seven times, and RotaTeq by ten times [40]. According to a meta-analysis of 11 studies, the first dose of the rotavirus vaccine increases the risk of intussusception by 3.5–8.5 times [41]. It is reported that the number of intussusception cases in the studies is most likely underestimated by 44% [19].

In Italy, two twins received the Rotarix vaccine. One week later, one of them developed intussusception symptoms and was urgently taken into surgery. A few hours after the surgery, the other twin started to experience the same symptoms, and he also underwent surgery, but not as urgently [42]. A two-month-old girl was vaccinated with Rotarix in Japan, and in ten days her two-year-old sister was hospitalized with severe gastroenteritis. It turned out that her sister infected her with a mutated vaccine strain of the virus [43]. A similar case with a RotaTeq vaccine has been reported in the US. A vaccinated infant infected his brother ten days post-vaccination with a rotavirus strain that was reassortant of two vaccine strains [44].

Immunodeficient infants can suffer from severe gastroenteritis for a long time after vaccination. However, at the age of two months, when the vaccination is given, it is still unknown whether the infant is immunodeficient or not [45].

In ten years, between 2008 and 2017, 539 deaths and more than 250 permanent disability cases due to rotavirus vaccine have been registered with VAERS. Prior to the introduction of vaccination, 20 deaths per year were estimated (i.e., 1:200,000). Considering that only 1–10% of all cases get registered with VAERS, the probability of dying after the vaccination is 27–270 times higher, than the probability of dying due to rotavirus.

Conclusions

Rotavirus has become scary only after the introduction of the vaccine. Exclusive breastfeeding decreases the risk of rotavirus infection.

There is evidence that those vaccinated infect those unvaccinated, which could be dangerous for immunocompromised people.

Vaccination increases the risk of intussusception by several times, and the probability of death following vaccination is tens of times higher than the probability of death from rotavirus.

Endnotes

1. Rotavirus. CDC Pink Book

2. Vesikari T et al. Effects of the potency and composition of the multivalent human-bovine (WC3) reassortant rotavirus vaccine on efficacy, safety and immunogenicity in healthy infants. *Vaccine.* 2006;24(22):4821-9

3. Ruiz-Palacios GM et al. Safety and efficacy of an attenuated vaccine against severe rotavirus gastroenteritis. *N Engl J Med.* 2006;354(1):11-22

4. Velázquez FR et al. Rotavirus infection in infants as protection against subsequent infections. *N Engl J Med.* 1996;335(14):1022-8

5. Molyneaux PJ. Human immunity to rotavirus. *J Med Microbiol.* 1995;43(6):397-404

6. Krawczyk A et al. Effect of Exclusive Breastfeeding on Rotavirus Infection among Children. *Indian J Pediatr.* 2016;83(3):220-5

7. Colgate ER et al. Delayed dosing of oral rotavirus vaccine demonstrates decreased risk of rotavirus gastroenteritis associated with serum zinc: a randomized controlled trial. *Clin Infect Dis.* 2016;63(5):634-41

8. Ho MS et al. Diarrheal deaths in American children. Are they preventable? *JAMA.* 1988;260(22):3281-5

9. Kilgore PE et al. Trends of diarrheal disease—associated mortality in US children, 1968 through 1991. *JAMA.* 1995;274(14):1143-8

10. Glass RI et al. The epidemiology of rotavirus diarrhea in the United States: surveillance and estimates of disease burden. *J Infect Dis.* 1996;174 Suppl 1:S5-11

11. Anderson EJ. Rotavirus vaccines: viral shedding and risk of transmission. *Lancet Infect Dis.* 2008;8(10):642-9

12. Rivera L et al. Horizontal transmission of a human rotavirus vaccine strain—a randomized, placebo-controlled study in twins. *Vaccine.* 2011;29(51):9508-13

13. Ye S et al. Multivalent rotavirus vaccine and wild-type rotavirus strain shedding in Australian infants: a birth cohort study. *Clin Infect Dis.* 2018;66(9):1411-8

14. Soares-Weiser K et al. Vaccines for preventing rotavirus diarrhoea: vaccines in use. *Cochrane Database Syst Rev.* 2012;11:CD008521

15. Correia JB et al. Effectiveness of monovalent rotavirus vaccine (Rotarix) against severe diarrhea caused by serotypically unrelated G2P[4] strains in Brazil. *J Infect Dis.* 2010; 201(3):363-9

16. Luchs A et al. Detection of the emerging rotavirus G12P[8] genotype at high frequency in brazil in 2014: successive replacement of predominant strains after vaccine introduction. *Acta Trop.* 2016;156:87-94

17. Cotes-Cantillo K et al. Effectiveness of the monovalent rotavirus vaccine in Colombia: a case-control study. *Vaccine.* 2014;32(25):3035-40

18. Snelling TL et al. Case-control evaluation of the effectiveness of the G1P[8] human rotavirus vaccine during an outbreak of rotavirus G2P[4] infection in central Australia. *Clin Infect Dis.* 2011;52(2):191-9

19. Ward RL et al. Lack of correlation between serum rotavirus antibody titers and protection following vaccination with reassortant RRV vaccines. *Vaccine.* 1995; 13(13):1226-32

20. Zaman K et al. Effectiveness of a live oral human rotavirus vaccine after programmatic introduction in Bangladesh: a cluster-randomized trial. *PLoS Med.* 2017;14(4):e1002282

21. Jeong S et al. Differentiation of RotaTeq vaccine strains from wild-type strains using NSP3 gene in reverse transcription polymerase chain reaction assay. *J Virol Methods.* 2016;237:72-8

22. Hemming M et al. Detection of rotateq vaccine-derived, double-reassortant rotavirus in a 7-year-old child with acute gastroenteritis. *Pediatr Infect Dis J.* 2014;33(6):655-6

23. Bucardo F et al. Vaccine-derived NSP2 segment in rotaviruses from vaccinated children with gastroenteritis in Nicaragua. *Infect Genet Evol.* 2012;12(6):1282-94

24. Rose TL et al. Evidence of vaccine-related reassortment of rotavirus, Brazil, 2008-2010. *Emerg Infect Dis.* 2013;19(11):1843-6

25. Markkula J et al. Detection of vaccine-derived rotavirus strains in nonimmuno-compromised children up to 3-6 months after RotaTeq vaccination. *Pediatr Infect Dis J.* 2015;34(3):296-8

26. Donato CM et al. Identification of strains of RotaTeq rotavirus vaccine in infants with gastroenteritis following routine vaccination. *J Infect Dis.* 2012;206(3):377-83

27. GabrielChodick. Rotavirus immunization and type 1 diabetes mellitus: a nested case–control study. *Pediatr Infect IDs.* 2014;6(4):147-9

28. Sella T et al. A retrospective study of the incidence of diagnosed Type 1 diabetes among children and adolescents in a large health organization in Israel, 2000-2008. *Diabet Med.* 2011;28(1):48-53

29. Michal-Teitelbaum C. Rotavirus vaccines in France: because of three infant death and too many serious side effects vaccines are no longer recommended for routine children immunization. *BMJ.* 2015:350:h2867/rr-1

30. Rotateq vaccine package insert

31. Rotarix vaccine package insert

32. Dixon K. Pneumonia deaths seen with Glaxo vaccine: FDA. *reuters.com.* 2008 Feb 15

33. VRBPAC meeting. Feb 20, 2008

34. Victoria JG et al. Viral nucleic acids in live-attenuated vaccines: detection of minority variants and an adventitious virus. *J Virol.* 2010;84(12):6033-40

35. Hewitson L et al. Screening of viral pathogens from pediatric ileal tissue samples after vaccination. *Adv Virol.* 2014;2014:720585

36. Vansickle J. Porcine circovirus grows more deadly. *National Hog Farmer.* 2008 Mar 15

37. Meng XJ. Spread like a wildfire—the omnipresence of porcine circovirus type 2 (PCV2) and its ever-expanding association with diseases in pigs. *Virus Res.* 2012;164(1-2):1-3

38. Yih WK et al. Intussusception risk after rotavirus vaccination in U.S. infants. *N Engl J Med.* 2014;370(6):503-12

39. Weintraub ES et al. Risk of intussusception after monovalent rotavirus vaccination. *N Engl J Med.* 2014;370(6):513-9

40. Carlin JB et al. Intussusception risk and disease prevention associated with rotavirus vaccines in Australia's National Immunization Program. *Clin Infect Dis.* 2013;57(10):1427-34

41. Kassim P et al. Risk of intussusception following rotavirus vaccination: an evidence based meta-analysis of cohort and case-control studies. *Vaccine.* 2017;35(33):4276-86

42. La Rosa F et al. Post-rotavirus vaccine intussusception in identical twins: a case report. *Hum Vaccin Immunother.* 2016;12(9):2419-21

43. Sakon N et al. An infant with acute gastroenteritis caused by a secondary infection with a Rotarix-derived strain. *Eur J Pediatr.* 2017;176(9):1275-8

44. Payne DC et al. Sibling transmission of vaccine-derived rotavirus (RotaTeq) associated with rotavirus gastroenteritis. *Pediatrics.* 2010;125(2):e438-41

45. Uygungil B et al. Persistent rotavirus vaccine shedding in a new case of severe combined immunodeficiency: a reason to screen. *J Allergy Clin Immunol.* 2010;125(1):270-1

Chapter Twenty-Two

HEPATITIS A

I am dying from the treatment of too many physicians.
— **Alexander the Great**

I f children and adults are vaccinated against pertussis in order to protect infants and infants are vaccinated against rubella in order to protect unborn infants, in the case of hepatitis A, infants get vaccinated in order to protect adults.

According to the CDC, in children younger than six years, 70% of infections are asymptomatic. In older children and adults, infection is usually symptomatic, with jaundice occurring in more than 70% of the patients.

Groups at risk for hepatitis A include homosexuals, users of illegal drugs, travelers to endemic countries, and persons working with infected primates. Two vaccines are available in the US: Havrix (GSK) and Vaqta (Merck), which were licensed in 1995–96, and have a 94–100% efficacy. There is also a combination vaccine with hepatitis B (Twinrix). All vaccines contain aluminum. Havrix contains aluminum hydroxide, and Vaqta contains AAHS (the same type of aluminum as Gardasil). The virus for both vaccines is grown on MRC-5 human diploid cell lines. Unlike hepatitis B and C, hepatitis A is an intestinal infection transmitted through the fecal-oral route and does not have a chronic form [1].

According to the WHO position paper, the incidence of hepatitis A is strongly correlated with socioeconomic indicators; the incidence of hepatitis A infection decreases with increasing incomes and access to clean water and adequate sanitation. In highly endemic countries, almost all persons are asymptomatically infected with hepatitis A in childhood, which effectively prevents clinical hepatitis A in adolescents and adults. The WHO does not recommend universal vaccination in these countries [2].

Seventy to 80 deaths from hepatitis A infection are reported in the US each year, and those are predominantly in people over 50 years old. Severe manifestations of hepatitis A infection are more likely in individuals with underlying alcoholic liver disease or with chronic hepatitis [3].

The indigenous population has been vaccinated against hepatitis A in Taiwan since 1995. One study found that the hepatitis A incidence decreased by more than three times due to vaccination, despite the fact that only 2% of the population was vaccinated, and most of them lived in mountain areas and isolated islands. Another study found that only 0.4% of the nonindigenous unvaccinated population had hepatitis A antibodies, which led the authors to conclude that it was the improvement of environmental sanitary conditions and hygiene, and not vaccination, that was responsible for the decline in hepatitis A occurrence. Improved sanitary conditions shifted hepatitis A incidence from childhood to young adults [4].

Israel became the first country in the world to introduce the hepatitis A vaccine into its national vaccination program in 1999. Within three years, hepatitis A incidence decreased by more than 98% among the vaccinated, and by 95% among the general population. Before the beginning of vaccination, 47% of the Jewish population had hepatitis A antibodies, and 12 years later, 67% had them. Among the Arab population, 83% had antibodies before the beginning of vaccination, and 88% had them 12 years later. That is, same as in Taiwan, it is not clear whether vaccination was the only factor responsible for reducing the incidence [5].

> As of 2020, only two European countries include hepatitis A vaccine in their national immunization schedule: Greece and Austria. Only in Greece is the vaccine funded by the National Health system.

A British study found that hepatitis A and typhoid vaccines for those who travel to endemic countries are not cost-effective. Only one in 2,000 people get infected with hepatitis A during travel, and in 90% of cases, the disease is mild [6].

Benefits Of Hepatitis A

Hepatitis A was an endemic disease in Italy during the 1970s, and it was usually contracted early in childhood, most commonly without inducing symptoms. Military students in Italy, who had antibodies for hepatitis A, suffered from asthma and allergic rhinitis two times less often than the students who did not have antibodies. Students, who had older siblings, also suffered from allergic diseases less frequently, which suggests that hepatitis A is not the only infection associated with low risk of atopic diseases. Other studies in recent decades also reveal an inverse relationship between hepatitis A antibodies and allergies in different countries. During the 1970s, the prevalence of hepatitis A antibodies in the United States was high in older people but low in younger people, whereas the opposite was true for atopic diseases [7].

In Turkey, children who did not have hepatitis A antibodies suffered from asthma and allergic rhinitis nine times more often. Those who did not have hepatitis B antibodies suffered from atopic diseases six times more often [8].

It is generally considered that hepatitis A superinfection (an infection that develops on top of another infection) in hepatitis B and C chronic patients leads to liver failure and high fatality rates. However, there is also evidence that hepatitis A infection can cause a full or temporary recovery from chronic hepatitis. The mechanisms of this phenomenon are unknown. A 2009 article describes a case of a 24-year-old intravenous drug user with chronic hepatitis. He ate raw fish and got infected with hepatitis A. After the symptoms resolved, he no longer had chronic hepatitis C. It was most likely due to the interferon gamma (a cytokine produced by Th1 cells), the level of which increased significantly after the infection [9]. Cases of hepatitis B suppression at the time of hepatitis A infection have also been reported [10, 11].

Until 1966, all types of hepatitis were simply called "viral hepatitis." A 1949 article describes three cases of viral hepatitis in Hodgkin's lymphoma patients. In two of them, lymphoma symptoms improved together with hepatitis A, but the third one died. Encouraged by this apparent improvement, the authors infected 21 volunteer Hodgkin's lymphoma patients with hepatitis. According to the preliminary results, 13 of them got hepatitis, and seven of those who got hepatitis had improvements in their lymphomas. At the time of writing the article, no one died [12].

Before the vaccine was licensed, the incidence of hepatitis A in the US was approximately one in 10,000, and the mortality rate was one in three million. In 1999, vaccination was introduced in 11 states, where the incidence was higher than one in 5,000. In 2006, the vaccine was added to the national immunization schedule. Hepatitis A incidence at the time was one in 100,000, and the mortality rate was one in 10 million [13, 14]. Almost all fatal cases were in people over 50 years of age with underlying conditions.

Hepatitis A cases in the US (1966-2017)

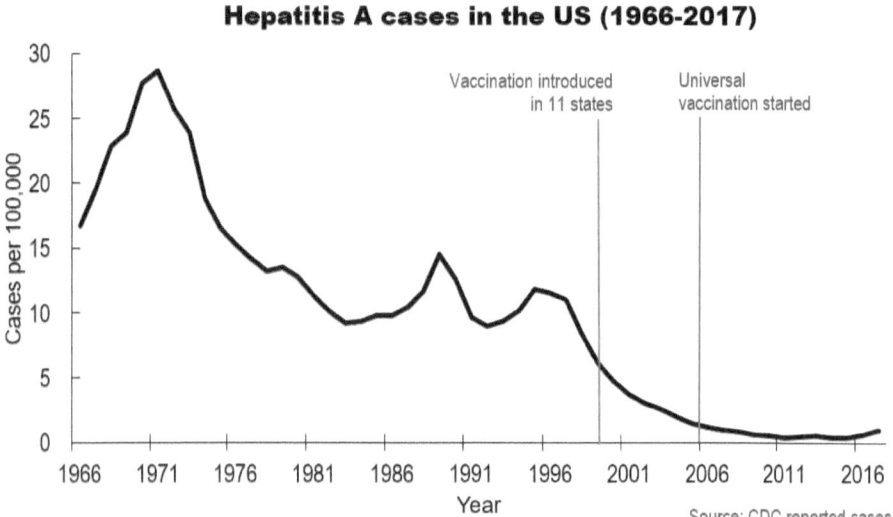

Source: CDC reported cases

Risk Factors

The number of hepatitis A cases in Germany, which was continuously decreasing, increased by 45% in 2015–16, and the median age of patients decreased significantly. It turned out to be because of the million asylum seekers that Germany hosted [15].

In 2001, the advisory committee of San Diego (California) highlighted the need for more public restrooms in the downtown area. A plan was developed in 2010 to fund four public toilets in downtown San Diego. Two units were installed in 2016, one of which was later removed because of the operating costs and concerns about crime. As of 2017, only one of the units has been installed and was in operation. Altogether, San Diego had a total of eight city restroom facilities, but only three were available 24 hours a day. San Francisco, on the other hand, another Californian city with a comparable homeless population, has 25 facilities open round the clock. In 2017, a hepatitis A outbreak began in the US, affecting mainly homeless people of San Diego, where more than 500 people were infected, and 20 people died. After that, 16 portable toilets and 78 hand-washing stations were installed in the city [16].

A pride parade (EuroPride), which attracted over half a million visitors, took place in Amsterdam in 2016. After that, the major European cities were swept by a wave of hepatitis A outbreaks among homosexuals. Thirty-seven cases were registered in England and 48 in the Netherlands [17, 18]. In most outbreaks, the detected strain was linked with the parade. Forty-six cases were registered in a Barcelona hospital. Ninety-six percent of them were male, and 67% identified themselves as homosexuals. The authors report that the main risk factor is the oral-anal contact during sex and that because of these outbreaks, hepatitis A was classified as a sexually transmitted disease [19].

In an outbreak in Berlin, out of 38 cases, 37 were men, of which 30 reported homosexual relationships. The woman also reported same-sex relationships. One of the patients was vaccinated 11 months before the disease onset [20]. In an outbreak in Rome, out of 513 cases, 87% were men [21]. In Tel Aviv, out of 19 cases, 17 were homosexuals [22]. In the Osaka outbreak, all 13 cases were homosexual, and the strain was linked to the Amsterdam pride parade [23]. Altogether, 1,500 cases of confirmed hepatitis A and 2,600 suspected cases, mainly among homosexuals, were reported in 16 European countries [24]. In the hepatitis A outbreak in Lyon in the first half of 2017, 46 cases were registered, 38 of them men, 33 homosexuals, and 15 HIV positive. Most of them have been vaccinated or had antibodies. It is also reported that since contracting hepatitis A is also possible from needle sharing, slamming (intravenous injection of recreational drugs along with anal intercourse), a practice that is gaining popularity among certain homosexual groups, can also increase the risk of infection [25].

In an outbreak of hepatitis A in Taiwan, out of more than 1,000 cases, 70% were homosexuals, 60% HIV positive, and over 60% also had syphilis, gonorrhea, or shigellosis [26]. There are no mentions of deaths from hepatitis A in any of these outbreaks.

Safety

According to a 2011 article, "There are no established criteria for diagnosing vaccine-related autoimmune disease. Postvaccination autoimmunity occurs quite a long time after vaccination, making it difficult to ascertain causality. Vaccines are composed of infectious agents, adjuvants, preservatives, and other ingredients. Each of these components might induce an immune response, which, in turn, could induce or aggravate autoimmunity." The authors vaccinated 40 healthy children against hepatitis A. Twenty-five percent of them developed autoantibodies (antibodies to own antigens), and one of them developed a temporary leukopenia (a decrease in the number of white blood cells). Two years after vaccination, two children still had autoantibodies [27].

In Vaqta vaccine clinical trials, aluminum was used as a placebo. In 1–10% of vaccinated children, conjunctivitis, otitis media, anorexia, insomnia, and other conditions were observed within 14 days after vaccination. Adults also experienced menstruation disorders and back pains. Serious adverse events were registered in 0.7% of those vaccinated, and 0.1% were judged to be vaccine-related by the study investigator [28]. In the Havrix clinical trials, the hepatitis B vaccine was used as a placebo. Serious adverse events were observed in 0.9% of the vaccinated with Havrix, together with other childhood vaccines [29].

As of 2019, over 150 death cases, 900 permanent disability cases, and over 4200 cases of serious adverse effects from hepatitis A vaccine have been registered with VAERS. In the pre-vaccine era, there were almost no cases of children dying from hepatitis A.

Conclusions

Hepatitis A is a mild disease in childhood, which is usually asymptomatic, especially in younger children. In developed countries in recent years it has mainly been affecting homosexuals.

Most countries do not vaccinate against hepatitis A.

Serious vaccination side effects, including death, are much more common than complications from hepatitis A.

Endnotes

1. Hepatitis A. *CDC Pink Book*

2. WHO position paper on hepatitis A vaccines – June 2012. *Wkly Epidemiol Rec.* 2012; 87(28/29):261–76

3. Lemon SM. Type A viral hepatitis: epidemiology, diagnosis, and prevention. *Clin Chem.* 1997;43(8 Pt 2):1494-9

4. Chen C et al. Hospitalization and mortality due to hepatitis A in Taiwan: a 15-year nationwide cohort study. *J Viral Hepat.* 2016;23(11):940-5

5. Bassal R et al. Seroprevalence of hepatitis A twelve years after the implementation of toddlers' vaccination: a population-based study in Israel. *Pediatr Infect Dis J.* 2017; 36(10):e248-51

6. Behrens RH et al. Is travel prophylaxis worth while? Economic appraisal of prophylactic measures against malaria, hepatitis A, and typhoid in travellers. *BMJ.* 1994;309(6959):918-22

7. Matricardi PM et al. Cross sectional retrospective study of prevalence of atopy among Italian military students with antibodies against hepatitis A virus. *BMJ.* 1997; 314(7086):999-1003

8. Kocabaş E et al. The prevalence of atopy in children with antibodies against hepatitis A virus and hepatitis B virus. *Turk J Pediatr.* 2006;48(3):189-96

9. Cacopardo B et al. Clearance of HCV RNA following acute hepatitis A superinfection. *Dig Liver Dis.* 2009;41(5):371-4

10. van Nunen AB et al. Suppression of hepatitis B virus replication mediated by hepatitis A-induced cytokine production. *Liver.* 2001;21(1):45-9

11. Davis GL et al. Acute type A hepatitis during chronic hepatitis B virus infection: association of depressed hepatitis B virus replication with appearance of endogenous alpha interferon. *J Med Virol.* 1984;14(2):141-7

12. Hoster HA et al. Studies in Hodgkin's syndrome; the association of viral hepatitis and Hodgkin's disease; a preliminary report. *Cancer Res.* 1949;9(8):473-80

13. Daniels D et al. Surveillance for acute viral hepatitis - United States, 2007. *MMWR.* 2009;58(3):1-27

14. Reported Cases and Deaths from Vaccine Preventable Diseases, United States

15. Michaelis K et al. Hepatitis A virus infections and outbreaks in asylum seekers arriving to Germany, September 2015 to March 2016. *Emerg Microbes Infect.* 2017;6(4):e26

16. Nelson R. Hepatitis A outbreak in the USA. *Lancet Infect Dis.* 2018;18(1):33-4

17. Beebeejaun K et al. Outbreak of hepatitis A associated with men who have sex with men (MSM), England, July 2016 to January 2017. *Euro Surveill.* 2017;22(5)

18. Freidl GS et al. Hepatitis A outbreak among men who have sex with men (MSM) predominantly linked with the EuroPride, the Netherlands, July 2016 to February 2017. *Euro Surveill.* 2017;22(8)

19. Rodríguez-Tajes S et al. Hepatitis A outbreak in Barcelona among men who have sex with men (MSM), January-June 2017: a hospital perspective. *Liver Int.* 2018;38(4):588-93

20. Werber D et al. Ongoing outbreaks of hepatitis A among men who have sex with men (MSM), Berlin, November 2016 to January 2017 - linked to other German cities and European countries. *Euro Surveill.* 2017;22(5)

21. Lanini S et al. A large ongoing outbreak of hepatitis A predominantly affecting young males in Lazio, Italy; August 2016 - March 2017. *PloS One.* 2017;12(11):e0185428

22. Gozlan Y et al. Ongoing hepatitis A among men who have sex with men (MSM) linked to outbreaks in Europe in Tel Aviv area, Israel, December 2016 - June 2017. *Euro Surveill.* 2017;22(29)

23. Tanaka S et al. Outbreak of hepatitis A linked to European outbreaks among men who have sex with men in Osaka, Japan, from March to July 2018. *Hepatol Res.* 2019; 49(6):705-710

24. Farfour E et al. Acute hepatitis A breakthrough in MSM in Paris area: implementation of targeted hepatitis A virus vaccine in a context of vaccine shortage. *AIDS.* 2018; 32(4):531-2

25. Charre C et al. Hepatitis A outbreak in HIV-infected MSM and in PrEP-using MSM despite a high level of immunity, Lyon, France, January to June 2017. *Euro Surveill.* 2017; 22(48)

26. Chen GJ et al. Hepatitis A outbreak among men who have sex with men in a country of low endemicity of hepatitis A infection. *J Infect Dis.* 2017;215(8):1339-40

27. Karali Z et al. Autoimmunity and hepatitis A vaccine in children. *J Investig Allergol Clin Immunol.* 2011;21(5):389-93

28. Vaqta vaccine package insert

29. Havrix vaccine package insert

Chapter Twenty-Three

TUBERCULOSIS

*The great tragedy of Science is the slaying
of a beautiful hypothesis by an ugly fact.*
— Thomas Huxley

B illions of people were vaccinated against tuberculosis with the BCG
vaccines since 1921—more than with any other vaccines. Despite
such a lengthy track record, BCG vaccination has generated at least
as much controversy as any other form of immunization. Its effectiveness
against tuberculosis is still debated since randomized clinical trials have
provided estimates ranging from 80% protection to no benefit at all.

Even though BCG vaccines are considered among the safest, the true
incidence of complications such as BCG-lymphadenitis or BCG-
osteomyelitis is unknown [1]. A BCG vaccine review published in 2002
reports that tuberculosis is caused by the bacterium *Mycobacterium
tuberculosis*. However, the vaccine contains other bacterium—*Mycobacterium
bovis*, which causes tuberculosis in cows.

> This is because Calmette and Guérin, after whom the vaccine is
> named (**B**acillus **C**almette–**G**uérin), originally developed it for
> cattle, and not for humans.

In order to prevent the bacteria from clumping together, Calmette added bile to the culture medium. Within a few months, an unusual colony type arose, which was less virulent for the guinea pigs. Calmette continued the process of growing these bacteria in the presence of bile for an astonishing 13 years, changing the culture medium every two weeks.

Since 1921, people started to receive the BCG vaccine. At that time, it was not possible to freeze-dry bacteria without destroying it; therefore, bacteria for BCG continued to be grown using the original method until 1961.

In 1924, BCG lots began to be distributed to various countries, where the attenuation of the bacteria continued for the same purpose—namely to prevent BCG from reverting to virulence while preserving an acceptable degree of what was called "potency." Thus, in different countries, daughter BCG strains were formed, which were named after the location of the laboratory (BCG Russia, Tokyo, etc.).

Presently, all BCG strains are prepared as lyophilized (freeze-dried) stocks that are resuspended before vaccination by adding water. In most BCG vaccines, 90–95% of bacteria are dead, but BCG-Tokyo is estimated to consist of 25% live bacteria. The importance of the proportion of viable bacteria in the vaccine is yet to be formally assessed. For example, do more dead bacteria compensate for less of the living ones? Science does not yet know the answer to this question.

The presence of antigens in the absence of virulence is an important factor for the attenuated vaccine. However, it is known that certain BCG strains have lost antigens compared to the original bacterium. In an experiment in Czechoslovakia, the BCG-Prague strain was replaced by BCG-Russia strain. Rates of disseminated BCG disease, including BCG osteitis, were greater with the Russian strain.

> In the 1970s, there was an epidemic of BCG osteitis in Sweden and Finland, after which Finland switched to another BCG strain, and Sweden halted the vaccination.

Have BCG strains evolved over time? The answer is clearly, yes. Does it matter? The answer depends on who this question is addressed to. A bacteriologist would be surprised if BCG has not changed considerably during the half-century of growth in the laboratory. For the person planning to administer BCG to an infant or for the public health official planning the vaccination of millions of newborns, more information is needed. Is there "the most protective BCG"? Is there "the safest BCG"? Are these necessarily different? Unfortunately, answers to these questions cannot yet be given. The author concludes that regardless of whether the future involves specific BCG strains, a genetically altered BCG, or a completely new vaccine, one hopes that those currently providing BCG vaccines will be prepared to validate laboratory observations in the field so that we are not once again left with the uncertainty of vaccinating millions each year without a clear understanding of its risks and benefits [1].

A 2011 review published in the *Lancet* reported that four billion people had been vaccinated with the BCG vaccine since 1921. More than 90% of children in the world today receive this vaccine. However, it has done little to contain the current tuberculosis pandemic. The worldwide number of new cases today is higher than at any other time in history.

Despite the evidence of confirmed efficacy against childhood tuberculous meningitis and miliary tuberculosis, protection induced by BCG can wane within a decade. Tuberculosis is still a disease of poverty and is inextricably associated with overcrowding and undernutrition. The authors conclude that our fundamental understanding of the pathogenesis of this disease is inadequate. Despite substantial progress in the worldwide tuberculosis control, it is unclear why tuberculosis incidence is falling only at a rate of less than 1% per year [2].

The authors of the 2017 article, who reviewed BCG studies of the last 20 years, write that the protective efficacy of BCG varies depending on the geographical location of where it was administered. They go on to say that we understand very little about why it protects when it does, or why it fails to protect in other cases. We are still unable to identify BCG-induced markers of protection in vaccinated infants. (*That is, if after other vaccines it is possible to test the level of antibodies, in case of BCG, it is impossible to establish whether the vaccine had any effect or not.*) BCG bacteria are still present in the vaccination site one month after vaccination, and for how long they survive is unknown. There have been case reports of long-term survival of BCG (for example, an HIV-infected individual developing disseminated BCG from the vaccine strain 30 years after the vaccination) [3].

At present, the World Health Organization estimates that approximately one-third of the world's population is infected with tuberculosis bacteria. However, only around 10% of all infected individuals, mainly those with lowered immunity, will ever develop an active disease.

Before antibiotics and other chemical therapies appeared, the typical treatment for tuberculosis involved increasing patient's immunity through improved nutrition, hygiene, and rest. All of these measures were used at sanatoria and resulted in the decline in mortality due to tuberculosis throughout the 19th century, long before antibiotics appeared. Antibiotics and other chemical therapies were introduced in the 1940s and 1950s, and their use caused the development of drug-resistant bacteria. In Peru, the incidence of tuberculosis was declining by 3.7% per year since 1996, but the incidence of cases caused by multiple-drug resistant strains has increased by 4.5%. In Belarus, 35% of newly diagnosed patients and 76% of previously treated patients had multiple-drug resistant tuberculosis. The authors of a 2014 study analyzed tuberculosis mortality in several countries and concluded that in Switzerland, England, and New York, the decline had occurred long before the introduction of anti-tuberculosis drugs. In Brazil and Japan, chemical therapy was coincident with the decline in tuberculosis mortality rates.

In Sierra Leone, the tuberculosis mortality rate had increased threefold in 20 years, despite the availability of antibiotics, which are ineffective. A sharp increase in mortality was observed in Japan in the late XIX – early XX centuries, during the time of heavy industrialization, and, most likely, the same happened in developed countries as well, before the statistics were collected [4].

In 1929, an incident occurred in the city of Lübeck in Germany, which was later called the "Lübeck disaster." Two hundred fifty-one neonates were given three doses of the new BCG vaccine orally, after which 90% developed tuberculosis, and 72 of them died. It was later determined that the vaccine had been contaminated with variable amounts of fully virulent M. tuberculosis. The authors of a study published in 2016 conclude three lessons from this incident. First, while the mortality was high (29%), the majority of neonates inoculated with M. tuberculosis eventually overcame the disease. This shows the high constitutional resistance of humans to the bacillus. Second, those who received a low dose of bacteria coped with the disease better than those who received a higher dose, which implies that the effectiveness of innate immunity depends on the dose of the bacteria. Third, two infants inoculated with the lowest dose died nevertheless, and their median time from inoculation to death was substantially shorter than for those who died after inoculation with higher doses. This suggests that some children are probably genetically susceptible to the disease [5].

264

Of the Western European countries, BCG is still officially included in the national immunization schedule only in Ireland. However, in practice, the vaccine stocks ran out in 2015, and since then, BCG in Ireland is not used.

Risk Factors

Active and passive smoking is associated with a twofold risk of tuberculosis [6]. In past and present smokers, the risk of infection, the risk of developing tuberculosis, the risk of complications, and the risk of death from tuberculosis are increased [7].

In underweight people, the risk of tuberculosis is 12 times higher compared to people with normal weight. In overweight people, the risk of tuberculosis is three times lower, and in obese people, it is five times lower. In the 1950s, it was found that men with low vitamin A and C levels had a higher tuberculosis incidence than men with adequate levels. The use of multivitamin-mineral supplements decreased tuberculosis incidence among family members of active tuberculosis cases. Since then, no adequate research has been carried out on the effect of nutrients on tuberculosis risk [8].

The association between diabetes and tuberculosis was documented by Avicenna, and we are re-discovering it today [9]. Diabetics contract tuberculosis three times more often and HIV carriers 20 times more often [2]. The risk of tuberculosis is also increased by the use of immunosuppressive drugs, such as corticosteroids. The association of drugs for rheumatological disorders with tuberculosis is an increasing problem in industrialized countries. According to the CDC, other risk factors include substance abuse, being homeless, or in prison. In 2015, 470 people died from tuberculosis in the United States.

Effectiveness

According to a systematic review published in 2014, the efficacy of the BCG vaccine for infants is 59%. Protection against meningeal and miliary tuberculosis was 90%. The further from the equator, the more effective the vaccine is. At an older age, the vaccine is less effective [10].

The largest double-blind, randomized controlled trial of BCG efficacy was conducted in south India and included 280,000 people, which were followed for 15 years. Two strains of BCG were used, both in high and low doses. The vaccine offered no overall protection in adults and a low level of overall protection (27%) in children, with no statistical significance. In the first years after the start of the trial, the vaccinated contracted tuberculosis more often than the unvaccinated. Then, in the period of five to 12 years after the vaccination, the unvaccinated contracted tuberculosis with higher incidence. After 12 years, tuberculosis was again occurring more in the vaccinated. The varying pattern of susceptibility by the period of follow up was observed in other trials as well [11].

A large double-blind, randomized controlled trial to evaluate the effectiveness of repeated BCG vaccination was conducted in northern Malawi (120,000 subjects). The vaccinated contracted leprosy 49% less often, but tuberculosis 69% more often. Other studies in Malawi and Venezuela also found that BCG does not protect against tuberculosis but protects against leprosy to some extent [12].

> The WHO recognized that there is no evidence of the effectiveness of revaccination and does not recommend it.

A controlled trial of BCG vaccination was conducted in 1950 in the USA. Throughout 14 years of observation, the efficacy of the vaccine was only 14%. Moreover, BCG vaccination had negative efficacy among the African American population. It was concluded that the protection offered by the vaccine was less than modest, relatively short-lived, and least effective among the segments of the population that needed it most. **Thus, BCG has never been introduced into the US vaccination schedule [13].**

The immunogenicity of tuberculosis vaccines is usually determined by the cytokine expression profile of T cells. However, a 2010 study found that the cytokine profile did not correlate with protection against tuberculosis [14].

A 2005 study found that a person who has previously been sick with tuberculosis has a four times higher risk of repeated infection than someone who hasn't been infected before. The authors conclude that "The failure of natural disease to protect against reinfection disease at a later point may partially explain the relative ineffectiveness of vaccination with BCG" [15].

And here is what the authors of a 2000 article titled "Is the development of a new tuberculosis vaccine possible?" write:

"Sadly, we are no closer to eliminating or even controlling tuberculosis (TB) today than we were when Koch first identified the causative agent, Mycobacterium tuberculosis. Although a meta-analysis of all vaccination data available has yielded a theoretical efficacy rate of 50%, it has been estimated that only 5% of all vaccine-preventable deaths caused by TB could have been prevented by BCG. Thus, BCG is not a satisfactory vaccine.

"In case of TB, the vaccinologists are faced with a difficult hurdle – to design a vaccine that is superior to the pathogen with regard to the immune response evoked. Given that T-cells are central to protection against TB, future vaccine design should focus on T-lymphocyte populations. Unfortunately, there is no precedent for this because all successful vaccines in use today work through antibodies rather than T-cells.

"Imagine the following scenario: one of the heroes in the TB field proclaims he has developed a therapeutic vaccine for TB based on his success in curing the disease in experimental animals. Because of the reputation of the scientist, and to proceed as fast as possible, controlled clinical trials comprising almost 2000 TB patients are immediately initiated by a governmental agency and the results already provided after 6 months. Due to great economic interest, the product is licensed to a pharmaceutical company, making the investigator a millionaire. The story is true. It occurred between August 1890 when Robert Koch, the highly respected discoverer of the TB bacillus, proclaimed at the 10th International Congress of Medicine that he had found a remedy for TB, and February 1891 when the official report on the clinical trials was published. Unfortunately, the report was crushing, with only 2% cured. We cannot risk such a fiasco again and it is therefore appropriate to ask whether the task of developing a TB vaccine is too formidable, even today" [16].

Safety

Until recently, it was believed that the uterus was sterile and that babies were born sterile. However, the latest evidence has refuted this paradigm. It turned out that the placenta is colonized by non-pathogenic bacteria and has its own microbiome (placentobiome) that performs metabolic functions and is different in premature and full-term infants.

L-forms are bacteria that lack a cell wall but still have the ability to develop. The BCG vaccine was found to contain L-form bacteria, which are able to multiply and form colonies. A study published in 2017, found that mothers vaccinated against tuberculosis in infancy, pass on the BCG bacteria L-forms to their newborn children through placenta. **Bacteria have been found in the placenta and umbilical cord blood of infants of 85% of the vaccinated mothers, and the infection occurred in the early stages of pregnancy.**

These transmitted mycobacterial L-forms originated from the maternal BCG vaccine and have a capacity to revert back to walled mycobacteria. Recent experiments have shown that L-forms can multiply indefinitely "as an alternative form of bacterial life."

Little is known of how long M. bovis BCG bacteria can survive in the vaccinated persons. Recently published data showed that conversion of bacteria to L-forms may often result in chronic infections, since L-forms remain dormant in the tissues for long periods, sequestering in protective regions of the body. Despite large amounts of literature published on L-forms, atypical bacterial forms have been neglected by clinicians for a very long time because of difficulty in identifying and proving them. However, they can survive for a significant length of time and can be the cause of latent, chronic, and recurrent infections, as well as the cause of diseases of unknown infectious-allergic or autoimmune origin [17].

According to a 2017 meta-analysis, BCG vaccination is associated with a 27% reduction in the risk of leukemia [18]. However, if all types of cancer were taken into account, BCG vaccination was associated with an increase in the risk of cancer by 13% [19].

After the BCG vaccination was discontinued on the southern island of New Zealand but continued on the northern island, the mortality rate from non-Hodgkin's lymphoma increased on the northern island and decreased on the southern island, even though it was the same level before. The authors conclude that proposals for using BCG vaccination against leukemia are unwise [20].

Non-Specific Effects

According to a 2006 review, when the BCG vaccine was introduced in the 1920s, it was suggested that BCG occasionally had nonspecific beneficial effects on mortality beyond the specific protection against tuberculosis. Considering that BCG has since then become the most used vaccine in the world, surprisingly few studies have been undertaken into the effect of BCG on general mortality and morbidity. Recent studies suggest that BCG has beneficial nontargeted effects on general infant morbidity and mortality in low-income countries, especially among girls. Apart from the anti-tetanus vaccination of pregnant women, none of the routine vaccines that are in use worldwide today were introduced as a result of trials focused on general mortality and morbidity as major outcomes [21].

According to a 2010 study, routine infant vaccines currently used in low-income countries were not tested in randomized trials for their impact on overall child survival before their introduction. It has been assumed that the impact of a vaccine on mortality is proportional to the vaccine's efficacy and the contribution of the target disease to overall mortality.

The previous 15 years of research, however, have shown that this assumption is not a tenable basis for vaccination policy as vaccines might have important non-specific effects. Measles and BCG vaccines, for example, are associated with a decrease in mortality, while DTP or a high titer measles vaccine is associated with an increase in mortality.

The authors investigated the efficacy of BCG revaccination in Guinea Bissau. The trial was stopped prematurely because of a **2.7-fold higher death rate among those vaccinated with BCG**. The authors believe that this was not related to the BCG vaccine, but to other vaccines, and to iron and vitamin A supplements that the children received during the study. In a study from Bangladesh, children who were vaccinated with BCG after nine months of age tended to have increased mortality. BCG, in general, was associated with a twofold increased mortality between nine months and five years of age [22].

According to observational studies, many African girls under the age of one year die every year from the nonspecific effects of DTP vaccination. In contrast, similar studies suggest that many African children may have their lives saved by the nonspecific immunological benefits of BCG. From an immunological point of view, this most likely happens because the immune reaction to DTP is shifted towards Th2 due to the aluminum adjuvant and because the intramuscular administration of the vaccine can cause chronic inflammation at the injection site. Unlike DTP, BCG shifts the immune reaction towards Th1, which probably has a beneficial effect [23].

Ten thousand infants participated in a study of the nonspecific effects of the vaccine in southern India. Among those who were vaccinated with one of the vaccines (DTP or BCG), mortality was lower compared to the unvaccinated. However, among those vaccinated with both vaccines, mortality was the same as among the unvaccinated. In girls who received both vaccines, mortality was 4.5 times higher than in those vaccinated with one vaccine. **The authors eliminated deaths in the first week, thinking they could not be due to non-specific effects of BCG vaccine, and that the high mortality in that first week might cloud relevant associations [24].**

Inspired by the non-specific effects of BCG in the Third World countries, the authors of the study published in 2016 decided to conduct a randomized BCG trial in Denmark, but they did not find non-specific effects. Vaccinated children did not get sick less than unvaccinated children [25].

According to several studies, systemic infections such as measles, hepatitis A and tuberculosis prevent allergies and asthma. This is explained by the fact that certain bacterial and viral infections shift the immune response towards Th1. BCG vaccination, however, does not prevent allergies and asthma [26]. BCG is, nonetheless, the most effective treatment for bladder cancer [27].

Vitamins C and D

In a 1933 study, guinea pigs were fed tuberculosis bacteria. Seventy percent of those who were maintained on a diet deficient in vitamin C developed intestinal tuberculosis. Among the animals whose diet was supplemented with an adequate amount of vitamin C (in the form of tomato juice or cabbage leaves), only 5% developed tuberculous. The authors conclude that the adequate supply of vitamin C protects guinea pigs from tuberculosis [28]. A protective effect of vitamin C against tuberculous infections in animals has been repeatedly described. Decreased resistance to tuberculous infection is observed in animals fed a vitamin C deficient diet and, conversely, increased susceptibility to acute scurvy is seen in infected animals. Tuberculosis patients excrete less vitamin C in urine than healthy people, which seems to indicate that there is an increased requirement for vitamin C during the infection [29]. According to a 2013 study, vitamin C levels in serum and cerebrospinal fluid of tuberculous meningitis cases was lower than in the control group. Among patients with complications, vitamin C levels were significantly lower compared to patients without complications [30]. In the same year, it was discovered that vitamin C kills tuberculosis bacteria in vitro [31]. According to a 2018 study, combining vitamin C with tuberculosis medications leads to faster recovery in mice [32].

In the pre-antibiotic era, high doses of vitamin D were widely used to treat tuberculosis patients. In 1854, Hermann Brehmer, a botany student who was suffering from TB, traveled to the Himalayan mountains to pursue his botanical studies and cured his TB. Low vitamin D levels have been associated with a fivefold increased risk of development of TB [33]. In a clinical study, the effects of two doses of vitamin D (600,000 IU) led to an improvement in symptoms [34]. In another clinical study, vitamin D supplementation did not reduce mortality. However, a dose of only 100,000 IU was used, which was probably insufficient, as the vitamin D levels in the participants did not significantly change during the study [35].

Statistics

In a 2008 study, tuberculosis incidence in different countries was compared with the gross domestic product (GDP). The study revealed that

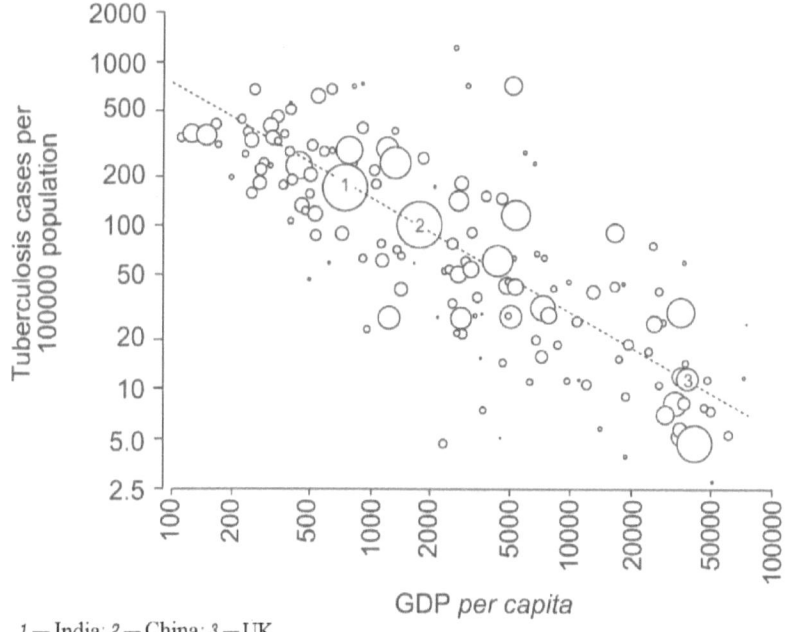

1 — India; 2 — China; 3 — UK

«Reproduced with permission of the © ERS 2019: European Respiratory Journal 32(5) 1415–1416; DOI: 10.1183/09031936.00078708 Published 31 October 2008»

the higher the income per capita is, the lower is the tuberculosis incidence in the country. The authors conclude: "To stop tuberculosis, we must fight poverty" [36].

The tuberculosis mortality rate in England decreased by 90% before antibiotics were introduced [4]. The same happened in the US. Before the vaccine development was initiated, tuberculosis mortality decreased by 98%.

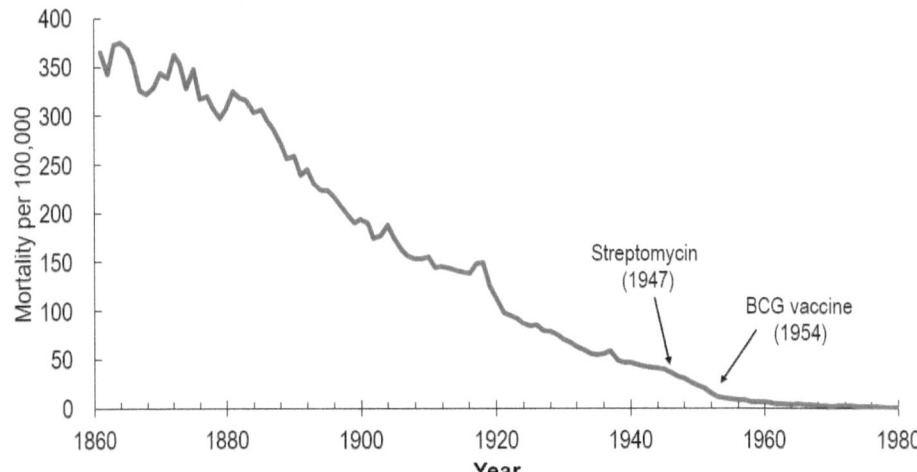

Tuberculosis mortality in the US (1860-1980)

Conclusions

Tuberculosis is the disease of poor countries. In developed countries, where there are no problems with good nutrition, tuberculosis is rare.

One-third of the world population is infected with Mycobacterium tuberculosis, but only 10% of them might develop the disease.

The tuberculosis vaccine is ineffective and probably causes more adverse events than tuberculosis.

Endnotes

1. Behr MA. BCG—different strains, different vaccines? *Lancet Infect Dis.* 2002;2(2):86-92

2. Lawn SD et al. Tuberculosis. *Lancet.* 2011;378(9785):57-72

3. Dockrell HM et al. What have we learnt about BCG vaccination in the last 20 years? *Front Immunol.* 2017;8:1134

4. Holloway KL et al. Lessons from history of socioeconomic improvements: a new approach to treating multi-drug-resistant tuberculosis. *J Biosoc Sci*. 2014;46(5):600-20

5. Fox GJ et al. Tuberculosis in newborns: the lessons of the "Lübeck Disaster". *PLoS Pathog*. 2016;12(1):e1005271

6. Lindsay RP et al. The Association between active and passive smoking and latent tuberculosis infection in adults and children in the united states: results from NHANES. *PloS One*. 2014;9(3):e93137

7. Hassmiller KM. The association between smoking and tuberculosis. *Salud Publica Mex*. 2006;48 Suppl 1:S201-16

8. Cegielski JP et al. Nutritional risk factors for tuberculosis among adults in the United States, 1971-1992. *Am J Epidemiol*. 2012;176(5):409-22

9. Restrepo BI. Convergence of the tuberculosis and diabetes epidemics: renewal of old acquaintances. *Clin Infect Dis*. 2007;45(4):436-8

10. Mangtani P et al. Protection by BCG vaccine against tuberculosis: a systematic review of randomized controlled trials. *Clin Infect Dis*. 2014;58(4):470-80

11. Fifteen year follow up of trial of BCG vaccines in south India for tuberculosis prevention. *Indian J Med Res*. 1999;110:56-69

12. Randomised controlled trial of single BCG, repeated BCG, or combined BCG and killed Mycobacterium leprae vaccine for prevention of leprosy and tuberculosis in Malawi. *Lancet*. 1996;348(9019):17-24

13. Comstock GW et al. Long-term results of BCG vaccination in the southern United States. *Am Rev Respir Dis*. 1966;93(2):171-83

14. Kagina BM et al. Specific T cell frequency and cytokine expression profile do not correlate with protection against tuberculosis after bacillus Calmette-Guérin vaccination of newborns. *Am J Respir Crit Care Med*. 2010;182(8):1073-9

15. Verver S et al. Rate of reinfection tuberculosis after successful treatment is higher than rate of new tuberculosis. *Am J Respir Crit Care Med*. 2005;171(12):1430-5

16. Kaufmann SH. Is the development of a new tuberculosis vaccine possible? *Nat Med*. 2000;6(9):955-60

17. Dimova T et al. Mother-to-newborn transmission of mycobacterial L-forms and Vδ2 T-cell response in placentobiome of BCG-vaccinated pregnant women. *Sci Rep*. 2017; 7(1):17366

18. Morra ME et al. Early vaccination protects against childhood leukemia: a systematic review and meta-analysis. *Sci Rep*. 2017;7(1):15986

19. Kendrick MA et al. BCG vaccination and the subsequent development of cancer in humans. *J Natl Cancer Inst*. 1981;66(3):431-7

20. Skegg DC. BCG vaccination and the incidence of lymphomas and leukaemia. *Int J Cancer*. 1978;21(1):18-21

21. Roth A et al. Bacillus Calmette-Guérin vaccination and infant mortality. *Expert Rev Vaccines*. 2006;5(2):277-93

22. Roth A et al. Effect of revaccination with BCG in early childhood on mortality: randomised trial in Guinea-Bissau. *BMJ*. 2010;340:c671

23. Claesson MH. Immunological Links to Nonspecific Effects of DTwP and BCG Vaccines on Infant Mortality. *J Trop Med*. 2011;2011:706304

24. Moulton LH et al. Evaluation of non-specific effects of infant immunizations on early infant mortality in a southern Indian population. *Trop Med Int Health*. 2005;10(10):947-55

25. Kjærgaard J et al. Nonspecific effect of BCG vaccination at birth on early childhood infections: a randomized, clinical multicenter trial. *Pediatr Res.* 2016;80(5):681-5

26. von Hertzen LC. Puzzling associations between childhood infections and the later occurrence of asthma and atopy. *Ann Med.* 2000;32(6):397-400

27. Fuge O et al. Immunotherapy for bladder cancer. *Res Rep Urol.* 2015;7:65-79

28. McConkey M et al. The relation of vitamin C deficiency to intestinal tuberculosis in the guinea pig. *J Exp Med.* 1933;58(4):503-12

29. Vitamin C and tuberculosis. *JAMA.* 1936;107(15):1225-6

30. Miric D et al. Changes in vitamin C and oxidative stress status during the treatment of tuberculous meningitis. *Int J Tuberc Lung Dis.* 2013;17(11):1495-500

31. Vilchèze C et al. Mycobacterium tuberculosis is extraordinarily sensitive to killing by a vitamin C-induced Fenton reaction. *Nat Commun.* 2013;4:1881

32. Vilchèze C et al. Vitamin C potentiates the killing of mycobacterium tuberculosis by the first-line tuberculosis drugs isoniazid and rifampin in mice. *Antimicrob Agents Chemother.* 2018;62(3)

33. Luong Kv et al. Impact of vitamin D in the treatment of tuberculosis. *Am J Med Sci.* 2011; 341(6):493-8

34. Salahuddin N et al. Vitamin D accelerates clinical recovery from tuberculosis: results of the SUCCINCT Study. A randomized, placebo-controlled, clinical trial of vitamin D supplementation in patients with pulmonary tuberculosis'. *BMC Infect Dis.* 2013;13:22

35. Wejse C et al. Vitamin D as supplementary treatment for tuberculosis: a double-blind, randomized, placebo-controlled trial. *Am J Respir Crit Care Med.* 2009;179(9):843-50

36. Janssens JP et al. An ecological analysis of incidence of tuberculosis and per capita gross domestic product. *Eur Respir J.* 2008;32(5):1415-6

Chapter Twenty-Four

MERCURY

*Medical science has made such tremendous progress
that there is hardly a healthy human left.*
— **Aldous Huxley**

A ccording to the WHO, mercury is one of the ten most dangerous chemicals. Mercury, states the WHO, is particularly dangerous to the development of the child in utero and in early life. Mercury is dangerous in elemental form (metal), as well as in inorganic (mercury chloride) and organic (methyl mercury) compounds. However, there is one organic compound of mercury, which is so safe, that infants and pregnant women can be safely injected with it. This compound is called **ethyl mercury** [1].

Thimerosal (*sodium ethylmercurithiosalicylate*) is a preservative that is added to multi-dose vaccine vials to prevent microbial contamination after opening the vial. Multi-dose vaccine vials are 2.5 times cheaper than single-dose vials. That is, a multi-dose vaccine costs 10 cents per dose, and a single-dose vaccine costs 25 cents. Moreover, single-dose vaccines occupy more space in refrigerators. These are the main reasons for using thimerosal. The concentration of thimerosal in vaccines is 0.01% or 25–50 mcg per dose. Mercury makes up 50% of the thimerosal weight, which means that one vaccine dose contains from 12.5 to 25 mcg of mercury [2].

Thimerosal was patented in 1928 under the trade name of "**Merthiolate**." It turned out that thimerosal is 40 times more effective as an antibacterial agent than phenol. Toxicity studies revealed that mice, rats, and rabbits, injected intravenously with thimerosal, had almost no reaction to it. They were only observed for one week [3].

A 1929 meningococcal infection epidemic in Indianapolis presented an opportunity to test the substance on humans. Twenty-two meningitis patients received a large dose of thimerosal intravenously, and it did not cause an anaphylactic shock in any of them. Researchers have concluded that thimerosal is safe. Subsequently, it turned out that all these 22 patients died [4]. This was the only clinical study, and since then, no more thimerosal safety studies have ever been conducted.

It was already known in 1943 that thimerosal is not ideal as a preservative and that microorganisms survive at a concentration used in vaccines. In 1982, the outbreaks of streptococcal abscesses resulting from DTP vaccines were observed. It turned out that streptococci survive in vaccines with thimerosal for two weeks. In another study, it turned out that thimerosal does not meet the European requirements for antibacterial effectiveness.

In 1999, the American Academy of Pediatrics (AAP) and the US Public Health Service called for the elimination of thimerosal from all vaccines in the US as soon as possible, as it turned out that its amount in vaccines exceeds the guidelines. In the early 2000s, more and more vaccines without thimerosal became available, and it was logical to expect that now children would be exposed to smaller amounts of mercury. However, this was not exactly what happened. Starting from 2002, the CDC began recommending influenza vaccines for infants, and the only vaccine licensed for children contained thimerosal. Then CDC extended recommendations of thimerosal-containing influenza vaccines to pregnant women. Since 2010, infants started to receive two doses of influenza vaccine initially (at six and seven months of age), and then one dose every year.

> Therefore, even though thimerosal was removed or almost removed from other vaccines, the amount of mercury children receive from vaccines remained approximately the same, and lifetime exposure to mercury from vaccines has more than doubled compared to the pre-2000 recommended schedule.

Thimerosal also remained in one of the meningococcal vaccines and in one tetanus and diphtheria vaccine [5]. Almost everywhere else in the world, thimerosal remained in other childhood vaccines as well. In 2012 the American Academy of Pediatrics and the WHO persuaded the United Nations not to ban the use of mercury in vaccines [6].

The Effect Of Vaccination On Mercury Levels

After vaccination with the hepatitis B vaccine, the blood concentration of mercury in preterm newborns increased more than 13-fold, and in full-term newborns, it increased 56-fold. The pre-vaccination level of mercury in preterm newborns was ten times higher than in full-term newborns, which suggests a higher maternal exposure to mercury of preterm newborns. Although 5–20 mcg/L is considered to be the normal level of mercury in the blood according to the HHS (Health & Human Services) guidelines, there are discrepancies in the published literature regarding what is considered normal and toxic levels. Furthermore, this data was derived entirely from adults with occupational exposure to mercury [7].

In a Brazilian study, mercury levels in the hair of infants, who received thimerosal vaccines, increased by 446% in the first six months. During the same time, mercury levels in the hair of their mothers decreased by 57% [8].

A study published in 2005 reported on newborn monkeys, one group of which received vaccines containing thimerosal in doses equivalent to those used for humans. The other group of monkeys received the same dose of methyl mercury through an oral tube. The half-life of mercury in the blood was much shorter for thimerosal (seven days) than for methyl mercury (19 days), and the concentration of mercury in the brain was three times lower in those who received thimerosal, as compared to those who got methyl mercury. However, 34% of mercury in the brain of thimerosal recipients was in an inorganic form, while for the methyl mercury recipients, this number was only 7%. **The absolute level of inorganic mercury in the brain was twice as high in thimerosal recipients than in methyl mercury recipients.** The level of inorganic mercury in the kidneys was also significantly higher in those who received thimerosal. It is known that inorganic mercury remains in the brain for years and decades [9]. The level of inorganic mercury in the brain did not change for a month after the last dose, unlike the level of organic mercury. Other studies also found that the level of inorganic mercury in the brain does not decrease.

"Results from an initial Institute of Medicine review (2001) of the safety of vaccines found that there was no sufficient evidence to render an opinion on the relationship between ethyl mercury exposure and developmental disorders in children. The IOM review did, however, note the possibility of such a relationship and recommended further studies to be conducted. However, a subsequent 2004 review abandoned the earlier recommendation as well as backed away from the AAP goal (to eliminate thimerosal from vaccines)." The authors conclude that "This approach is difficult to understand, given our current limited knowledge of the toxicokinetics and developmental neurotoxicity of thimerosal, a compound that has been (and will continue to be) injected in millions of newborns and infants" [10].

Hamsters that were given thimerosal injection in doses equivalent to those used for humans had lower brain and body weight, smaller stature, decrease in neuronal density, neuronal necrosis, demyelination and necrosis of the Purkinje cells, which is characteristic of ASD [11]. Male voles that had mercury or cadmium added to their water started showing autism symptoms [12].

Ethyl-, Methyl- And Inorganic Mercury

A CDC review article, published in 2017, analyzes studies of ethyl mercury and methyl mercury, and concludes that both forms are equally toxic. Among other things, both cause DNA damage, impair DNA synthesis, alter intracellular calcium homeostasis, disrupt cell division mechanism, lead to oxidative stress, disrupt glutamate homeostasis and decrease glutathione activity, which, in turn, further weakens the protection against oxidative stress [13].

In a 2012 Croatian study, newborn rats were divided into two groups. The first group received thimerosal injections, and the second group received inorganic mercury ($HgCl_2$) injections. They were observed for six days. Thimerosal receiving rats had a much higher brain and blood concentration of mercury than the inorganic mercury recipients [14]. In another study, newborn rats, which received thimerosal injections, had 1.5 times higher brain concentration and 23 times higher blood concentration of mercury, compared to rats that received inorganic mercury injections.

According to the authors, "This confirms the fact that ethyl mercury, which is a metabolic product of thimerosal, more easily passes the blood–brain barrier" [15].

According to an Italian study, ethyl mercury is 50 times more toxic for cells than methyl mercury [16]. Ethyl mercury also crosses the placenta easier than methyl mercury [17].

Thimerosal Toxicity

In a 2010 Polish study, newborn rats were injected with thimerosal in doses equivalent to those used for vaccination of human infants. Ischemic degeneration of neurons in the prefrontal and temporal cortex, diminished synaptic reactions, atrophy in the hippocampus and cerebellum, and pathological changes of the blood vessels in the temporal cortex were observed [18]. In another study, newborn rats that were injected with thimerosal started showing characteristic ASD symptoms, such as impaired locomotion, increased anxiety, and antisocial behavior [19]. Newborn rats that were injected with 20 times the dose of thimerosal of the Chinese immunization schedule exhibited developmental delays, social interaction deficiency, and inclination to depression, synaptic dysfunction, endocrine system disorders, and autistic-like behavior [20].

In a study at Harvard University, pregnant and nursing rats were injected with thimerosal. Newborn rats showed a delayed startle response, decreased motor learning, and a significant increase in cerebellar levels of oxidative stress [21]. In a 2010 study, premature rats were injected with different doses of thimerosal after birth. Impaired memory function, decreased learning ability and increased apoptosis (cell death) in the prefrontal cortex of the brain were observed. The authors conclude that this and previous studies "raised serious concerns about adverse neurodevelopmental disorder such as autism in humans following the ongoing worldwide routine administration of thimerosal containing vaccines to infants" [22].

According to a 2012 study, mice that were injected with thimerosal had high levels of glutamate and aspartate in the prefrontal cortex, which are associated with the death of nerve cells. The authors conclude that "Exposure to thimerosal leads to neurotoxic changes in the developing brain, arguing for urgent and permanent removal of this preservative from all vaccines for children (and adults) since effective, less toxic and less costly alternatives are available. The stubborn insistence of some vaccine manufacturers and health agencies on continuation of use of this proven neurotoxin in vaccines is testimony of their disregard for both the health of young generations and for the environment" [23].

A 2011 review analyzed the studies of the effects of low doses of thimerosal. The author concluded that all studies found that thimerosal is toxic for brain cells and that thimerosal exposure similar to the one that infants get from the vaccines can potentially affect human neurodevelopment [24].

In another review article, German scientists report the following facts:

1. Despite the fact that thimerosal has been used for 70 years, and amalgam fillings for 170 years, no controlled randomized studies of their safety have been conducted so far.

2. The safety of ethyl mercury is usually justified only by the fact that the blood concentration of mercury decreases much faster than in the case of methyl mercury. However, it does not mean that mercury is quickly removed from the body: it is simply absorbed by the organs much quicker. In studies of rabbits injected with thimerosal and radioactive mercury, the level of mercury in the blood decreased by 75% within six hours of the injection, but it increased significantly in the brain, liver, and kidneys.

3. Thimerosal at very low (nanomolar) concentrations inhibits phagocytosis. Phagocytosis is the first step of the innate immune system, and it seems likely that injection of thimerosal would, therefore, inhibit infants' immune system as they only have the innate system until the acquired immune system gets built up with age.

4. Thimerosal leads to strong autoimmunity in genetically metal-susceptible mice, compared to methyl mercury.

5. Epidemiological studies do not consider genetic susceptibility factors, autoimmunity reactions, and mercury exposure during pregnancy (amalgam, thimerosal), and thus are not able to detect a statistically significant effect, even if there is one [25].

Acrodynia And Kawasaki Syndrome

Kawasaki disease (inflammation of blood vessels throughout the body) was first described in 1967 in Japan. Its cause is still unknown. In 1985–90, when the amount of thimerosal received through vaccination increased significantly, Kawasaki disease incidence increased by ten times, and by 1997 it increased by 20 times. Since 1990, 88 cases of patients developing Kawasaki Disease with the onset a few days after vaccination have been reported to the CDC, and in 19% of cases, the symptoms manifested on the same day. Countries with vaccination programs similar to the one in the US, but with lesser thimerosal, experience a significantly lower incidence of Kawasaki disease.

Another disease with an unknown cause was **acrodynia**. It was considered a mysterious, systemic disorder, mainly affecting children under the age of five. At its epidemic height (1880–1950), it affected about one in 500 children in industrialized nations. Acrodynia is characterized by high fever, rash, swollen lymph nodes, pink swollen hands and feet, etc. Neurological, cutaneous, and cardiovascular symptoms are most commonly seen. In 1953, mercury from teething powders, baby powders, and diapers treated with calomel (85% mercurous chloride) was accepted as the cause of acrodynia. After a federal ban on these mercury-containing products in 1954, acrodynia disappeared. It was also reported that in some cases, acrodynia occurred after vaccination.

Diagnostic criteria and clinical presentation are similar for both Kawasaki disease and acrodynia. Symptoms and laboratory test results, which are seen in Kawasaki disease, were also described in mercury poisoning. Kawasaki disease affects males two times more often than females. This may be explained by in vitro studies on human cells, which have shown that **testosterone increases the toxicity of mercury**, while estrogen protects against mercury toxicity.

> According to the Environmental Protection Agency (EPA), about 8–10% of American women have mercury levels sufficiently high to cause neurological disorders in their children.

Another similar disease was the **Minamata disease**, which appeared in 1956 in Japan. In 1959, it was found that Minamata disease was caused by industrial mercury waste dumped into Minamata Bay, which was transformed into organic methyl mercury after bioaccumulating in the local fish and seafood. It is remarkable that both acrodynia and Minamata disease were long suspected to be caused by infectious agents, until mercury was established as the cause several years or decades later. The cause of Kawasaki disease is still unknown, but it is also believed that it might be caused by infection, despite the fact that it is not contagious and has a recurrence rate of 1% to 5%, while recurrences of infectious diseases are very rare [26].

Calomel (Hg$_2$Cl$_2$), a type of mercury, which was responsible for acrodynia, is 100 times less toxic to neurons than ethyl mercury [25].

Even though the use of mercury was widespread in the first half of the 20th century, only some children developed acrodynia. Similarly, only some children develop ASD nowadays.

The authors of the Australian study decided to test the hypothesis that autism, like acrodynia, is a consequence of hypersensitivity to mercury. They checked the prevalence rate of autistic children among the grandchildren of people who survived acrodynia, and it turned out that the incidence of ASD among them was seven times higher than the national average (1:25 vs. 1:160) [27].

A 2003 article describes the story of an 11-month-old Swiss boy that started showing symptoms resembling ASD. He no longer laughed or played, was becoming more and more restless, and slept only one to two hours every night. He was no longer able to crawl and stand up, and he lost weight. He had multiple check-ups but could not be diagnosed. Three months later, he was admitted into a hospital. After numerous repeated tests, and only when the parents were specifically asked, it turned out that four weeks before the onset of symptoms, a thermometer had been broken in the house. Mercury had spilled onto the living room carpet, which had been vacuum cleaned only. The boy was diagnosed with mercury poisoning (acrodynia) [28].

Aluminum And Mercury

A 2018 study reported that **aluminum and mercury** are toxic to the neuronal-glial cells of the central nervous system and cause an inflammatory reaction. It turned out that they have a synergistic effect and **enhance each other's toxicity**. For example, at a concentration of 20nM, aluminum and mercury enhance the inflammatory response by four and two times, respectively, and together, at the same concentration, by nine times. At a concentration of 200nM, aluminum and mercury enhance the inflammatory response by 21 and 5.6 times, respectively, and by 54 times if given together [29].

To achieve an aluminum concentration of 20 nM in the brain, assuming equal distribution, it is enough for just 0.04% of aluminum from only one dose of DTP vaccine or 0.2% from one dose of hepatitis B vaccine to get into the brain. And if equal distribution is not assumed, a much lower dose is enough to achieve toxic concentration.

Tic Disorder And Developmental Delays

Vaccination with thimerosal is associated with an increased risk of tic disorder. Although tic disorder was once considered rare, today it is considered the most common movement disorder. The first case of tics due to mercury poisoning was described in 2000. Subsequently, a series of epidemiological studies revealed a significant association between thimerosal in vaccines and an increased risk of tics in children, and several studies even observed a significant dose-dependent relationship [30].

According to a 2014 study, each microgram of mercury in vaccines is associated with an increase in the odds of a pervasive developmental disorder by 5.4%, the risk of specific developmental delay by 3.5%, tic disorder by 3.4%, and hyperkinetic syndrome by 5% [31].

Hepatitis B vaccine with thimerosal is associated with a twofold increase in the risk of specific delays in development. For those who received three doses of such vaccine, the risk of specific delays was three times higher, as compared to those who received the vaccine without thimerosal [32]. The same vaccine is also associated with a tenfold increase in the need for special education for boys [33].

The risk of premature puberty was five times higher in children who received 100 mcg of mercury from vaccines in the first seven months of life. Premature puberty was found in one in 250 children in this 2010 study, which is a 40-fold increase from previous estimates [34].

Mercury And Autism

According to a 2001 article, autism symptoms are similar to mercury intoxication symptoms [35]. A 2009 Canadian study found that thimerosal is three times more toxic to males than it is to females. At doses of 38–76 mg/kg, male mice die, while female mice continue to live [36].

In a 2001 study, the authors measured the amount of mercury in the hair from the first haircut of 94 children with autism and found that the concentration of mercury in their hair was seven times lower than in the hair of the control group. The mothers in the autistic group had significantly higher levels of mercury exposure through Rho D immunoglobulin injections and amalgam fillings than control mothers. Hair mercury levels among controls were significantly correlated with the number of the mothers' amalgam fillings and their fish consumption as well as the exposure to mercury through childhood vaccines. These correlations were absent in the autistic group. The authors concluded that the results "support a hypothesis that these infants were **retaining mercury in tissue** at a higher rate than control infants. The lack of mercury in the hair of autistics may be due to a decrease in blood mercury levels feeding the hair follicles. This decrease is likely caused by the retention of the mercury inside the cells where it most likely causes its major biological damage" [37].

According to a Korean study published in 2017, higher levels of mercury in the blood of mothers at late pregnancy and the levels of mercury in the umbilical cord are associated with autistic behaviors in children at five years of age [38]. A 2017 systematic review and meta-analysis of 44 studies found that children with ASD have a significantly higher level of mercury in the blood and brain than healthy children, while the level of mercury in the hair of children with ASD is significantly lower [39].

In a 2007 study, children with autism had twofold higher levels of mercury in baby teeth, but similar levels of lead and zinc when compared to neurotypical children. Children with autism also had significantly higher usage of oral antibiotics during their first year of life (mainly due to otitis media). The authors write that "Antibiotic use is known to almost completely inhibit excretion of mercury in rats due to alteration of gut flora. Thus, higher use of oral antibiotics in the children with autism may have reduced their ability to excrete mercury, and hence may partially explain the higher level in baby teeth. Higher usage of oral antibiotics in infancy may also partially explain the high incidence of chronic gastrointestinal problems in individuals with autism" [40].

Glutathione is an antioxidant produced by cells, which plays a role against mercury-induced poisoning. Children with autism have significantly lower levels of glutathione than neurotypical children [41].

The level of porphyrins in the urine is an indirect biomarker of the presence of heavy metals in the body. A study of Parisian children determined that children with autism had elevated porphyrin levels in urine compared to control groups [42]. Subsequently, similar results were obtained in the studies in the USA, Australia, Korea, and Egypt [43–45].

According to a 2011 study in the US, the higher the mercury concentration in ambient air, the higher the risk of autism [46]. In Texas, for every 1,000 pounds of environmentally released industrial mercury, there was a 43% increase in the rate of special education services and a 61% increase in the rate of autism. The number of children with autism was 437% higher in cities and 255% higher in the suburbs compared to rural areas [47].

The authors of a 2013 study analyzed the VAERS database and found that the risk of ASD was two times higher in infants who received the DTaP vaccine with thimerosal compared to those who received a mercury-free vaccine. An analysis of Vaccine Safety Datalink (VSD), another database, showed that the hepatitis B vaccine with thimerosal is associated with a threefold increase in the risk of ASD [48]. In another study, newborn boys vaccinated against hepatitis B had a threefold higher risk of developing autism, as compared to the unvaccinated boys, or boys vaccinated at least one month after birth [49]. In a third study, those vaccinated against hepatitis B had a ninefold risk of developmental delay compared to the unvaccinated [50].

The Other Side

An article published in 2014 reported that there had been over 165 studies to date that focused on thimerosal and found it to be harmful. Of these studies, 16 were conducted to specifically examine the effects of thimerosal on human infants and/or children, who have had outcomes of death, acrodynia, poisoning, allergies, malformations, autoimmune reactions, developmental delays, and neurodevelopmental disorders, including tics, speech and language delays, attention deficit disorder, and ASD. However, the CDC still insists that there is "no relationship between thimerosal-containing vaccines and autism rates in children." This is a puzzling conclusion because a study conducted directly by the CDC found a 7.6-fold increased risk of autism from exposure to thimerosal during infancy. The same study found that the risk of nonorganic sleep disorders was five times higher, the risk of speech disorders was two times higher, and the risk of neurologic development disorders was 1.8 times higher.

The CDC's current stance is based primarily on six specific epidemiological studies that the CDC has completed, funded, and/or cosponsored since the late 1990s. All these studies are analyzed in the above-mentioned article:

1. **Madsen, 2003.** The authors analyzed the data from psychiatric clinics in Denmark from 1971 to 2000 and concluded that after the removal of thimerosal from the vaccines (in 1992), the incidence of ASD increased. However:

a) estimates of total autism cases in Denmark were based on diagnoses occurring just during inpatient visits from 1971 to 1994, and then from 1995 to the last year of the study, they included both inpatient and outpatient visits. Thus, the inclusion criteria were greatly expanded two years after the phaseout of thimerosal from infant vaccines in Denmark, creating an "artificial increase" in autism prevalence. The authors conceded that "The proportion of outpatient to inpatient activities was about 4 to 6 times as many outpatients as inpatients." However, in an earlier publication, the same authors had stated regarding this same data, "in our cohort, 93.1% of the children were treated only as outpatients," meaning there were 13 times as many outpatients as inpatients. In addition, the authors stated that the Danish registry, which was used to count cases, did not include a large Copenhagen clinic before 1993. This clinic accounted for as many as 20% of the autism cases nationwide, which would again artificially inflate the autism incidence observed in Denmark after the phaseout of thimerosal was initiated in 1992. The authors do not mention this change in inclusion criteria, and neither do they attempt to adjust their analysis in accordance with the anomaly;

b) the diagnostic criteria for autism changed within the course of the study. From 1971 to 1993, the ICD-8 standard was used, and from 1994 to 2000, the ICD-10 standard was used. This could result in as much as a 25-fold increase in cases as due to this change the instantaneous increase in autism prevalence in Denmark went from a low of 1.2/10,000 to a high of 30.8/10,000;

c) the 2001 data, which showed a decline in the autism rate since 1999, was included in the first version of the article that was submitted to *JAMA*. *JAMA* rejected the article, and the authors submitted it to the journal *Pediatrics*. One of the reviewers at *Pediatrics* noticed that the authors do not discuss the decrease in the autism incidence, which could point to the possibility that removal of thimerosal could have played a role in it. In response to this criticism, the authors removed the 2001 incidence numbers, and the article was published. The authors' decision to withhold this data resembles scientific fraud, especially when coupled with the previously discussed problematic methods for counting autism cases. If the 2001 data had been included in the final publication, the results would have been consistent with a more recent CDC study, according to which, the ASD prevalence in Denmark after 1992 decreased from a high of 1.5% in 1994–95 to a low of 1% in 2002–4.

2. **Stehr-Green, 2003.** This study was conducted in response to a California study, which showed a correlation between thimerosal and autism. The authors compared the data from three geographical areas (Denmark, Sweden, and California). Danish data was the same as in the previous study. The data from Sweden was based on inpatient (hospital) visits only (that is, on just a small fraction of all autism cases). The data from California included only part of all ASD cases. The study was problematic in its attempt to combine ecological data from three different countries that, relative to each other, demonstrated different vaccination policies and widely different thimerosal exposure levels.

3. **Hviid, 2003.** The authors stated that the mean age of autism diagnosis was 4.7 years. However, cases and controls as young as one year of age were included in the analysis. In addition, rather than counting persons within the cohort, the authors counted "person-years of follow up." With this technique, each age group (one-year-olds, two-year-olds, etc.) was considered equally, despite the fact that younger age groups were much less likely to receive an autism diagnosis.

4. **Andrews, 2004.** A retrospective study in the United Kingdom. It has the same issues as the previous study. Very young children, who could not possibly be diagnosed yet, were included in the study. The authors did not release the raw data, so it could not be analyzed properly.

5. **Verstraeten, 2003.** This study was conducted in at least five separate phases. After conducting the final phase (the results of which are reported in the publication), the authors stated that there was no relationship between thimerosal exposure in vaccines and autism incidence. However, no data is reported in the published study to support this conclusion.

The first phase of this study, released in an internal presentation, showed that infants who received more than 25 mcg of mercury in vaccines and immunoglobulins at the age of one month, were 7.6 times more likely to have an autism diagnosis, than those not exposed to any injection-derived mercury.

The second phase of the study showed that infants who received 62 mcg of mercury before three months of age, were 2.5 times more likely to have autism diagnosis compared to those exposed to less than 37.5 mcg.

In the third phase of the study, in which more data stratification methods and different inclusion/exclusion criteria were applied to the analysis, the relative risk of autism for children at three months, exposed to thimerosal, dropped to 1.69. Apparently, the author had been under pressure, since he wrote in an internal CDC correspondence: "I do not wish to be the advocate of the anti-vaccine lobby and sound like being convinced that thimerosal is or was harmful, but at least I feel we should use sound scientific argumentation and not let our standards be dictated by our desire to disprove an unpleasant theory."

The fourth and fifth phases of the study were based on partial data only and included children at the ages of zero to three years old, even though the average age for an autism diagnosis at the time was 4.4 years. Nevertheless, the study still found a significantly increased risk for tics and language delay among those vaccinated with thimerosal.

6. **Price, 2010**. A case-control study in the US in which the control group received the same vaccines. This is called *overmatching*, and it is impossible to draw conclusions from this kind of study. Moreover, their initial report found that prenatal exposure to thimerosal correlated with an eightfold increase in the risk of ASD, but for some reason, this data was excluded from the publication.

Five out of the six studies were directly commissioned by the CDC, raising the possible issue of conflict of interests or research bias, since vaccine promotion is a central mission of the CDC [51].

The third phase of the Verstraeten study was presented at the CDC secret conference in 2000, which was dedicated to thimerosal (Simpsonwood meeting). Among other things, Dr. Clements, the vaccine advisor at the WHO, stated: "Perhaps this study should not have been done at all, because the outcome of it could have, to some extent, been predicted and we have all reached this point now where we are left hanging, even though I hear the majority of the consultants say to the Board that they are not convinced there is a causality direct link between thimerosal and various neurological outcomes. I know how we handle it from here is extremely problematic."

A 2016 article analyzed all the studies about the possible relationship between mercury and autism published between 1999 and 2016. The authors found 91 studies, and **74% of them support the existence of a link between mercury and ASD [52]**.

Endnotes

1. WHO. Thimerosal in vaccines. www.who.int/vaccine_safety/committee/topics/thimerosal /questions/en/
2. Drain PK et al. Single-dose versus multi-dose vaccine vials for immunization programmes in developing countries. *Bull World Health Organ.* 2003;81(10):726-31
3. Baker JP. Mercury, vaccines, and autism: one controversy, three histories. *Am J Public Health.* 2008;98(2):244-53
4. Powell H et al. Merthiolate as a germicide. *Am J Epidemiol.* 1931;13(1):296-310
5. Geier DA et al. Thimerosal: clinical, epidemiologic and biochemical studies. *Clin Chim Acta.* 2015;444:212-20
6. Ban on all mercury-based products would risk global immunization efforts, says AAP, WHO. *AAP News.* 2012 Jun 1
7. Stajich GV et al. Iatrogenic exposure to mercury after hepatitis B vaccination in preterm infants. *J Pediatr.* 2000;136(5):679-81
8. Marques RC et al. Hair mercury in breast-fed infants exposed to thimerosal-preserved vaccines. *Eur J Pediatr.* 2007;166(9):935-41
9. Rooney JP. The retention time of inorganic mercury in the brain—a systematic review of the evidence. *Toxicol Appl Pharmacol.* 2014;274(3):425-35
10. Burbacher TM et al. Comparison of blood and brain mercury levels in infant monkeys exposed to methylmercury or vaccines containing thimerosal. *Environ Health Perspect.* 2005;113(8):1015-21
11. Laurente J et al. Neurotoxic effects of thimerosal at vaccine doses on the encephalon and development in 7 days-old hamsters. *An Fac Med Lima.* 2007;68
12. Curtis JT et al. Chronic metals ingestion by prairie voles produces sex-specific deficits in social behavior: an animal model of autism. *Behav Brain Res.* 2010;213(1):42-9
13. Risher JF et al. Alkyl mercury-induced toxicity: multiple mechanisms of action. *Rev Environ Contam Toxicol.* 2017;240:105-49
14. Blanuša M et al. Mercury disposition in suckling rats: comparative assessment following parenteral exposure to thimerosal and mercuric chloride. *J Biomed Biotechnol.* 2012;2012:256965
15. Orct T et al. Comparison of organic and inorganic mercury distribution in suckling rat. *J Appl Toxicol.* 2006;26(6):536-9
16. Guzzi G et al. Effect of thimerosal, methylmercury, and mercuric chloride in Jurkat T Cell Line. *Interdiscip Toxicol.* 2012;5(3):159-61
17. Léonard A et al. Mutagenicity and teratogenicity of mercury compounds. *Mutat Res.* 1983;114(1):1-18
18. Olczak M et al. Lasting neuropathological changes in rat brain after intermittent neonatal administration of thimerosal. *Folia Neuropathol.* 2010;48(4):258-69

19. Olczak M et al. Persistent behavioral impairments and alterations of brain dopamine system after early postnatal administration of thimerosal in rats. *Behav Brain Res.* 2011; 223(1):107-18

20. Li X et al. Transcriptomic analyses of neurotoxic effects in mouse brain after intermittent neonatal administration of thimerosal. *Toxicol Sci.* 2014;139(2):452-65

21. Sulkowski ZL et al. Maternal thimerosal exposure results in aberrant cerebellar oxidative stress, thyroid hormone metabolism, and motor behavior in rat pups; sex- and strain-dependent effects. *Cerebellum.* 2012;11(2):575-86

22. Chen YN et al. Effect of thimerosal on the neurodevelopment of premature rats. *World J Pediatr.* 2013;9(4):356-60

23. Duszczyk-Budhathoki M et al. Administration of thimerosal to infant rats increases overflow of glutamate and aspartate in the prefrontal cortex: protective role of dehydroepiandrosterone sulfate. *Neurochem Res.* 2012;37(2):436-47

24. Dórea JG. Integrating experimental (in vitro and in vivo) neurotoxicity studies of low-dose thimerosal relevant to vaccines. *Neurochem Res.* 2011;36(6):927-38

25. Mutter J et al. Mercury and autism: accelerating evidence? *Neuro Endocrinol Lett.* 2005; 26(5):439-46

26. Mutter J et al. Kawasaki's disease, acrodynia, and mercury. *Curr Med Chem.* 2008; 15(28):3000-10

27. Shandley K et al. Ancestry of pink disease (infantile acrodynia) identified as a risk factor for autism spectrum disorders. *J Toxicol Environ Health A.* 2011;74(18):1185-94

28. Chrysochoou C et al. An 11-month-old boy with psychomotor regression and auto-aggressive behaviour. *Eur J Pediatr.* 2003;162(7-8):559-61

29. Alexandrov PN et al. Synergism in aluminum and mercury neurotoxicity. *Integr Food Nutr Metab.* 2018;5(3)

30. Geier DA et al. Thimerosal exposure and increased risk for diagnosed tic disorder in the United States: a case-control study. *Interdiscip Toxicol.* 2015;8(2):68-76

31. Geier DA et al. A dose-response relationship between organic mercury exposure from thimerosal-containing vaccines and neurodevelopmental disorders. *Int J Environ Res Public Health.* 2014;11(9):9156-70

32. Geier DA et al. Thimerosal-containing hepatitis B vaccination and the risk for diagnosed specific delays in development in the United States: a case-control study in the vaccine safety datalink. *N Am J Med Sci.* 2014;6(10):519-31

33. Geier DA et al. A Cross-Sectional Study of the Association between Infant Hepatitis B Vaccine Exposure in Boys and the Risk of Adverse Effects as Measured by Receipt of Special Education Services. *Int J Environ Res Public Health.* 2018;15(1)

34. Geier DA et al. Thimerosal exposure & increasing trends of premature puberty in the vaccine safety datalink. *Indian J Med Res.* 2010;131:500-7

35. Bernard S et al. Autism: a novel form of mercury poisoning. *Med Hypotheses.* 2001; 56(4):462-71

36. Branch DR. Gender-selective toxicity of thimerosal. *Exp Toxicol Pathol.* 2009; 61(2):133-6

37. Holmes AS et al. Reduced levels of mercury in first baby haircuts of autistic children. *Int J Toxicol.* 2003;22(4):277-85

38. Ryu J et al. Associations of prenatal and early childhood mercury exposure with autistic behaviors at 5years of age. *Sci Total Environ.* 2017;605-606:251-7

39. Jafari T et al. The association between mercury levels and autism spectrum disorders: a systematic review and meta-analysis. *J Trace Elem Med Biol.* 2017;44:289-97

40. Adams JB et al. Mercury, lead, and zinc in baby teeth of children with autism versus controls. *J Toxicol Environ Health A*. 2007;70(12):1046-51

41. James SJ et al. Metabolic biomarkers of increased oxidative stress and impaired methylation capacity in children with autism. *Am J Clin Nutr*. 2004;80(6):1611-7

42. Nataf R et al. Porphyrinuria in childhood autistic disorder: implications for environmental toxicity. *Toxicol Appl Pharmacol*. 2006;214(2):99-108

43. Austin DW et al. An investigation of porphyrinuria in Australian children with autism. *J Toxicol Environ Health A*. 2008;71(20):1349-51

44. Youn S et al. Porphyrinuria in Korean children with autism: correlation with oxidative stress. *J Toxicol Environ Health A*. 2010;73(10):701-10

45. Khaled EM et al. Altered urinary porphyrins and mercury exposure as biomarkers for autism severity in Egyptian children with autism spectrum disorder. *Metab Brain Dis*. 2016;31(6):1419-26

46. Blanchard KS et al. The value of ecologic studies: mercury concentration in ambient air and the risk of autism. *Rev Environ Health*. 2011;26(2):111-8

47. Palmer RF et al. Environmental mercury release, special education rates, and autism disorder: an ecological study of Texas. *Health Place*. 2006;12(2):203-9

48. Geier DA et al. A two-phase study evaluating the relationship between Thimerosal-containing vaccine administration and the risk for an autism spectrum disorder diagnosis in the United States. *Transl Neurodegener*. 2013;2(1):25

49. Gallagher CM et al. Hepatitis B vaccination of male neonates and autism diagnosis, NHIS 1997-2002. *J Toxicol Environ Health A*. 2010;73(24):1665-77

50. Gallagher C. Hepatitis B triple series vaccine and developmental disability in US children aged 1–9 years. *Toxicol Environ Chem*. 2008;90(5):997-1008

51. Hooker B et al. Methodological issues and evidence of malfeasance in research purporting to show thimerosal in vaccines is safe. *Biomed Res Int*. 2014;2014:247218

52. Kern JK et al. The relationship between mercury and autism: a comprehensive review and discussion. *J Trace Elem Med Biol*. 2016;37:8-24

Chapter Twenty-Five

AUTISM

Whenever you find yourself on the side of the majority,
it is time to pause and reflect.
— **Mark Twain**

S ince the 1990s, the prevalence of autism spectrum disorder (ASD) has increased by several orders of magnitude. The cause of autism is still unknown, which does not stop the CDC from confidently stating that vaccines do not cause autism. But is it really so? Given that most scientists are absolutely certain that vaccines are not associated with autism, it is logical to assume that studies comparing vaccinated and unvaccinated children have been conducted and that they showed the ASD incidence for both groups to be the same. However, this is not the case. **Studies comparing vaccinated and unvaccinated children in the context of autism have not been conducted.** In all studies, which supposedly prove that the vaccines are not associated with autism, a comparison has been made between the groups of vaccinated children.

Well, not exactly all the studies. In fact, one study comparing vaccinated and completely unvaccinated children was published in 2017, and it found that **vaccinated children develop autism four times more often than unvaccinated children.** This study has many flaws: it was retrospective, based on anonymous surveys, and only 660 homeschooled children participated in it. However, no other similar studies have been conducted yet [1].

A Little Bit Of History

Childhood autism was first described in 1943. The author, Leo Kanner, describes 11 cases of a previously unknown disease. It is accompanied by symptoms such as extreme desire to be alone, temper tantrums, verbal rituals, strict adherence to a daily routine, obsessiveness, inappropriate statements, echolalia (uncontrollable, automatic repetition of words), and a mania for spinning round things. These children do not pay attention to people but are interested in objects, especially the ones that could be spun. Some made the impression of silent wisdom. Others differed by showing good mechanistic memory and early development. For example, Kanner describes an 18-months-old boy, who was able to distinguish between 18 symphonies only by their first sounds. All the children were born into highly intelligent families. Four of the fathers were psychiatrists, nine of the 11 mothers were college graduates. The oldest girl, described by Kanner, was born in 1931. This is the year when mercury was first added to the vaccines, and a year later, aluminum was added [2].

Kanner probably stole the discovery of autism from Hans Asperger, a Vienna pediatrician. Even though Asperger published an article describing children with similar symptoms a year after Kanner, he was giving lectures about such children as early as 1938. Kanner denied knowing about Asperger's work, but this was unlikely to be true since the chief diagnostician in Asperger's clinic came to work with Kanner in 1938 [3]. However, autism was actually discovered by an almost unknown Soviet scientist Grunya Sukhareva, who described autism symptoms back in 1925 and named it with the same word [4]. Kanner knew about Sukhareva's work since he quoted her in his 1949 article.

Regressive Autism

When a child develops normally and then loses speech and social skills at the age of 12–24 months, it is called **regressive autism**. The first case, similar to regressive autism, was described in Kanner's article in 1943. The boy was vaccinated against smallpox at the age of 12 months. Around this time, mental regression started, and he stopped imitating word sounds. The article, of course, does not associate this regression with the vaccine. Kanner emphasizes that in all the 11 cases that he had seen, signs of autism were observed in children from birth. In 1976, a case of regressive autism in a 15-month-old boy was described, which the author associated with smallpox vaccination. He believes that a causal relationship between vaccination and ASD is unlikely, but acknowledges that the vaccine has triggered the onset of autism [5].

In 1987, half of the autism cases were of regressive form [6]. However, up until the mid-2000s, there was a debate about whether regressive autism actually existed, or whether parents simply idealized their children so much that they did not pay attention to early symptoms of ASD. Albeit, it is known that parents, regardless of their educational background or parental experience, are able to accurately identify developmental problems in their children [7]. In a 2005 study, the authors analyzed home videos and concluded that regressive autism does exist [8]. According to a 2018 study, **88% of the ASD cases were classified as regressive**. The authors conclude that regressive autism may be more of a rule than an exception [9]. Parents of children with regressive autism usually believe that ASD in their children was caused by vaccines [10].

In a study published in 2008, MMR vaccination at the time of a disease was associated with a 17-fold increase in the risk of regressive autism [11]. To date, the CDC does not consider mild diseases, such as common cold or varicella, to be a contraindication for MMR or any other vaccine. The authors believe that the relationship between autism and vaccination during illness needs to be further studied, and the guidelines may need to be revised. (*If MMR during a mild illness increases the risk of ASD, could it be that for some children, infection with several viruses at a time could cause too strong of an inflammation and that MMR or MMRV, which contain three to four viruses, could increase the risk of autism, as compared to monovalent vaccines or natural infections? Science has not yet given answers to these questions.*)

Autism Prevalence

The DSM-5 (5th edition of the Diagnostic and Statistical Manual of Mental Disorders, published in 2013) combined infantile (Kanner) autism, pervasive developmental disorder not otherwise specified (PDD-NOS), and Asperger syndrome, into a single diagnosis called **autism spectrum disorder (ASD)**. The DSM-5 was supposed to result in a decrease in the number of autism cases by 30% [12]. In 2012, 46% of ASD cases were attributable to infantile autism, 44% to PDD-NOS, and 10% to Asperger syndrome. From this point on, the term autism refers to ASD.

In 1970 in the US, autism occurred in one in 10,000 children. In 1987 in one in 3,000. In 2007 in one in 91. In 2012 in one in 68. In 2014 in one in 45 [13–17]. **In 2016, 2.76% of children aged three to 17 years old in the US had autism spectrum disorder (one in 36).** Seven percent (one in 14) show developmental disabilities [18]. Those diagnosed with ADHD are 10.2%, as compared to 6% in 1998 [19]. Same as with autism, ADHD is three times more common in boys than in girls [20]. According to another study, developmental disabilities were observed in one out of six children in the US in 2008. These disorders include ASD, ADHD, cerebral palsy, learning disorders, etc. [21]

> Among those born in 1931 in California, one out of 100,000 had autism. Among those born in 2012, it was one in 85. The prevalence started to increase gradually in the 1940s and then increased sharply for those born in 1980, 1990, and 2007 [22].

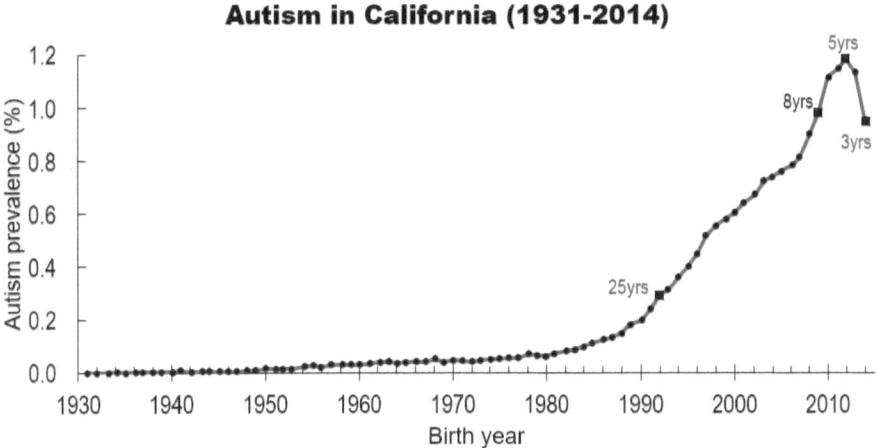

Autism in California (1931-2014)

Is There An Epidemic?

Some scientists believe that there is no autism epidemic, but rather that the diagnostic criteria have changed and that there have always been that many people with ASD, but no one noticed them [23]. However, the calculations of these scientists are usually wrong, which they subsequently acknowledge themselves [24]. Others suggest that the ASD epidemic is explained by replacing the intellectual disability diagnosis. It is not the case, however. Intellectual disability prevalence stayed relatively constant, while ASD prevalence rose sharply [25].

> According to a study published in 2014, 75–80% of the increase in the autism incidence is due to an actual increase in the disorder rather than to changing diagnostic criteria.

Among the suspected toxins, polybrominated diphenyl ethers (fire-retardant materials that almost all mattresses and sofas are filled with today), aluminum adjuvants, and glyphosate correlate with autism [26].

There are also other studies according to which the autism epidemic is real and is not a consequence of changes in criteria [27, 28].

There has been a trend in the media towards the normalization of ASD in recent years. Sesame Street added a doll with ASD. Movies and TV shows are released, which portray people with autism as ordinary people, who are just a little asocial but instead are better than ordinary people in other skills. We are told that ASD should be "welcomed" because people with autism are not sick. They are regular people, just a little different. In reality, ASD is a serious illness in the vast majority of cases. In 28% of cases, people with ASD exhibit self-injurious behaviors [29]. Fifty percent of them are non-verbal, up to 80% are intellectually challenged, and 30% of children also have a seizure disorder. The risk of accompanying diseases, such as otitis media, asthma, allergies, gastrointestinal disorders, etc., is much higher for people with ASD [30]. The cost of supporting an individual with an ASD and intellectual disability during his or her lifespan in the United States and the United Kingdom is over $2 million, and for ASD without intellectual disability, it is 1.4 million [31]. Only a small percentage of people with ASD are the way they are being portrayed in the media—gifted with extreme artistic, intellectual, or technical ability [30].

Aluminum

In a 2015 Egyptian study, the level of aluminum in the hair of autistic patients was found to be five times higher than that of the control group

[32]. Similar results were obtained in studies in Japan, Saudi Arabia, and other countries [33–34]. According to a study published in 2018, mice pups, injected with aluminum hydroxide in the amount equivalent to what children receive from vaccines, subsequently showed diminished social interest. These mice also gained less weight, which has been demonstrated in other studies as well. The authors note that the half-life of oral aluminum is relatively short (24 hours). Aluminum in adjuvants, however, takes much longer to be eliminated because of its exceptional affinity to the various antigens [35].

A 2017 review reports that "There is good evidence to suggest that immunization may accelerate or precipitate the transition between subclinical and overt symptomatic autoimmune conditions within the first 30 days post-immunization" [36]. Aluminum exposure is associated with increased productions of pro-inflammatory cytokines, induction of chronic oxidative stress, mitochondrial dysfunction, microglial activation, and functional dysregulation of microglia (immune system cells in the brain). These changes, in turn, are linked to ASD.

The authors of the already mentioned 2011 study found that children from countries with the highest ASD prevalence appear to have the highest exposure to aluminum from vaccines [37]. According to a 2018 study, autistic people have very high levels of aluminum in their brains. Judging by the place of aluminum detection, it enters the brain through the lymphatic system. This study had no control group since no suitable brain samples had been found. Therefore, the authors compared the levels of aluminum with that found in other studies. The levels of aluminum in the brains of young people with ASD were higher than in the brains of older people suffering from Alzheimer's [38].

The author of a 2011 study analyzed the vaccination coverage of US states between 2001 and 2007 and found that a 1% increase in the vaccination coverage is associated with a 1.7% increase in ASD and speech impairment {39}.

Inflammation And Immune Activation

Pregnant women that received the influenza vaccine had significantly elevated levels of C-reactive protein (inflammation marker) for at least two days after vaccination. Inflammation during pregnancy significantly increases the risk of preeclampsia and preterm birth [40]. Elevated levels of C-reactive protein during pregnancy are associated with an increased risk of autism in children [41].

According to a study published in 2018, typhoid vaccination induced systemic low-grade inflammation. The level of **IL-6 cytokines** (pro-inflammatory cytokines produced by Th2 cells) increased by more than 400% but without fever or sickness symptoms. This systemic inflammation significantly reduces the ability to interpret the mental state of other people. The authors conclude that systemic inflammation can contribute to socio-cognitive deficits. Other studies have also shown that **social interactions are more difficult for people with inflammation.** In this study, IL-6 levels only increased by five times. In the studies using endotoxin, IL-6 levels increased by 100-1000 times [42].

In a 2007 study, pregnant rats were injected with the cytokine IL-6, and ASD symptoms were observed in their pups [43]. According to a 2014 study, maternal immune activation during pregnancy in rhesus monkeys led to ASD symptoms in their offsprings [44]. In 2018, it was discovered that immune activation in mice, a few days after birth, led to symptoms similar to those of ASD and to other neuropsychiatric conditions [45]. In another study, the authors analyzed the brain tissue of people with autism and found active neuroinflammatory processes in their brains. (These people did not die of infection, but of heart attacks and other causes) [46]. Increased inflammatory processes in the brain (*microglial activation*) were also found in living people with ASD. The authors conclude that **autism is caused by immune abnormalities** [47]. According to another study, elevated levels of IL-6 cytokine are observed in people with autism. Mice with elevated IL-6 in the brain display many autistic features [48].

According to a 2013 study, aluminum increases the IL-6 levels in rats [49]. The hepatitis B vaccine (which contains aluminum), administered to newborn rats, also increases the levels of IL-6 in the hippocampus, while the BCG vaccine lowers them. The IL-6 levels were not elevated immediately but were elevated in adulthood [50]. In another study of the same group, it is reported that in mice vaccinated against hepatitis B in infancy, neurobehavioral disorders were observed in adulthood as a consequence of pro-inflammatory processes in the hippocampus induced by the immune system bias towards Th2 [51]. **Aluminum in nanomolar concentrations causes inflammation in brain cells. That is, it is enough for 0.01% of the aluminum contained in the vaccines to enter the brain to induce inflammation** [52].

298

Summarizing these and other studies, a group of independent scientists, running the VaccinePapers.org site, concludes the following: aluminum from vaccines enters the brain through the lymphatic system, where it causes an increase in IL-6 cytokine levels and chronic immune activation, which, in turn, cause autism and other neurological disorders.

But why do the ASD symptoms often start right after the MMR vaccine, even though it does not contain aluminum? One of the possible explanations is that MMR, being the first live vaccine given to a child, causes a strong immune reaction, and increases the levels of **MCP-1 cytokine** (*macrophage chemoattractant protein*) in the brain [53]. This cytokine, as its name implies, attracts macrophages. Inflammation, even when not in the brain, increases the levels of MCP-1 [54]. Increased levels of MCP-1 cause the macrophages from the entire body to rush to the brain, even if the inflammation is not there. These macrophages carry aluminum from previous vaccines. This way, MMR helps aluminum to get into the brain, which, in turn, leads to an increase in the levels of IL-6 and ASD. From a 2017 study, it is known that MCP-1 levels are elevated in people with autism [55]. Also, newborns, who became subsequently autistic, had elevated levels of MCP-1 after birth [56].

Mitochondrial Dysfunction

The case of Hannah Poling was described in 2006. A 19-month-old girl was given a series of vaccines. Forty-eight hours later, she developed a fever, inconsolable crying, irritability, lethargy, and refused to walk. Four days later, she was waking up multiple times in the night, and could no longer normally climb stairs. For the next three months, she was irritable and increasingly less responsive verbally, after which the family noted clear autistic behaviors, such as spinning, gaze avoidance, disrupted sleep/wake cycle, and fixation on specific television programs. She continued to have diarrhea, poor appetite, and did not gain weight for six months. Evaluation at 23 months showed atopic dermatitis, slow hair growth, toe walking, and the autism diagnosis was given. From 30 months of age, she took vitamin supplements, and her symptoms improved. She was diagnosed with **mitochondrial dysfunction**. It is unclear whether the mitochondrial dysfunction was the result of a primary genetic abnormality, atypical development of essential metabolic pathways, or other factors. **The authors conclude that young children with mitochondrial dysfunction** might be more prone to undergo autistic regression if they have infections and immunizations at the same time [57].

There is nothing special about this case, except for the fact that the girl's father, Jon Poling, is a neurologist who documented all the tests he ran on his daughter. Moreover, Poling worked with Andrew Zimmerman, one of the prominent neurologists in the US, who appeared as an expert witness in vaccine courts, where he argued that there is no connection between MMR and autism. Zimmerman was the co-author of the above-mentioned article, and in his expert opinion stated that in the case of Hanna Poling, there was a connection between vaccination and autism.

Hannah Poling was initially one of several participants in a class-action lawsuit (Omnibus Autism Proceeding) on the link between vaccination and autism, representing 5,500 children. HHS removed this case form the Proceeding and paid the family, that signed a non-disclosure agreement, $20 million. The Omnibus Autism Proceeding, however, was rejected. The fact that Zimmerman changed his opinion in the process, and gave different expert opinions in the Proceeding and Hanna Poling case, was unknown at the time since the Hanna Poling case was sealed. This information was only revealed after the attorney leaked it to a journalist. After his conclusion in the Hanna Poling case, Zimmerman was no longer invited to be an expert witness in vaccine court, but his expert opinion, written before he changed it, was used as an argument to dismiss the Omnibus Autism Proceeding.

Mitochondrial dysfunction is not something rare. According to a 2012 study, it is observed in 5% of autism cases, and according to a 2018 study, in 16% of autism cases [58, 59].

In a 2011 study, the authors analyzed 1,300 cases of compensation for post-vaccination complications that were heard in court and found that although vaccines do not cause autism officially, and the Omnibus Autism Proceeding was dismissed, compensation to people with autism was paid in at least 83 cases. Most of the compensation cases are sealed, so a group was created to phone the people who went to the vaccine court [60]. It is also known that parents, who used the word "encephalopathy" in their lawsuit in the vaccine court, won the case and received compensation. Those, who went to court with similar symptoms but used the word "autism," lost, and their case was dismissed [61].

Genetics

When compared to genetic studies of the nature of autism, studies of environmental risk factors are in their infancy and have significant methodological limitations [62]. Ten to 20 times more research dollars are spent on studies of the genetic causes of autism than on the environmental ones [63]. Almost all genetic risk factors for ASDs can be found in unaffected individuals. Hence it follows that without the environmental factor, genetic risk remains a risk only, and autism does not develop [64].

According to a 2004 study, the risk of pervasive developmental disorder in children of Ethiopian immigrants born in Israel was much lower than in native Israelis. However, among the Ethiopian-born children, there was not a single case of pervasive developmental disorder (among 11,800 children). The authors conclude that childbirth in Israel, an industrialized country, is a marker of an environmental risk of autism [65].

The authors of a 2017 study proposed a hypothesis that stem cells, contained in the umbilical cord blood, can suppress the inflammation observed in the brain of people with ASD. They injected autistic children intravenously with their own umbilical cord blood, stored at birth. These children showed a significant improvement in symptoms [66]. If stem cells of people with ASD, contained in their own blood at birth, can improve their ASD symptoms, it might indicate that autism is not a congenital or genetic condition.

Acrodynia And Autism

Since there are no studies, which compare vaccinated and unvaccinated children in the context of autism (or rather, there is one that indicated that they are linked), **the statement that vaccines do not cause autism is false**. All the other studies on autism, were first of all, only epidemiological, and secondly, focused only on one vaccine (MMR), and on one vaccine component (thimerosal). There is not a single study examining the possible role of any vaccine other than MMR in the autism epidemic. Therefore, if anything can be concluded from the existing studies, it is only that MMR does not cause autism, and that thimerosal does not cause autism. Studies on thimerosal were analyzed in the previous chapter, so here I will analyze some studies that allegedly prove that MMR is not linked with autism.

First, to understand why epidemiological studies may not reveal the link between vaccines and autism, even if there is one, let's return to acrodynia. Acrodynia was caused by mercury in tooth powder, diapers, and various medications, and affected one in every 500 children in the first half of the 20th century. A 1950 review article analyzes various possible causes of acrodynia. Infection, diet deficiency, allergy, fungus, or arsenic poisoning are listed among the suspected causes. Possible mercury poisoning is also mentioned—this hypothesis was first expressed in 1846. However, according to the author's opinion, acrodynia is a form of encephalopathy, which is caused by psychological and emotional factors [67].

It was only in 1953 that mercury was established to be the cause of acrodynia, and it was done on the basis of a case series study of 28 children. That is, on the basis of the exact same study design that Andrew Wakefield conducted, when he linked MMR and autism. The authors explain that some medications, which are tolerated well by most, might be dangerous to some people after all. They mention mercury diuretics, "thousands of injections are given without untoward effects but occasionally a therapeutic dose results in sudden death" [68].

A 1966 article, dedicated to the already eradicated acrodynia, reports that this disease presented a fascinating enigma to a generation of pediatricians. The theory of mercury as a cause of acrodynia was accepted slowly, after hesitation, opposition, and even ridicule. Acrodynia disappeared only after the ban on mercury, without fanfare and festivities. At the end of the article, the author, who determined the final relationship between mercury and acrodynia 16 years earlier, asks the following question: "Is there scientific proof that the theory is correct? We early believers collected shreds of evidence and then predicted that the disease would disappear when mercury was withdrawn as a common household remedy and medical panacea. And acrodynia did disappear. But, does this constitute scientific proof? So much has changed since the 1950's that we could possibly give credit to the wrong measure. And the believers in an acrodynogenic virus may say: Viral epidemics come and go, and we are now in a period of natural decline of the disease. Virologists sometimes use this argument in their discussions. It would take many years to refute this opinion and there are no virologists willing to spend their time on a dead disease. Thus, the anti-mercurialists have won by default and we remain with the question: What constitutes scientific proof? Can it ever be achieved in medicine?" [69]

Acrodynia affected only children susceptible to mercury, and there were only 0.2% of such children. ASD also only affects susceptible children, and there are less than 3% of those, as of today. Even when assuming that vaccines can cause autism, epidemiological studies, which do not take this susceptibility into account, might not reveal an association. Moreover, since all the existing epidemiological studies are focused only on MMR or thimerosal, they would not be able to even theoretically identify an association, if other components or other vaccines might cause autism as well.

> The assumption that only MMR can cause autism, and other vaccines cannot, is similar to an assumption that only Marlboro can cause lung cancer, and other brands of cigarettes cannot.

Epidemiological studies of acrodynia, most likely, could not have detected this link. Firstly, due to the low susceptibility to the disease, and secondly, because mercury was widely used at the time. These studies certainly could not have revealed a link if scientists had suggested that acrodynia was caused only by tooth powders, and had not considered that acrodynia could also be caused by diapers, mercury anthelmintic chocolates, or broken thermometers. If a disease similar to acrodynia were to appear today, no one would have banned mercury on the basis of the data available by 1953. The evidence based on a group of 28 children and other anecdotal cases would have been regarded by the scientific community as laughable, and mercury would have kept killing children susceptible to it for many more decades, while the scientific community would have spent billions of dollars testing for genetic causes of acrodynia (and, of course, finding them), and would have conducted large epidemiological studies, the design of which is inherently unsuitable to identifying mercury as a cause of such disease. This is exactly what has been happening with autism since the 90s. To date, there is much more scientific evidence on the association between vaccination and autism, than there was in 1953 on the association between mercury and acrodynia.

303

The Other Side

Studies that are most often cited as proof that vaccines do not cause autism:

1. Madsen, 2002. A Danish study, according to which, those vaccinated with MMR had a 17% lower risk of autism than those unvaccinated. That is, the vaccine had a protective effect against autism [70]. In his 2003 article, professor of epidemiology calculated that if only 10% are susceptible to regressive autism, then with the given design of the study, it will turn out, that MMR is associated with four times higher risk of regressive autism. However, if all types of autism were to be analyzed together, given the same design, there would be no association, and even a protective effect would appear [71].

Also, this study analyzes person-years instead of cases, which is logical for epidemiological studies but is not logical in cases of chronic diseases, such as autism. As a result, cases of early diagnosis (and they are a minority) have more weight than cases of later diagnosis. Additionally, the average age in the "unvaccinated" group was five years, and the average age of the vaccinated was 3.7 years. Therefore, the probability of having been diagnosed was much lower for the vaccinated group. The average age for autism diagnosis in Denmark was five years, so about half of the children were too young to be diagnosed.

Poul Thorsen, one of the authors of this and other Danish studies, is accused of stealing over a million dollars from the CDC and has been awaiting extradition to the USA since 2011. Although, for some reason, no one seems to be in a hurry to arrest him, even though he is not hiding and continues to publish articles.

2. Taylor, 1999. A British study, according to which, the autism prevalence did not increase drastically after the introduction of MMR in 1988 but grew gradually [72]. This study does not account for the fact that older children received MMR as part of the "catch-up vaccination program." Hence, the authors mistakenly conclude that since children born before 1988 also have autism, MMR has nothing to do with it. Despite all this, the authors found a clustering of autism diagnoses within six months of MMR vaccination. They conclude that when parents do not remember the exact age of the onset of symptoms, they just randomly say 18 months (MMR vaccine is given at 12 months). Therefore, they discard all the cases of the onset of symptoms at 18 months, analyze the data again, and the statistical significance disappears.

3. DeStefano, 2004. A case-control study in Atlanta. The authors found that by the age of three years, more children had been vaccinated with MMR in the autism group than in the control group. Among children in the three to five years age group, this association was significantly higher. However, the authors concluded that children with autism were probably vaccinated at a younger age since vaccination is required to enroll in early intervention programs for ASD correction [73].

That is, the previous two studies actually found a possible link between MMR and ASD, however, they are widely cited as evidence of the lack of correlation.

4. Jain, 2015. This study found that among children who had an older sibling with ASD, MMR was not associated with autism [74].

This study (like all the others) does not account for the "healthy user bias," although it does mention it. That is, the parents of these children, who already have one child with ASD, and whose risk of ASD is higher a priori, refuse vaccination more often, fearing its consequences. Again, in this and all the other studies, "unvaccinated" refers only to those who have not received the MMR vaccine, but might have been vaccinated with all other vaccines. In addition, the authors of these studies have conflicts of interest. This is also a good point to look back at what Cochrane states in its systematic review: "The design and reporting of safety outcomes in MMR vaccine studies, both pre- and post-marketing, are largely inadequate" [75].

In 2004, the CDC published the above-mentioned study (DeStefano), which did not find a link between the MMR vaccine and autism. **William Thompson, one of the authors, later admitted that he and his colleagues found that African Americans, who received the MMR vaccine before the age of 36 months, were at an increased risk for autism, but this data was never published, and the evidence was destroyed [76].** Thompson first told Dr. Brian Hooker, a researcher on autism, about the manipulation of the data. Hooker analyzed the raw data from the CDC study afresh. He confirmed that the risk of autism among African American children vaccinated before the age of two years was 340% higher than among those vaccinated later. Hooker published his findings in a peer-reviewed open-access journal. However, within hours of CNN publishing the story of the CDC whistle-blower, Hooker's article was removed from the journal website. It was stated that the journal and publisher "believe that its continued availability may not be in the public interest." Later, the article was retracted due to "undeclared competing interests" [77].

> However, the article of the author, who admitted data manipulation, was not retracted. Moreover, it is still used as an argument that vaccines do not cause autism.

Conclusions

Although the media and health authorities claim that there is no link between vaccination and autism, this statement is not supported by the scientific data. The only study comparing vaccinated children to the completely unvaccinated, found the risk of autism to be four times higher in those vaccinated.

Epidemiological studies have focused only on one vaccine (MMR) and one vaccine component (thimerosal). All of these studies had gross methodological errors, yet some of them still found an increased risk of autism in those vaccinated. Moreover, epidemiological studies, which do not account for the genetic susceptibility to the disease (as in the case of acrodynia), may not reveal a correlation even if there is one.

There is much more evidence that vaccination can cause autism (through immune activation) than there is evidence of the contrary.

Endnotes

1. Mawson AR. Pilot comparative study on the health of vaccinated and unvaccinated 6- to 12- year old U.S. children. *J Transl Sci.* 2017:10.15761/JTS.1000186

2. Kanner L. Autistic disturbances of affective contact. *Nervous Child.* 1943;2:217-50

3. Baron-Cohen S. Leo Kanner, Hans Asperger, and the discovery of autism. *Lancet.* 2015; 386(10001):1329-30

4. Manouilenko I et al. Sukhareva—prior to Asperger and Kanner. *Nord J Psychiatry.* 2015; 69(6):479-82

5. Eggers C. Autistic syndrome (Kanner) and vaccination against smallpox. *Klin Padiatr.* 1976;188(2):172-80

6. Hoshino Y et al. Clinical features of autistic children with setback course in their infancy. *Jpn J Psychiatry Neurol.* 1987;41(2):237-45

7. Glascoe FP. Using parents' concerns to detect and address developmental and behavioral problems. *J Soc Pediatr Nurs.* 1999;4(1):24-35

8. Werner E et al. Validation of the phenomenon of autistic regression using home videotapes. *Arch Gen Psychiatry.* 2005;62(8):889-95

9. Ozonoff S et al. Onset patterns in autism: variation across informants, methods, and timing. *Autism Res.* 2018;11(5):788-97

10. Goin-Kochel RP et al. Emergence of autism spectrum disorder in children from simplex families: relations to parental perceptions of etiology. *J Autism Dev Disord.* 2015; 45(5):1451-63

11. Schultz ST et al. Acetaminophen (paracetamol) use, measles-mumps-rubella vaccination, and autistic disorder: the results of a parent survey. *Autism.* 2008; 12(3):293-307

12. Kulage KM et al. How will DSM-5 affect autism diagnosis? A systematic literature review and meta-analysis. *J Autism Dev Disord.* 2014;44(8):1918-32

13. Christensen Dea. Prevalence and characteristics of autism spectrum disorder among children aged 8 years - autism and developmental disabilities monitoring network, 11 sites, United States, 2012. *MMWR Surveill Summ.* 2018;65(13):1-23

14. Treffert DA. Epidemiology of infantile autism. *Arch Gen Psychiatry.* 1970;22(5):431-8

15. Burd L. A prevalence study of pervasive developmental disorders in North Dakota. *J Am Acad Child Adolesc Psychiatry.* 1987;26(5):700-3

16. Kogan MD et al. Prevalence of parent-reported diagnosis of autism spectrum disorder among children in the US, 2007. *Pediatrics.* 2009;124(5):1395-403

17. Zablotsky B et al. Estimated prevalence of autism and other developmental disabilities following questionnaire changes in the 2014 national health interview survey. *Natl Health Stat Report.* 2015(87):1-20

18. Zablotsky B et al. Estimated prevalence of children with diagnosed developmental disabilities in the United States, 2014-2016. *NCHS Data Brief.* 2017(291):1-8

19. Xu G. Twenty-year trends in diagnosed attention-deficit/hyperactivity disorder among US children and adolescents, 1997-2016. *JAMA Netw Open.* 2018;1(4):e181471

20. Skogli EW et al. ADHD in girls and boys—gender differences in co-existing symptoms and executive function measures. *BMC Psychiatry.* 2013;13:298

21. Boyle CA et al. Trends in the prevalence of developmental disabilities in US children, 1997-2008. *Pediatrics.* 2011;127(6):1034-42

22. Nevison C et al. California autism prevalence trends from 1931 to 2014 and comparison to national ASD data from IDEA and ADDM. *J Autism Dev Disord.* 2018;48(12):4103-17

23. Croen LA et al. The changing prevalence of autism in California. *J Autism Dev Disord.* 2002;32(3):207-15

24. Croen LA. Response: a response to Blaxill, Baskin, and Spitzer on Croen et al. (2002), "The changing prevalence of autism in California". *J Autism Dev Disord.* 2003;33(2):227-9

25. Nevison CD et al. Diagnostic substitution for intellectual disability: a flawed explanation for the rise in autism. *J Autism Dev Disord.* 2017;47(9):2733-42

26. Nevison CD. A comparison of temporal trends in United States autism prevalence to trends in suspected environmental factors. *Environ Health.* 2014;13:73

27. Hertz-Picciotto I et al. The rise in autism and the role of age at diagnosis. *Epidemiology.* 2009;20(1):84-90

28. Gurney JG et al. Analysis of prevalence trends of autism spectrum disorder in Minnesota. *Arch Pediatr Adolesc Med.* 2003;157(7):622-7

29. Soke GN et al. Brief report: prevalence of delf-injurious behaviors among children with autism spectrum disorder - a population-based study. *J Autism Dev Disord.* 2016; 46(11):3607-14

30. Long B. Autism Basics, Central California Diagnostic Center. www.dcc-cde.ca.gov/af/afbasic.htm

31. Buescher AV et al. Costs of autism spectrum disorders in the United Kingdom and the United States. *JAMA Pediatr.* 2014;168(8):721-8

32. Mohamed FE et al. Assessment of hair aluminum, lead, and mercury in a sample of autistic egyptian children: environmental risk factors of heavy metals in autism. *Behav Neurol.* 2015;2015:545674

33. Yasuda H et al. Assessment of infantile mineral imbalances in autism spectrum disorders (ASDs). *Int J Environ Res Public Health.* 2013;10(11):6027-43

34. Al-Ayadhi L. Heavy metals and trace elements in hair samples of autistic children in Central Saudi Arabia. *Neurosciences (Riyadh).* 2005;10(3):213-8

35. Sheth SK et al. Is exposure to aluminium adjuvants associated with social impairments in mice? A pilot study. *J Inorg Biochem.* 2018;181:96-103

36. Morris G et al. The putative role of environmental aluminium in the development of chronic neuropathology in adults and children. How strong is the evidence and what could be the mechanisms involved? *Metab Brain Dis.* 2017;32(5):1335-55

37. Tomljenovic L et al. Do aluminum vaccine adjuvants contribute to the rising prevalence of autism? *J Inorg Biochem.* 2011;105(11):1489-99

38. Mold M et al. Aluminium in brain tissue in autism. *J Trace Elem Med Biol.* 2018;46:76-82

39. Delong G. A positive association found between autism prevalence and childhood vaccination uptake across the U.S. population. *J Toxicol Environ Health A.* 2011; 74(14):903-16

40. Christian LM et al. Inflammatory responses to trivalent influenza virus vaccine among pregnant women. *Vaccine.* 2011;29(48):8982-7

41. Brown AS et al. Elevated maternal C-reactive protein and autism in a national birth cohort. *Mol Psychiatry.* 2014;19(2):259-64

42. Balter LJ et al. Low-grade inflammation decreases emotion recognition - evidence from the vaccination model of inflammation. *Brain Behav Immun.* 2018;73:216-21

43. Smith SE et al. Maternal immune activation alters fetal brain development through interleukin-6. *J Neurosci.* 2007;27(40):10695-702

44. Bauman MD et al. Activation of the maternal immune system during pregnancy alters behavioral development of rhesus monkey offspring. *Biol Psychiatry.* 2014;75(4):332-41

45. Missig G et al. Perinatal immune activation produces persistent sleep alterations and epileptiform activity in male mice. *Neuropsychopharmacology.* 2018;43(3):482-91

46. Vargas DL et al. Neuroglial activation and neuroinflammation in the brain of patients with autism. *Ann Neurol.* 2005;57(1):67-81

47. Suzuki K et al. Microglial activation in young adults with autism spectrum disorder. *JAMA Psychiatry.* 2013;70(1):49-58

48. Wei H et al. Brain IL-6 elevation causes neuronal circuitry imbalances and mediates autism-like behaviors. *Biochim Biophys Acta.* 2012;1822(6):831-42

49. Viezeliene D. Selective induction of IL-6 by aluminum-induced oxidative stress can be prevented by selenium. *J Trace Elem Med Biol.* 2013;27(3):226-9

50. Li Q et al. Neonatal vaccination with bacillus Calmette-Guérin and hepatitis B vaccines modulates hippocampal synaptic plasticity in rats. *J Neuroimmunol.* 2015;288:1-12

51. Yang J et al. Neonatal hepatitis B vaccination impaired the behavior and neurogenesis of mice transiently in early adulthood. *Psychoneuroendocrinology.* 2016;73:166-76

52. Lukiw WJ et al. Nanomolar aluminum induces pro-inflammatory and pro-apoptotic gene expression in human brain cells in primary culture. *J Inorg Biochem.* 2005; 99(9):1895-8

53. Jensen KJ et al. A randomized trial of an early measles vaccine at 4½ months of age in Guinea-Bissau: sex-differential immunological effects. *PloS One.* 2014;9(5):e97536

54. D'Mello C et al. Cerebral microglia recruit monocytes into the brain in response to tumor necrosis factoralpha signaling during peripheral organ inflammation. *J Neurosci.* 2009;29(7):2089-102

55. Han YM et al. Distinct Cytokine and Chemokine Profiles in Autism Spectrum Disorders. *Front Immunol.* 2017;8:11

56. Zerbo O et al. Neonatal cytokines and chemokines and risk of Autism Spectrum Disorder: the Early Markers for Autism (EMA) study: a case-control study. *J Neuroinflammation.* 2014;11:113

57. Poling JS et al. Developmental regression and mitochondrial dysfunction in a child with autism. *J Child Neurol.* 2006;21(2):170-2

58. Rossignol DA et al. Mitochondrial dysfunction in autism spectrum disorders: a systematic review and meta-analysis. *Mol Psychiatry.* 2012;17(3):290-314

59. Varga NÁ et al. Mitochondrial dysfunction and autism: comprehensive genetic analyses of children with autism and mtDNA deletion. *Behav Brain Funct.* 2018;14(1):4

60. Holland M et al. Unanswered Questions from the Vaccine Injury Compensation Program: a Review of Compensated Cases of Vaccine-Induced Brain Injury. *Pace Envtl L Rev.* 2011;28(480)

61. Attkisson S. Vaccines, autism and brain damage: what's in a name? *CBS News.* 2010 Sep 14

62. Modabbernia A et al. Environmental risk factors for autism: an evidence-based review of systematic reviews and meta-analyses. *Mol Autism.* 2017;8:13

63. UC Davis M.I.N.D. Institute study shows California's autism increase not due to better counting, diagnosis. 2009 Feb 18

64. Robinson EB et al. Genetic risk for autism spectrum disorders and neuropsychiatric variation in the general population. *Nat Genet.* 2016;48(5):552-5

65. Kamer A et al. A prevalence estimate of pervasive developmental disorder among immigrants to Israel and Israeli natives- a file review study. *Soc Psychiatry Psychiatr Epidemiol.* 2004;39(2):141-5

66. Dawson G et al. Autologous Cord Blood Infusions Are Safe and Feasible in Young Children with Autism Spectrum Disorder. *Stem Cells Transl Med.* 2017;6(5):1332-9

67. Leys D. A review of infantile acrodynia ('pink disease'). *Arch Dis Child.* 1950; 25(123):302-10

68. Warkany J et al. Acrodynia and mercury. *J Pediatr.* 1953;42(3):365-86

69. Warkany J. Acrodynia - Postmortem of a Disease. *Am J Dis Child.* 1966;112(2):146-56

70. Madsen KM et al. A population-based study of measles, mumps, and rubella vaccination and autism. *N Engl J Med.* 2002;347(19):1477-82

71. Spitzer WO. Measles, mumps, and rubella vaccination and autism. *N Engl J Med.* 2003;348(10):951-4

72. Taylor B et al. Autism and measles, mumps, and rubella vaccine: no epidemiological evidence for a causal association. *Lancet.* 1999;353(9169):2026-9

73. DeStefano F et al. Age at first measles-mumps-rubella vaccination in children with autism and school-matched control subjects: a population-based study in metropolitan atlanta. *Pediatrics.* 2004;113(2):259-66

74. Jain A et al. Autism occurrence by MMR vaccine status among US children with older siblings with and without autism. *JAMA*. 2015;313(15):1534-40

75. Demicheli V et al. Vaccines for measles, mumps and rubella in children. *Cochrane Database Syst Rev*. 2012(2):CD004407

76. Chhawchharia R et al. Commentary—Controversies surrounding mercury in vaccines: autism denial as impediment to universal immunisation. *Indian J Med Ethics*. 2014; 11(4):218-22

77. Hooker BS. Measles-mumps-rubella vaccination timing and autism among young African American boys: a reanalysis of CDC data. *Transl Neurodegener*. 2014;3:16

EPILOGUE

The only thing necessary for the triumph of evil
is for good men to do nothing.
— **Edmund Burke**

In 1938, a leading expert in the field of infectious diseases, Charles Cyril Okell, wrote in his article for the *Lancet* journal:

"When Jenner and Pasteur developed the idea of artificial immunisation they did something more than make a scientific discovery; they founded a faith and as so often happens with faith came an offset of superstition and charlatanry. Neither of these great innovators approached the matter as entirely unprejudiced and impersonal observers. They aspired to be missionaries as well as scientists.

"Yet the immunisation of the masses has been undertaken with almost a religious fervour. The enthusiast rarely stopped to wonder where it would all finish or whether the fulsome promises made to the public in the form of "propaganda" would ever be honoured. Without propaganda there can, of course, be no large-scale immunisation, but how perilous it is to mix up propaganda with scientific fact. If we baldly told the whole truth it is doubtful whether the public would submit to immunisation.

"On the whole diphtheria immunisation has proved a fairly safe affair, but suppose we included in our propaganda a candid account of the various untoward accidents which have accompanied the procedure. No method involving a parenteral injection is without a significant risk. When injecting a healthy individual with anything we are always skating on thin ice. Sick people for the most part are quite prepared to take a risk in trying out a remedy, but the main desire of well people is to preserve their status quo. If you knock them out in an effort to protect them from a disease there is no knowing they will ever get, there is the devil to pay. Accidents and mistakes must inevitably happen and when they take place what might have been a highly instructive lesson is usually suppressed or distorted out of recognition. Those who have had to take detailed notice of the immunisation accidents of the past few years know that to get the truth of what really went wrong generally calls for the resources of something like a secret service...

"Compulsory vaccination which once had the suffrage of the nation has now hardly a serious supporter. We are ashamed to jettison the idea completely and perhaps afraid that if we did the accident of some future epidemic might put us in the wrong. We prefer to let compulsory vaccination die a natural death and are relieved that the general public is not curious enough to demand an inquest" [1].

Almost nothing has changed in the 80 years since these words were written. Vaccination is still being supported by widespread propaganda, and almost all deaths or serious adverse effects caused by vaccination are hushed up. The only thing that has changed is the attitude towards mandatory vaccination. Eighty years ago, most developed countries discontinued mandatory vaccination, but now we are witnessing its return. Each year more and more countries pass laws requiring parents to vaccinate their children or laws restricting unvaccinated children from attending childcare facilities and schools, and these laws are widely approved by the community.

Hitler wrote that "people more readily fall victims to the big lie than the small lie, since they themselves often tell small lies in little matters but would be ashamed to resort to large-scale falsehoods. It would never come into their heads to fabricate colossal untruths, and they would not believe that others could have the impudence to distort the truth so infamously. Even though the facts which prove this to be so may be brought clearly to their minds, they will still doubt and waver and will continue to think that there may be some other explanation. For the grossly impudent lie always leaves traces behind it."

Today, when more and more vaccines are being added to the immunization schedule, many parents begin to doubt whether their children need all these vaccines. They think that some vaccines are more important, but some perhaps should be avoided. I used to think the same way at one point, but not being able to find a simple answer to this question, I began to study the scientific research myself. Having analyzed statistics and scientific data about each vaccine on the immunization schedule, I did not find a single vaccine the potential benefit of which exceeds the risk. Nonetheless, for a very long time, I could not believe that vaccination was just a "big lie." I could not shake off the feeling that it was simply impossible and that there were probably more studies, which I just do not know about yet. Only when I went through about a thousand studies did the vaccination finally become the "big lie" to me.

> If propaganda was able to convince parents that injecting toxic substances into their healthy infants is good and will only make them healthier—it means that people can be convinced of anything with no exception. Having realized this, any sensible person should ask themselves if there is anything else that they've perceived as an indisputable fact without delving deep enough into the topic.

For example, could other areas of medicine also be lies? Marcia Angell worked as an editor and editor-in-chief of the most prestigious medical journal, *The New England Journal of Medicine*, for 20 years. She wrote in 2009: *"It is simply no longer possible to believe much of the clinical research that is published, or to rely on the judgment of trusted physicians or authoritative medical guidelines. I take no pleasure in this conclusion, which I reached slowly and reluctantly over my two decades as an editor of The New England Journal of Medicine. The pharmaceutical industry has gained enormous control over how doctors evaluate and use its own products. Its extensive ties to physicians, particularly senior faculty at prestigious medical schools, affect the results of research, the way medicine is practiced, and even the definition of what constitutes a disease"* [2].

Richard Horton, editor-in-chief of the second most prestigious medical journal *The Lancet*, expresses similar ideas in his 2015 article: *"Much of the scientific literature, perhaps half, may simply be untrue. Afflicted by studies with small sample sizes, tiny effects, invalid exploratory analyses, and flagrant conflicts of interest, together with an obsession for pursuing fashionable trends of dubious importance, science has taken a turn towards darkness"* [3].

One could argue that editors-in-chief of the most influential medical journals are the most important people in the field of medicine in the world. They are basically the people who decide what will or will not become a part of medical science. They openly say that they believe neither the clinical studies that they publish nor the science which results from those studies. They consider medicine to be completely corrupt. These articles, however, went by almost completely unnoticed and were quickly forgotten. Neither the media nor the health authorities will remind you of them.

This book presents a lot of research, but the key topic in the case of vaccination is not the studies that *do exist,* but rather the studies that *do not exist.* No vaccines from the immunization schedule have been through safety studies that compare vaccinated children with children who received an inert placebo. (This does not mean that such studies do not exist at all. Some clinical studies use saline as a placebo, but they are not the studies of the vaccines from the immunization schedule.) There are also no studies that compare the health of vaccinated and completely unvaccinated children. Both kinds of studies are easy to conduct, but pharmaceutical companies and health authorities oppose them by all means possible.

Unfortunately, the health of the public is not a priority for the health authorities today, and the health of your children is solely your responsibility. Going against the recommendations is a brave step, which is not always easy to take. However, only when a significant number of parents will fight for their children's right to health, something might begin to change.

Endnotes

1. Okell C. From a bacteriological back-number. *Lancet.* 1938;231(5966):48-9
2. Angell M. Drug companies & doctors: a story of corruption. *nybooks.com.* 15/1/2009
3. Horton R. What is medicine's 5 sigma? *Lancet.* 2015;385(9976):1380

www.ingramcontent.com/pod-product-compliance
Lightning Source LLC
Chambersburg PA
CBHW021349210526
45463CB00001B/45